Springer Japan KK

K. Tanikawa, T. Ueno (Eds.)

# Liver Diseases and Hepatic Sinusoidal Cells

With 241 Figures

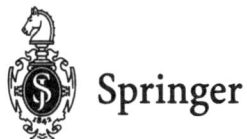 Springer

Kyuichi Tanikawa, M.D.
Professor Emeritus
Kurume University School of Medicine
and
President
International Institute for Liver Research
Kurume Research Center
2432-3 Aikawa-machi, Kurume
Fukuoka 839-0861, Japan

Takato Ueno, M.D.
Assistant Professor
The Second Department of Internal Medicine
and
Division Chief
Liver Cancer Research Division
Research Center for Innovative Cancer Therapy
Kurume University School of Medicine
67 Asahi-machi, Kurume
Fukuoka 830-0011, Japan

ISBN 978-4-431-68012-3       ISBN 978-4-431-67935-6 (eBook)
DOI 10.1007/978-4-431-67935-6

Library of Congress Cataloging-in-Publication Data

Liver diseases and hepatic sinusoidal cells / K. Tanikawa, T. Ueno.
    p.   cm.
    Includes bibliographical references and index.
    ISBN-13: 978-4-431-68012-3
    1. Liver—Pathophysiology.   2. Liver—Cytopathology.   3. Liver
cells.   I. Tanikawa, Kyuichi, 1932–   II. Ueno, T. (Takato), 1951–
    RC847 .L62   1999
    616.3'62071—dc21
                                                    98-45747
                                                    CIP
Printed on acid-free paper

© Springer Japan 1999
Originally published by Springer-Verlag Tokyo in 1999
Softcover reprint of the hardcover 1st edition 1999

SPIN: 10682058

# Preface

I first recognized the existence of hepatic sinusoidal cells and became very much interested in them almost 40 years ago when I was a graduate student at Chiba University and studied intrahepatic cholestasis by electron microscopy. Later, in 1973, when an international conference on collagen metabolism in the liver was held in Freiburg, Germany, I was invited to talk on the fine structure of hepatic fibrosis. During the preparation of my presentation I had noted numerous Ito cells (hepatic stellate cells) in fibrous tissue and also fibrous bundles around Ito cells in normal liver. From these observations I presented in my talk the important role of Ito cells in hepatic fibrogenesis. In that conference no well-known pathologist or hepatologist, except Prof. Hans Popper, agreed with my talk. Today no one disputes the important role of Ito cells in hepatic fibrosis. Since that Freiburg conference I have been deeply involved in the study of hepatic sinusoidal cells.

Recently we reported on the important role played by the contraction and relaxation of Ito cells in the control of hepatic sinusoidal circulation. As described above, we recognized the importance of the hepatic sinusoidal cell in the function of the liver and pathogenesis of various liver diseases and therefore organized the Japanese Meeting of Hepatic Sinusoidal Cell Study at the end of each year. Japanese studies on these cells have progressed remarkably since the first meeting was held in 1987.

A meeting was held last year on the occasion of my retirement from Kurume University, and the authors of this monograph were speakers at the meeting. I very much hope that the hepatic sinusoidal cell will be more actively studied by hepatologists everywhere for the better understanding of liver function and pathogenesis of liver diseases.

I would like to sincerely thank Prof. K. Noguchi for his efforts in the management of the Japanese Meeting of Hepatic Sinusoidal Cell Study over such a long period of time, and Dr. T. Ueno for his efforts in editing this monograph.

K. Tanikawa, M.D.
Professor Emeritus, Kurume University
President, International Institute for Liver Research
President, Japan Society of Hepatology

# Contents

## Liver Tumor and Hepatic Sinusoidal Cells

## Liver Transplantation and Hepatic Sinusoidal Cells

## Others

# List of Contributors

Arai, M.    242
Arii, S.    318

Braet, F.    17

De Zanger, R.B.    17

Ebe, Y.    66
Eddouks, M.    17
Empsen, C.    17
Enzan, H.    219

Fujiwara, K.    101, 114

Gondo, K.    156

Hagiwara, S.    128
Hamada, H.    296
Hanaki, K.    318
Harada, M.    337
Hasegawa, G.    66
Hayashi, Y.    219
Hijioka, T.    209
Hikiba, Y.    296
Hiroi, M.    219
Hozawa, S.    242

Ichida, T.    307
Imamura, M.    318
Ishii, K.    199
Itoh, Y.    190

Kamada, T.    209

Kamegaya, Y.    141
Kanai, F.    296
Kanaoka, H.    190
Kaneda, K.    76
Kasukawa, R.    91
Kawada, N.    232
Kawaguchi, M.    337
Kawahara, T.    327
Kawano, S.    209
Kim, K.    252
Kin, M.    168, 274
Kiyoku, H.    219
Kojima, S.    232
Konstandoulaki, M.    17
Kumashiro, R.    199, 327
Kuroda, N.    219
Kuromatsu, R.    288

Luo, D.    17

Maruyama, K.    242
Mitsuyama, M.    66
Miyakawa, K.    128
Miyazaki, E.    219
Mochida, S.    101, 114
Mori, A.    318
Mori, T.    190
Moriga, T.    318
Moriwaki, H.    232
Moriyama, H.    296
Muto, Y.    232

Nagase, S.    232

# Part I
# Introduction

# The Intestine, Spleen, and Liver

Kyuichi Tanikawa

*Summary.* Blood from the intestine and the spleen flows directly into the liver. Numerous antigenic substances, including endotoxin, are absorbed from the intestine and go to the liver. The spleen, which contains at least one-third of the lymphatic tissue in the body, responds to antigenic substances, including endotoxin, and produces numerous cytokines, antibodies, and antigen-specific T cells which first flow into the liver. Thus, the intestine and spleen strongly affect the liver, and endotoxin seems to play an important role in modulating the effect of both organs. This chapter investigates the importance of these organs in the pathogenesis of various liver diseases, including alcoholic hepatitis, obstructive jaundice, and primary biliary cirrhosis.

*Key words.* Intestine, Spleen, Endotoxin, Liver disease, Alcoholic hepatitis

In liver function and the pathogenesis of liver diseases, it is important to consider the effect of neighboring organs on the liver. The intestine and spleen are the most important because blood from both organs flows directly into the liver (Fig. 1). Thus, changes in these organs have a large effect on the liver.

Various nutrients absorbed from the small intestine are transfered to the liver. Water and numerous antigenic substances, including endotoxin absorbed from the colon, also go to the liver through the portal vein. Of these, the most important antigenic substances is endotoxin, the outer cell membrane component of gram-negative bacteria, which flows into the liver in increased amounts when endotoxin is overproduced in the colon or absorbed in large quantities from the colon. Endotoxin entering the hepatic sinusoid is generally first taken up by Kupffer cells. However, a recent study indicated that one-quarter of lipopolysaccharide (LPS) injected into the portal vein is directly taken up by hepatocytes and excreted into the bile [1]. Thus, the

The Second Department of Internal Medicine, Kurume University School of Medicine, 67 Asahi-machi, Kurume, Fukuoka 830-0011, Japan
Present Address: International Institute for Liver Research, Kurume Research Center, 2432-3 Aikawa-machi, Kurame, Fukuoka 839-0861, Japan

4    K. Tanikawa

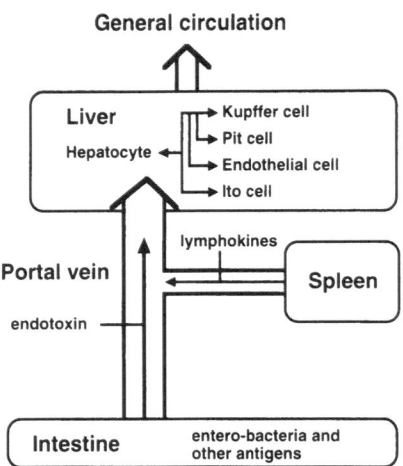

General circulation

Liver — Kupffer cell
Hepatocyte — Pit cell
— Endothelial cell
— Ito cell

lymphokines

Portal vein          Spleen

endotoxin

Intestine    entero-bacteria and
other antigens

FIG. 1. Schematic presentation of the relationship between the liver and the intestine and spleen

hepatocytes play an important role in the clearance of endotoxin in the circulation, as do the Kupffer cells.

Endotoxemia, which occurs without gram-negative bacteria infection in the body, is termed endogenous. Thus the "endogenous endotoxemia" seen in some liver diseases occurs in the following conditions: (1) increased absorption of endotoxin from the colon (2) dysfunction of Kupffer cells (3) dysfunction of hepatocytes, and (4) shunt formation between the portal system and the general circulation.

We examined the absorption of LPS injected into the colon of rats with various experimental liver injuries by measuring the concentration of LPS in the portal vein, and we found a large increase in LPS absorption from the colon in liver cirrhosis, alcohol abuse [2], and extrahepatic obstruction [3].

In these pathologic conditions we examined the mechanism of endotoxin absorption in the colonic epithelium by immune electron microscopy using antibody against LPS, and found LPS particles passing through colonic epithelial cells (Fig. 2).

The spleen plays an important role in taking up antigenic substances in the circulation, and in the production of antibodies, antigen-specific T cells, and numerous cytokines. There are many macrophages in the red pulp of the spleen, and these take up antigenic materials in the circulation and release cytokines which stimulate splenic lymphocytes. In order to clarify the difference in function between splenic macrophages and Kupffer cells, we investigated the production of TNFα in cultured cells of these two types when they were stimulated by LPS, and found that splenic macrophages produce more TNFα than Kupffer cells (Fig. 3) [4]. In an in vivo study, serum TNFα levels were much higher in control rats than in splenectomized rats after intravenous injection of LPS (Fig. 4). These studies indicate that the activity of TNFα production differs between splenic macrophages and Kupffer cells, and that splenic macrophages are oriented more to the production of cytokines which stimulate lymphocytes in the spleen. Our studies also demonstrated that Ia antigens are expressed more on the surface of splenic macrophages than on Kupffer cells. On the other hand, testing the uptake of latex particles in vivo and in vitro showed that phagocytic ability was much higher in Kupffer cells than in splenic macrophages.

Fig. 2. Immune electron micrograph of endotoxin passing through a colonic epithelial cell. Electron-dense particles of lipopolysaccharides (LPS) injected into the colon are shown in a colonic epithelial cell using antibody against LPS (Pfizer Pharmaceuticals, New York, USA). ×15000

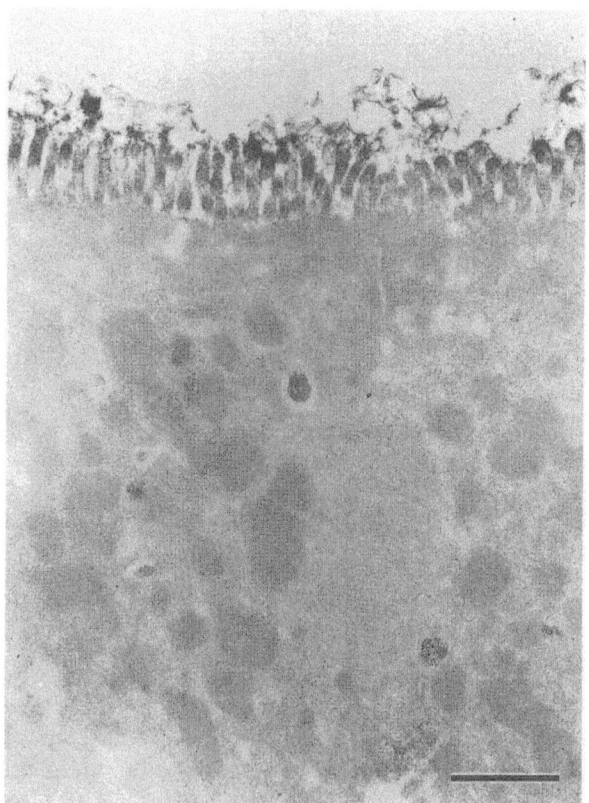

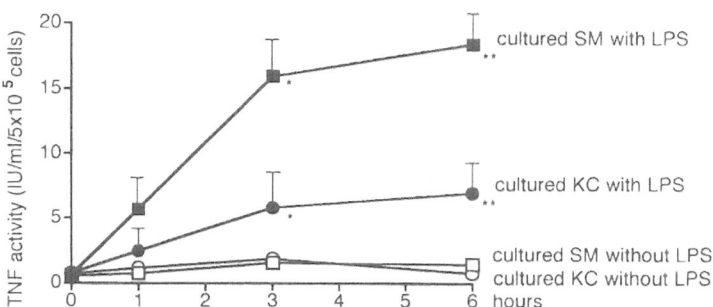

Fig. 3. TNF levels in the culture medium of splenic macrophages and Kupffer cells. Isolated rat splenic macrophages (*SM*) and Kupffer cells (*KC*) were stimulated with and without 1 μg/ml of LPS for different lengths of time (0, 1, 3, and 6h) and the activities of TNFα in the culture medium were determined by bioassay. *VS*P < 0.05, **VS**P < 0.01 (Student's *t*-test)

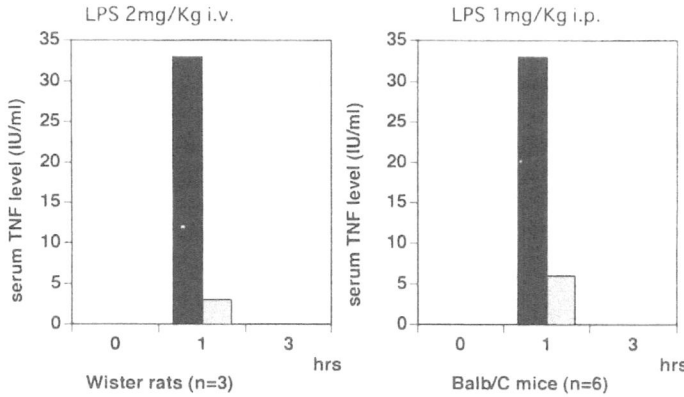

F<small>IG</small>. 4. Effect of splenectomy on serum TNF levels after LPS elicitation. A remarkable rectuction in TNFα levels in serum was noted in splenectomized rats and mice after intravenous injection of LPS (2 mg/kg). *Black columns*, control group; *shaded columns*, splenectomized group

From our studies, it is important to note that large amounts of cytokines, including TNFα produced in the spleen by the stimulation of antigenic substances such as endotoxin, flow into the liver and first affect the sinusoidal cells. In addition, sensitized lymphocytes or antibodies produced in the spleen also enter directly into the liver.

The spleen has been investigated in association with portal hypertension, and thrombocytopenia seen in portal hypertension has been considered to be due to splenomegaly because the spleen is an organ which stores thrombocytes. Therefore, we performed partial splenic embolization for thrombocytopenia associated with liver cirrhosis. It is of interest to note that liver function improved after a reduction in spleen size [5]. This indicates that the spleen has some control over liver function. Our study has shown a close association between liver regeneration after partial hepatectomy and the size of the spleen [6] (Fig. 5), and liver regeneration after partial hepatectomy for hepatocellular carcinoma was better in patients with a small spleen than in those with a large one. TGFβ produced within the spleen might be involved in this phenomenon.

One of the leading causes of portal hypertension is an increased inflow of blood into the portal system due to a hyperdynamic state. A hyperdynamic state is probably caused by peripheral arterial dilatation, which occurs most prominently in the splanchnic area [7]. In addition, the most important factor for such peripheral arterial dilatation has been considered to be NO produced in the arterial endothelium by endotoxin. For these reasons, intestinal factors also seem to be deeply involved in portal hypertension.

The reason why the spleen is located in close contact with the liver is unknown. However, this association could be a worthwhile subject for future research.

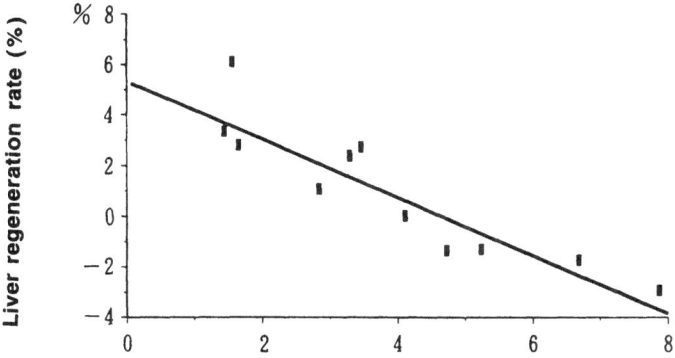

FIG. 5. Relationship between liver regeneration and spleen volume. Regeneration of the liver after resection of a hepatocellular carcinoma associated with liver cirrhosis showed a close relationship with the size of the spleen, and poor regeneration was noted in patients with a larger spleen

## Alcoholic Hepatitis

It is important to clarify the causes of endotoxemia, which is often seen in alcoholic liver diseases, especially in alcoholic hepatitis.

Our study showed a large increase in LPS in the portal blood after injection of LPS into the colon of rats fed with a liquid alcohol diet (Fig. 6), suggesting alcohol abuse to be a cause of increased endotoxin absorption.

It has also been found that the uptake of latex particles by Kupffer cells is strongly inhibited in rats fed with a liquid alcohol diet, and also in cultured Kupffer cells taken

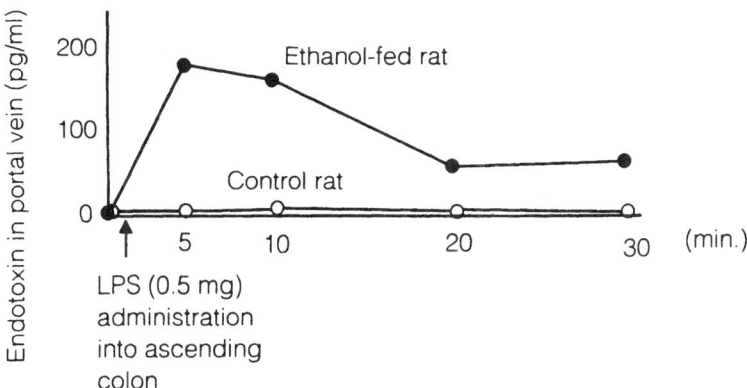

FIG. 6. Endotoxin concentration in portal blood after LPS administration to the ascending colon in chronic ethand-fed rats. Endotoxin levels in the portal vein were significantly higher in ethanol-fed rats

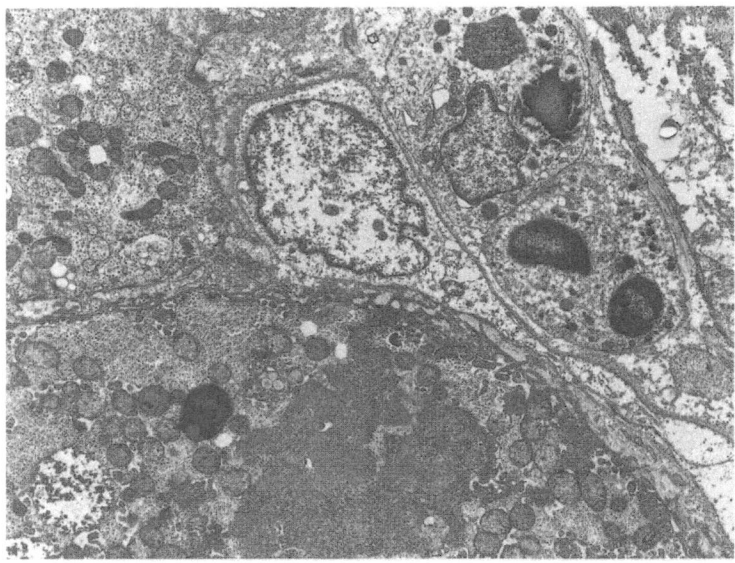

FIG. 7. Electron micrograph of the liver from a patient with alcoholic hepatitis. Many PMN cells are in close contact with the endothelial cell. Note a hepatocyte with a large Mallory body. ×3600

from rats fed the same diet [8]. These studies indicate an impairment of the phagocytic function of Kupffer cells over a long period of alcohol intake. In fact, a strongly impaired uptake of colloidal particles for a liver scintigram is often observed in alcoholic hepatitis, and a clearance study using CsFe colloidal particles infused intravenously also demonstrated uptake to be seriously impaired. This clinical evidence agrees with experimental studies. In addition, immune microscopy shows poor staining in Kupffer cells of alcoholic hepatitis patients using an antibody against LPS.

An elevated IgA level in the serum is well known in alcoholic liver injuries, and our study revealed an elevated IgA class anti-LPS antibody in alcoholic liver injuries, suggesting that an elevated serum IgA is probably due to an increased absorption of antigenic substances including endotoxin from the colon.

Although the impairment of intrahepatocyte transport of endotoxin in alcoholic liver injuries has not been explained in the literature, it seems very clear that endotoxemia seen in alcoholic liver injuries is mainly caused by an increased absorption of endotoxin from the intestine and a dysfunction of Kupffer cells.

Endotoxemia, manifested or subclinical, probably plays an important role in the pathogenesis of alcoholic liver injuries because splenic macrophages stimulated by endotoxin produce large amounts of cytokines, including TNFα, which first flow into the liver.

Alcoholic hepatitis is histologically characterized by a remarkable infiltration of polymorphonuclear (PMN) cells, which probably play an important role in the pathogenesis of alcoholic hepatitis. In this study, electron microscopy showed that numerous PMN cells appeared to be in close contact with sinusoidal endothelial cells (Fig. 7). They had also infiltrated through the sinusoidal wall toward hepatocytes,

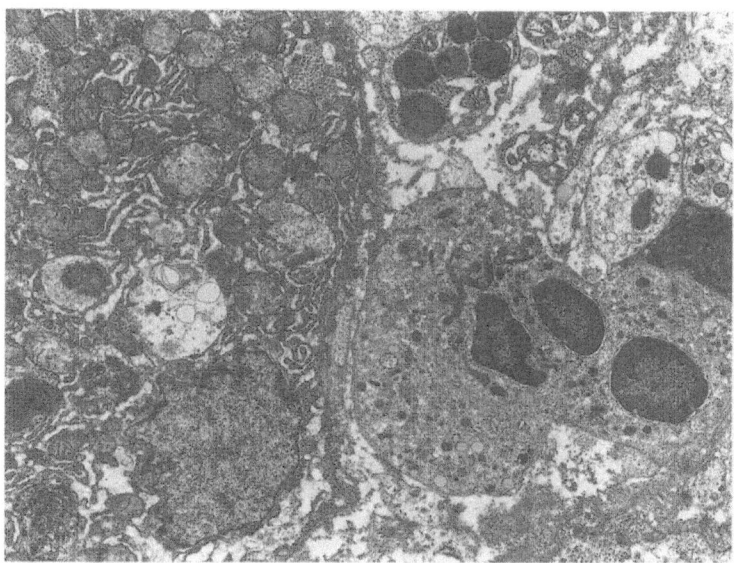

FIG. 8. Electron micrograph of the liver from a patient with alcoholic hepatitis. A PMN cell infiltrating through the endothelial wall is reaching toward a hepatocyte which appears markedly degenerated. ×5000

which appeared to have degenerated (Fig. 8), suggesting an expression of adhesion molecules on the sinusoidal endothelial cells as well as the pathogenetic processes of alcoholic hepatitis. We have previously demonstrated an enhanced expression of ICAN-1 on the cultured sinudoial endothelial cells induced by TNFα or IL-1 [9].

Thus, adhesion molecules on the sinusoidal endothelial cells seem to be expressed mainly by cytokines such as TNFα flowing into the liver from the spleen. On the other hand, production of IL-8 in the liver is necessary for an accumulation of PMN cells. Our study has shown an increased induction of IL-8 in the liver tissue by TNFα. In fact, the numbers of infiltrated PMN cells in liver biopsy specimens and the serum IL-8 values are shown to be well correlated [2] (Fig. 9), and serum values of IL-8 and TNFα are important predictive factors in the prognosis of alcoholic hepatitis.

Putting these data together, the mechanism of alcoholic hepatitis is suggested to be as follows. First, an increased absorption of endotoxin in the colon and a depressed uptake by Kupffer cells during alcohol abuse cause endotoxemia. Second, splenic macrophages stimulated by endotoxin release cytokines, including TNFα, which flow into the liver. The expression of adhesion molecules on the surface of sinusoidal endothelial cells or PMN cells is enhanced by TNFα and other cytokines coming from the spleen. On the other hand, IL-8 is produced by TNFα in the liver. This causes an accumulation of PMN cells in the liver, which adhere to the sinusoidal cells. Adhesion of PMN cells to the sinusoidal endothelial cells results in PMN passing through the sinusoidal wall and reaching the hepatocytes, and also in circulatory disturbance of the sinusoid. These are probably pathogenetic processes of alcoholic hepatitis [2] (Fig. 10).

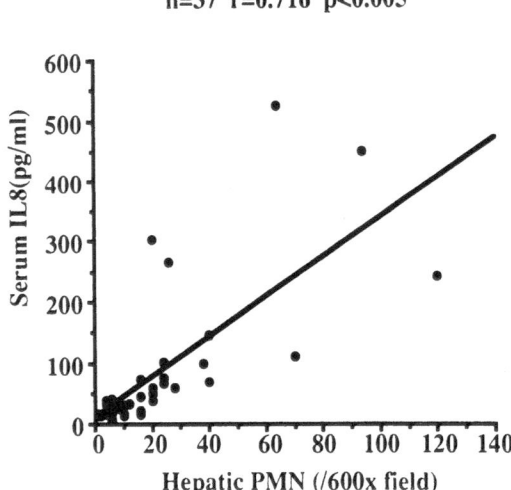

n=37  r=0.716  p<0.005

FIG. 9. Correlation of serum IL-8 and hepatic neutrophils in alcoholic liver diseases. Serum IL-8 levels and the number of PMN cells in the liver tissue are well correlated

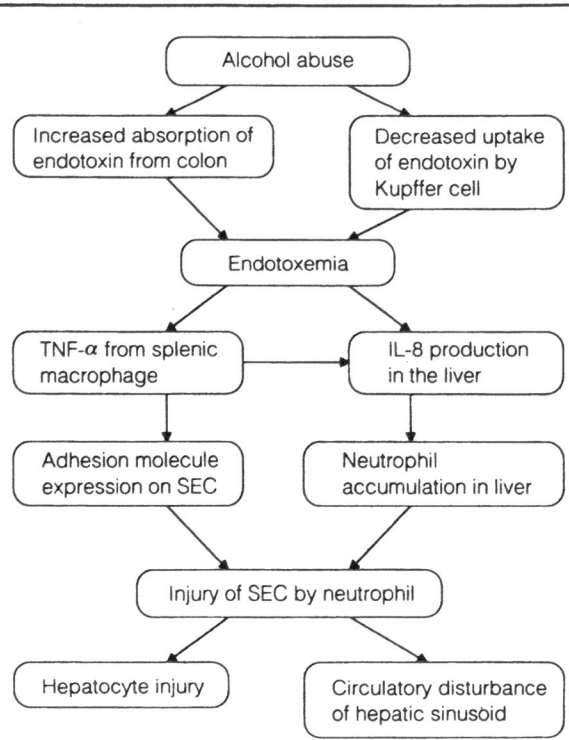

Neutrophil-mediated liver cell injury in alcoholic hepatitis

FIG. 10. Proposed pathogenesis of alcoholic hepatitis

# Obstructive Jaundice

Endotoxemia is often observed clinically in patients with obstructive jaundice without an accompanying infection of gram-negative bacteria.

Our experimental study has demonstrated that compared with control rats, rats with extrahepatic obstructive jaundice show a large elevation of LPS in the portal vein after an injection of LPS into the colonic lumen [3], suggesting an increased absorption of endotoxin through the colonic wall in such pathological conditions.

It is known that most toxic substances in the blood of patients with obstructive jaundice are increased levels of bile acids, and among the various bile acids, chenodeoxycholic acid has the most inhibitory effect on the phagocytosis of cultured Kupffer cells, and ursodeoxycholic acid has no effect on the function of Kupffer cells [10].

This experimental study indicates a dysfunction of Kupffer cells in obstructive jaundice. In fact, a CsFe colloid clearance study revealed that if clearance was clinically delayed (Fig. 11), then the overloading of electron-dense materials in the cytoplasm of Kupffer cells, as demonstrated by electron microscopy, would be a cause of dysfunction (Fig. 12).

In obstructive jaundice, impaired excretion of endotoxins by hepatocytes because of bile duct obstruction would be another factor in endotoxemia, in addition to an increased intestinal absorption of endotoxin and Kupffer cell dysfunction.

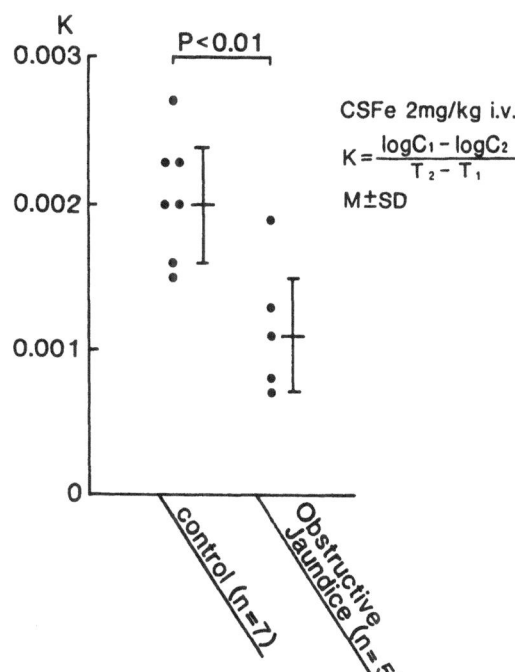

FIG. 11. Colloidal CSFe clearance in patients with obstructive jaundice is strongly impaired

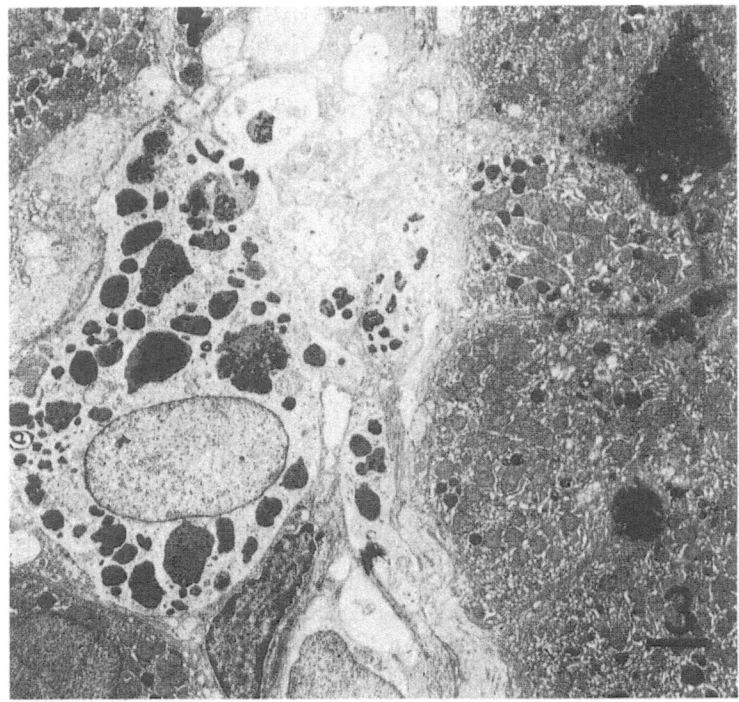

FIG. 12. Electron micrograph of the liver from a patient with obstructive jaundice. A Kupffer cell is seen to be enlarged and full of electron-dense material, representing a state of over-loading. ×2000

## Primary Biliary Cirrhosis

Primary biliary cirrhosis (PBC) is a progressive disease of medium-sized intrahepatic bile ducts, which is characterized by positive mitochondrial antibody and elevated IgM in the serum.

In order to clarify the mechanism of elevated IgM in the serum, we investigated IgM-class anti-LPS antibody, which was shown to be significantly elevated [3] (Fig. 13). This finding suggests an increased absorption of antigenic substances, including endotoxin. In addition, although we have described the importance of hepatocytes in the excretion of endotoxin, we have also demonstrated a remarkable accumulation of endotoxin in the intrahepatic bile duct, which disappeared after unsodeoxycholic acid (UDCA) administration [11].

It is not clear whether or not the accumulation of endotoxin in the intrahepatic bile duct is a primary cause of PBC. However, an accumulation of lymphocytes around the intrahepatic bile duct may be caused by a leak of endotoxin accumulated in the bile duct to the portal areas. Our study has also shown numerous IgM-positive plasma cells accumulated around the bile duct in PBC, suggesting that endotoxin leakage to the portal area is the cause of elevated IgM-class anti-LPS antibody in this disease.

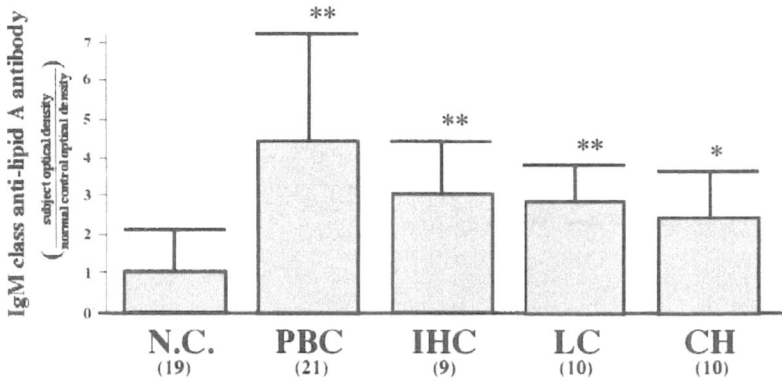

FIG. 13. IgM class anti-lipid A antibody in various liver diseases. The antibody was strongly elevated in PBC. The number of patients is shown in parentheses. *N.C.*, normal control; *PBC*, primary biliary cirrhosis; *IHC*, intrahepatic cholestasis; *LC*, liver cirrhosis; *CH*, chronic hepatitis. *$P < 0.05$; **$P < 0.01$

# Conclusion

The important roles of the intestine and the spleen have been shown by demonstrating examples of alcoholic hepatitis, obstructive jaundice, and primary biliary cirrhosis, and endotoxin seems to play a key role in the pathogenesis of these diseases. Future research into liver disease should pay more attention to the neighboring organs.

## References

1. Mimura Y, Sakisaka S, Harada M, et al. (1995) Role of hepatocytes in direct clearance of lipopolysaccharide in rats. Gastroenterology 109:1969–1976
2. Kumarhiso R, Sakisaka S, Noguchi K, et al. (1997) Liver cell death in alcoholic hepatitis. In: Okita K (ed) Frontier in hepatology '97. Springer, Tokyo, pp 67–79
3. Tanikawa K, Noguchi K, Sasatomi K (1996) Role of cytokines and adhesion molecules in the pathogenesis of biliary liver diseases. In: Berg PA, Leuschner U (eds) Bile acids and immunology. Kluwer, Dordrecht, pp 86–93
4. Shimauchi Y, Tanaka M, Yoshitake M, et al. (1993) Functional differences between rat Kupffer cells and splenic macrophages. In: Knook DL, Wisse E (eds) Cells of the hepatic sinusoid, vol 4. Kupffer Cell Foundation, pp 198–200
5. Sakata K, Hirai K, Tanikawa K (1996) A long term investigation of transcatheter splenic embolization for hypersplenism. Hepato-Gastroenterology 43:309–318
6. Sato K, Tanaka M, Tanikawa K (1995) The effect of spleen volume on liver regeneration after hepatectomy. A clinical study of liver and spleen volumes by computed tomography. Hepato-Gastroenterology 42:961–965
7. Iwao T, Oho K, Sakai T, et al. (1997) Splanchnic and extrasplanchnic arterial hemodynamics in patients with cirrhosis. J Hepatol 27:817–823
8. Tanikawa K, Noguchi K, Sata M (1991) Ultrastructural features of Kupffer cells and endothelial cells in chronic ethanol-fed rats. In: Wisse E, Knook DL, McCuskey RS (eds) Cells of the hepatic sinusoid, vol 3. Kupffer Cell Foundation, Leiden, pp 445–448

9. Ohira H, Ueno T, Shakado S, et al. (1994) Cultured rat hepatic sinusoidal endothelial cells express intercellular adhesion molecule-1 (ICAM-1) by tumor necrosis factor-$\alpha$ or interleukin-1$\alpha$ stimulation. J Hepatol 20:729–734

10. Tanikawa K (1989) Kupffer cell function in cholestasis. In: Wisse E, Knook DL, Decker K (eds) Cells of the hepatic sinusoid, vol 2. Kupffer cell Foundation, Rijswijk, pp 288–292

11. Sasatomi K, Noguchi K, Sakisaka S, et al. (1998) Abnormal accumulation of endotoxin in biliary epithelial cells in primary biliary cirrhosis and primary sclerosing cholangitis. J Hepatol, in press

# Part II
# Hepatic Sinusoidal Cells:
# Characteristics and Special Topics

# Endothelial Cells of the Hepatic Sinusoids: A Review

E. Wisse, F. Braet, D. Luo, D. Vermijlen, M. Eddouks,
M. Konstandoulaki, C. Empsen, and R.B. De Zanger

*Summary.* Hepatic sinusoidal endothelial cells differ from other endothelial cells. They possess open fenestrae that are grouped in sieve plates and lack a basal lamina. Fenestrae measure about 150 nm, occur at a frequency of 9–13/mm$^2$, and occupy 6%–8% of the endothelial surface (porosity). These filter characteristics determine the exchange between the blood and the parenchymal cells, and are influencing the transport of lipoproteins including cholesterol and vitamin A. Forced sieving and endothelial massage are thought to enhance the passage of lipoproteins and to refresh the fluids in the space of Disse. Alcohol, nicotine, and other agents affect fenestrae in different ways and contribute either to fatty liver or hyperlipidemia. Furthermore, sinusoidal endothelial cells have: 1) a large capacity for pinocytosis via coated pits and macropinocytotic vesicles, 2) a variety of adhesion molecules, and receptors (scavenger, hyaluronan, collagen, Fc), and 3) a large capacity to digest material by numerous lysosomes. Endothelial cells secrete a limited amount of cytokines, but are vulnerable to products released by Kupffer cells, as in the case of endotoxemia or liver preservation. Capillarization of sinusoids includes the loss of fenestrae and the formation of a basal lamina and occurs in pathological conditions.

## Introduction

Investigations by transmission (TEM and scanning SEM) electron microscopy have resulted in detailed descriptions of sinusoidal cells of the liver, together with their reactions in normal and experimental conditions [93, 217, 221–225]. Biochemical studies implied isolation, purification, and culture of these cells [111–113]. At present, studies are focused on the molecular biology and the clinical aspects of this intriguing class of cells [54, 204, 205, 209], making it clear that a number of important hepatic functions and pathogenetic mechanisms reside in sinusoidal cells.

In the 1960s and 1970s, textbooks of histology described sinusoids as bordered by undifferentiated endothelial lining cells, able to differentiate into Kupffer cells when activated by a proper stimulus. Electron microscopy in combination with the method

Laboratory for Cell Biology and Histology, Free University of Brussels (VUB), Laarbeeklaan 103, 1090 Brussels-Jette, Belgium

17

of perfusion fixation clarified this situation and provided evidence that a normal hepatic sinusoid is inhabited by four different types of cells [234]: endothelial cells [190, 222], Kupffer cells [223, 224], fat-storing cells [92, 93, 217, 218], and pit cells [225, 233, 235, 236]. These cells are located in and around the hepatic sinusoid; each cell type has its own identity, as expressed in different morphology and function in experiments and disease. Transitional forms between the cells have never been observed and are supposed to be absent.

Endothelial cells of the hepatic sinusoid have been characterized morphologically by TEM [221, 222] and on the molecular level by their content of enzymes, mRNA, surface antigens, receptors, adhesion molecules, and recognition by specific antibodies [52, 151]. There have been suggestions for further subdivision of hepatic endothelial cells on the basis of size, density, support for the development of hemopoietic cells [31], and interleukin-1 (IL-1) binding capacity [9]. One must take into account, however, that the liver harbors many different types of endothelial

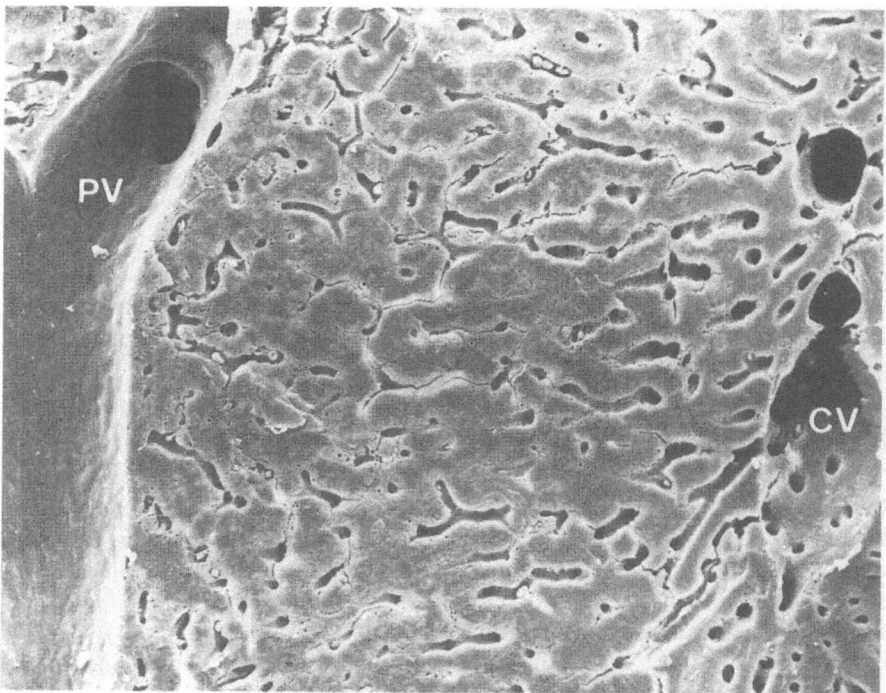

FIG. 1. The hepatic liver lobule in a glutaraldehyde-perfusion fixed rat liver, dehydrated in alcohol and freeze-fractured in alcohol at the temperature of liquid nitrogen, then critical point-dried and sputter-coated with gold. To the *left side*, a branch of the portal vein (*PV*); to the *right* a branch of the central vein (*CV*). Notice the absence of connections (inlets) to sinusoids in the portal vein, and the abundance of sinusoidal connections in the central vein. Sinusoids close to the portal vein are narrow and tortuous, whereas the sinusoids close to the central vein become more straight and parallel. (×340)

cells in different locations, i.e., arteria, portal vein, sinusoids, central vein (Fig. 1), and lymphatic vessels, meaning that endothelial cells are involved in the microcirculation and in lining the large vessels. Once endothelial cells are isolated from the liver, it is not unthinkable that endothelial cells from these different locations are collected in suspension. Endothelial cells in different types of vessels in the liver, however, seem to share positive staining for vimentin [119].

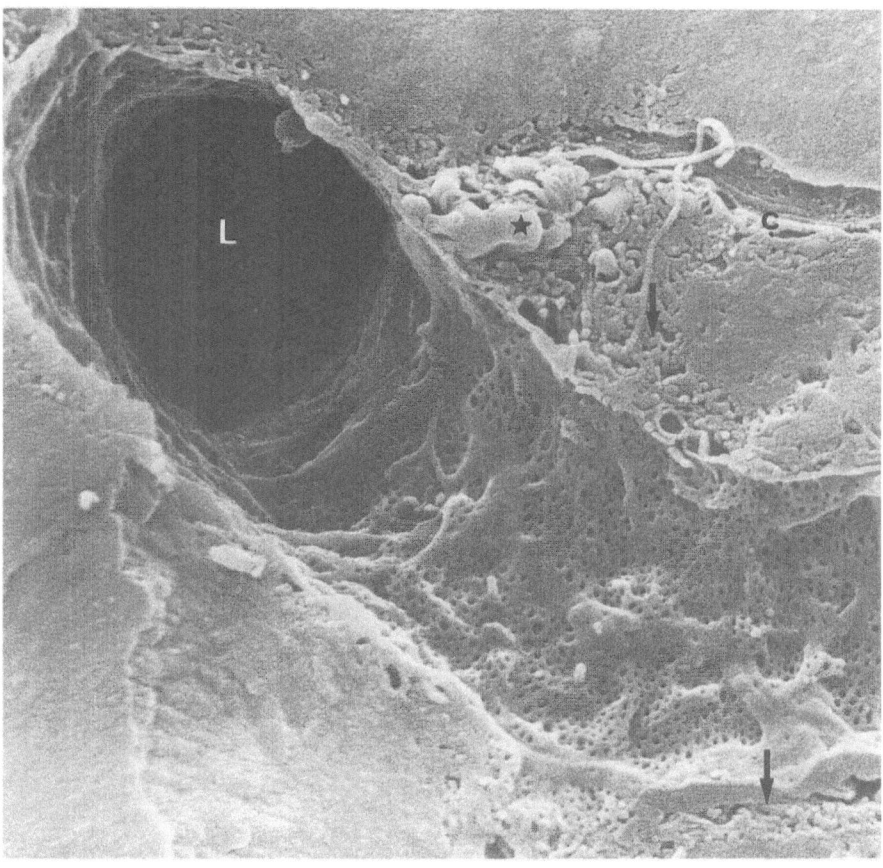

FIG. 2. Scanning electron microscope micrograph (SEM) of a rat liver sinusoid, prepared as in Fig. 1. The endothelial lining shows numerous fenestrae. Within the space of Disse, microvilli can be seen (*arrows*). At the *top right*, a bundle of collagen fibrils (*c*) is lying close to droplets (*asterisk*), probably fat droplets of a fat-storing cell. Within the frozen-fractured parenchymal cells, organelles are barely seen. *L*, lumen of the sinusoid. ($\times$11 700)

# Description of Endothelial Cells

Endothelial cells of the hepatic sinusoid are flat cells, forming the lining of the sinusoidal wall. Their thin, flat processes of cytoplasm are spread out and contain fenestrae, clustered in groups to form sieve plates (Fig. 2). Thicker cytoplasmic arms, containing pinocytotic vesicles, mitochondria, lysosomes, and other organelles, are interspersed between these thin, flat parts. The endothelial cells encircle the

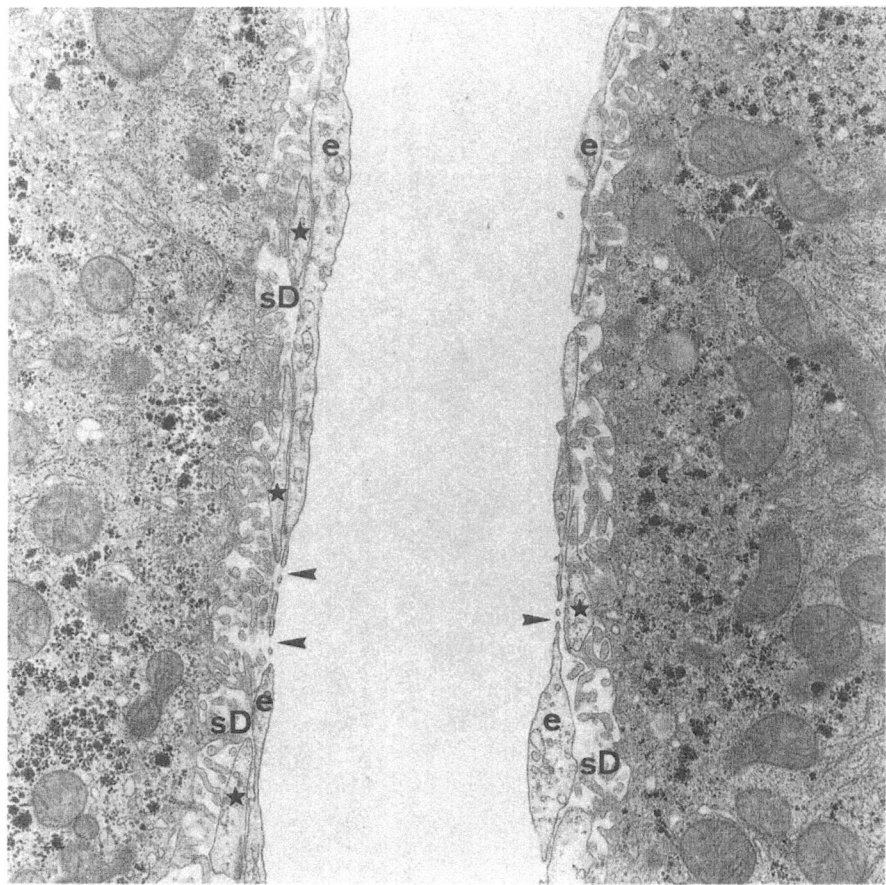

FIG. 3. A hepatic sinusoid of rat liver, fixed by perfusion fixation with glutaraldehyde, postfixed in osmium, dehydrated in alcohol, and embedded in Epon. The lumen of the sinusoid (L) is lined by the endothelium (e), showing the presence of fenestrae (arrowheads). The space of Disse (sD) contains numerous microvilli of the parenchymal cells together with small pieces of cytoplasm of fat-storing cells (asterisks). Within the parenchymal cells, different organelles can be seen, such as mitochondria, cisternae of the rough endoplasmic reticulum, and glycogen. (×17 125)

sinusoidal lumen and form cylindrical structures all by themselves, and are arranged as single cells in a row to form the typical liver capillary, the sinusoid. The term "sinusoid" seems to stem from a French embryology study performed in the last century, giving the liver capillaries this particular and lasting name. There is reason enough to maintain the special name, because the structure and function of this capillary differs from all other capillaries in the body. Other organs, such as the spleen and the bone marrow which are often mentioned together with the liver as reticuloendothelial system (RES) organs, might contain comparable sinusoids, but this is not clear at the moment.

There are, in normal conditions, certainly no discontinuities or open spaces between sinusoidal endothelial cells. Free access of fluid, solutes, droplets, and particles from the lumen toward the space of Disse and vice versa is solely provided by fenestrae (Fig. 3). Membrane contacts between endothelial cells are not showing any peculiar structure; cells touch and are apparently glued together by adhesion molecules without any visible structural component such as a zonula or macula adherens. Cell membrane contacts occur between thin rims of cytoplasm; they are therefore also very limited in contact surface and probably do not provide enough space for gap junctions. Obviously, endothelial cells are supported by branched arms of fat-storing cells [233, 246], which are closely apposed to the backside of endothelial cells by flat surfaces of their branched cytoplasmic arms, which surround the endothelial cells as (contractile) pericytes. It is therefore believed that hepatic endothelial cells are not very firmly attached to other cells in the tissue and are not metabolically coupled to each other as endothelial cells elsewhere are.

Although minute amounts of basal lamina components can be detected within the space of Disse by immunocytochemistry [39], a clear basal lamina structure is missing [221, 222, 230]. Sometimes small fragments of basal lamina-like material can be seen, mostly in between endothelial cells and fat-storing cells. Kupffer cells and pit cells attach to endothelial cells without showing specialized cell junctions. Kupffer cells and pit cells are mobile and motile cells, being able to change their shape and also to attach to endothelial cells and actively move away from a particular position. Also, they are able to (partly) replace endothelial cells by inserting themselves into the endothelial lining. Kupffer cells and pit cells might even extravasate and penetrate the space of Disse or the tissue, as occurs in some experiments or diseases.

In addition to fenestrae, other specialized structures of hepatic sinusoidal endothelial cells are the pronounced components of the vacuolar apparatus, showing a variety of vacuolar and vesicular structures, such as bristle-coated pinocytotic vesicles, uncoated vesicles of comparable size, bristle-coated Golgi vesicles, macropinocytotic vacuoles, electron lucent vacuoles, and vacuoles of the same size with increasing electron density up to and including numerous electron-dense lysosomes (Fig. 4). By morphometry it was determined that hepatic endothelial cells possess about 45% of the volume of pinocytotic vesicles in the liver, which points to an extreme specialization, because the cells take only about 3% of the tissue volume [21]. The lysosomes of endothelial cells contribute 17% to the total lysosomal volume [21]. Compared with other endothelial cells in the body, the hepatic endothelial cells are extremely specialized in pinocytosis and digestion and can therefore be considered members of the RES.

Uptake by bristle-coated vesicles and macropinocytotic vesicles of endothelial

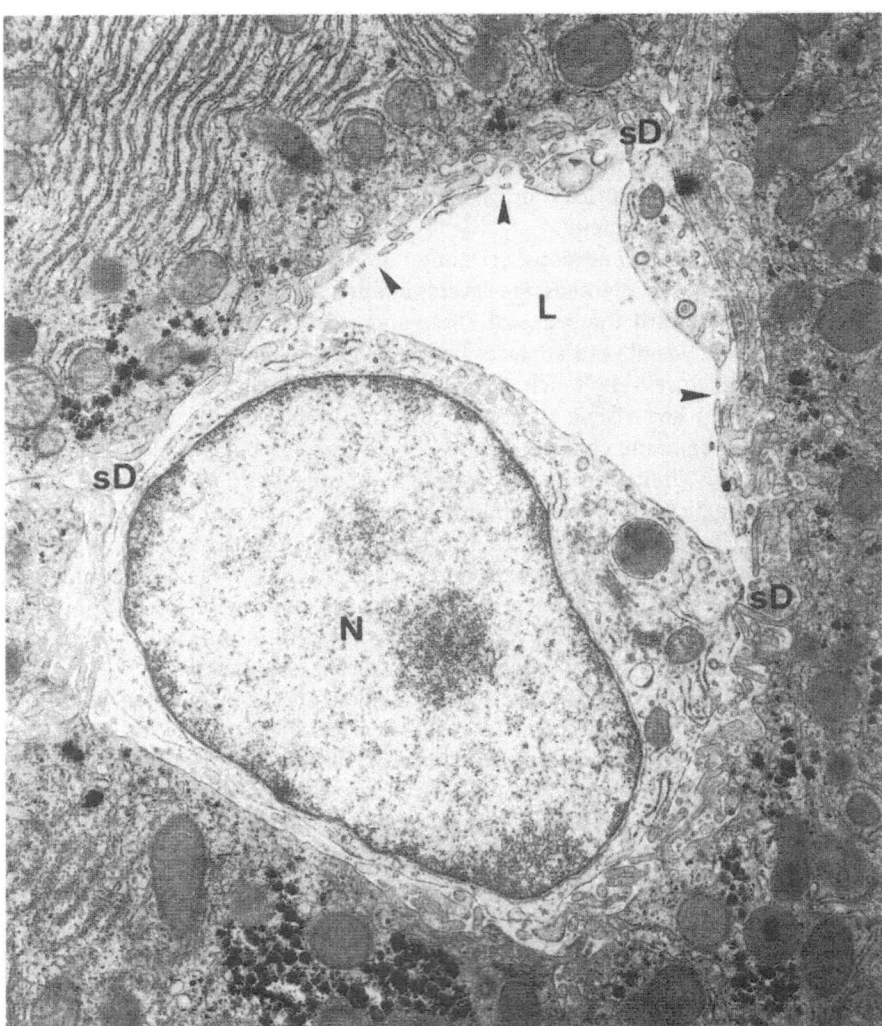

FIG. 4. Transmission electron microscope (TEM) micrograph of an endothelial cell in rat liver. Apart from the large nucleus (*N*), we observe a small Golgi apparatus, cisternae of the rough endoplasmic reticulum, a dense body (lysosome), and thin processes containing fenestrae (*arrowheads*). In the parenchymal cells, packed cisternae of rough endoplasmic reticulum are present, next to mitochondria, peroxisomes, and glycogen. *L*, lumen of the sinusoid; *sD*, space of Disse. (×17 125)

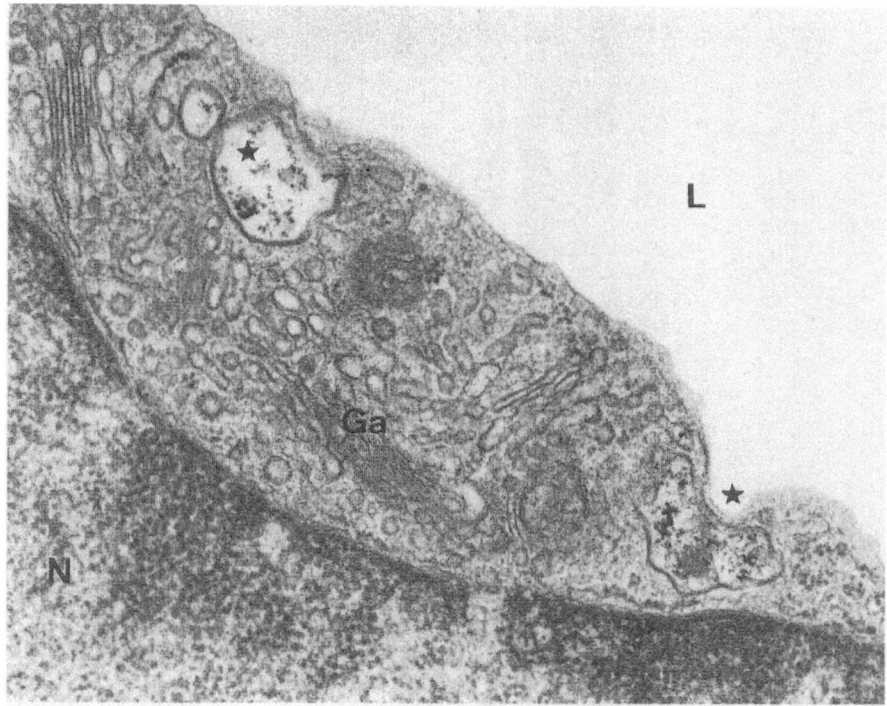

FIG. 5. Macropinocytotic vacuoles (*asterisks*) of endothelial cells, 3 min after i.v. injection of particles consisting of ferric oxyhydroxide citrate (Ami-25, see [231]), showing the presence of these particles within their lumen. The peculiar shape and position of the vacuole at the *right side* is typical for early stages of macropinocytotic vacuole formation. It is thought that these vacuoles are not a product of the fusion of bristle-coated micropinocytotic vesicles, because the vacuoles already contain particles 3 min after injection. This time interval seems too short to form such vacuoles by fusion of bristle-coated micropinocytotic vesicles. Other organelles in this micrograph are several Golgi apparatuses (*Ga*) and a part of the nucleus (*N*). *L*, lumen of the sinusoid. (×48 000)

cells (Figs. 5–7) has been demonstrated for a number of small, colloidal particles, such as thorotrast, saccharated iron oxide, ferric oxyhydroxide citrate (Ami-25), latex (<0.1 μm), colloidal gold, antimony sulfide, and horseradish peroxidase [222, 226]. In a period of 10 to 30 min after the initial uptake, particles are found in round electron lucent vacuoles, which gradually fuse or develop into vacuoles with increasing density, until particles are found in real electron-dense lysosomes. In conditions of particle overload, when large amounts of circulating small colloidal particles are ingested by the RES, endothelial cells can show images of extensive storage. This storage consists of rounded conglomerates of particles with a diameter comparable to

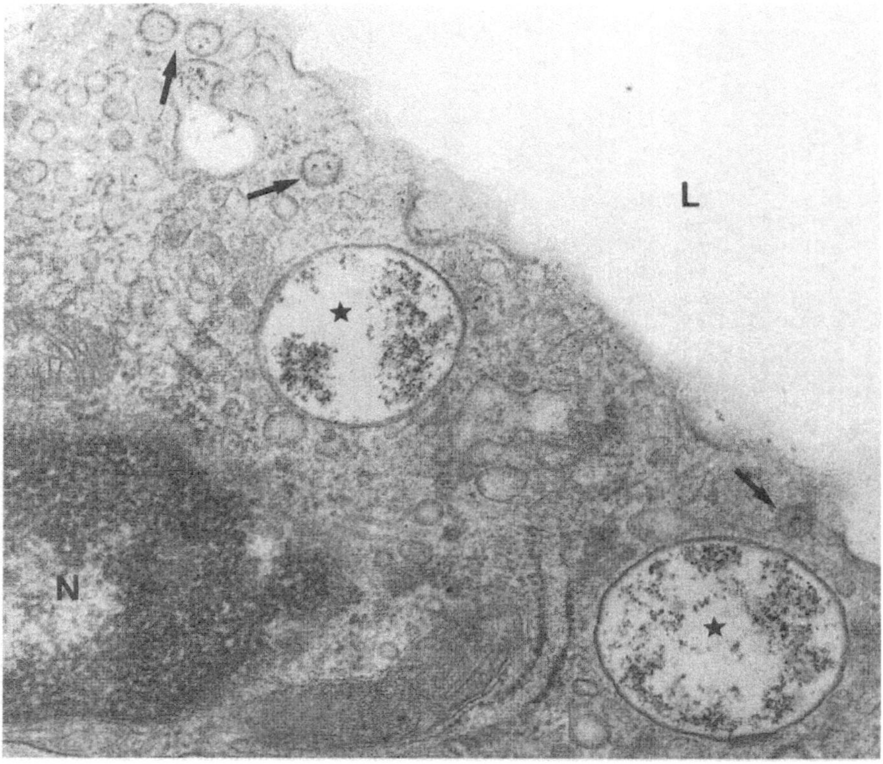

24    E. Wisse et al.

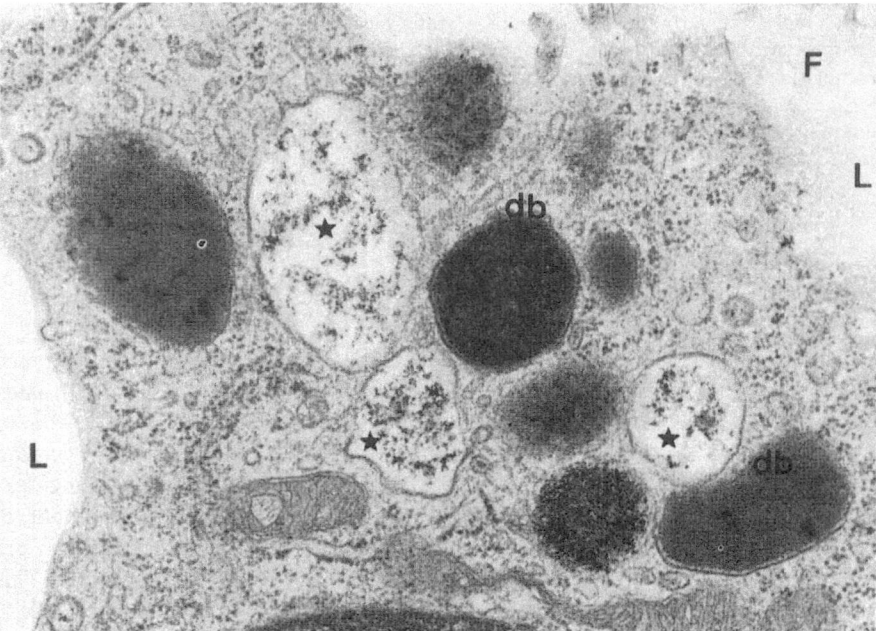

6

7

FIG. 6. Two macropinocytotic vacuoles (*asterisks*) at 15 min after i.v. injection of the particles shown in Fig. 5. More particles have accumulated and have formed condensed material in the vacuoles, which have become rounded. Some bristle-coated micropinocytotic vesicles also contain particles (*arrows*). L, lumen of the sinusoid. (×74 000)

FIG. 7. TEM micrograph of an endothelial cell, showing macropinocytotic vacuoles (*asterisks*) near vacuoles with increasing electron density and dense bodies (*db*, lysosomes). F, fenestrae; L, lumen of the sinusoid. (×50 000)

◀──────────────────────────────────────────────────────────────

the size of lysosomes; the conglomerates aggregate in membrane-bound clusters (Fig. 8). These conglomerates are larger than regular lysosomes and are supposed to represent residual bodies [222, 226]. Significant differences in long-term handling of these substances occur between Kupffer cells and endothelial cells [232]. Other substances, taken up by endothelial cells, include fluorescently labeled collagen [84], acetyl-low density lipoprotein (LDL) [10], and Ox-LDL [44]. In the case of degradable sub-

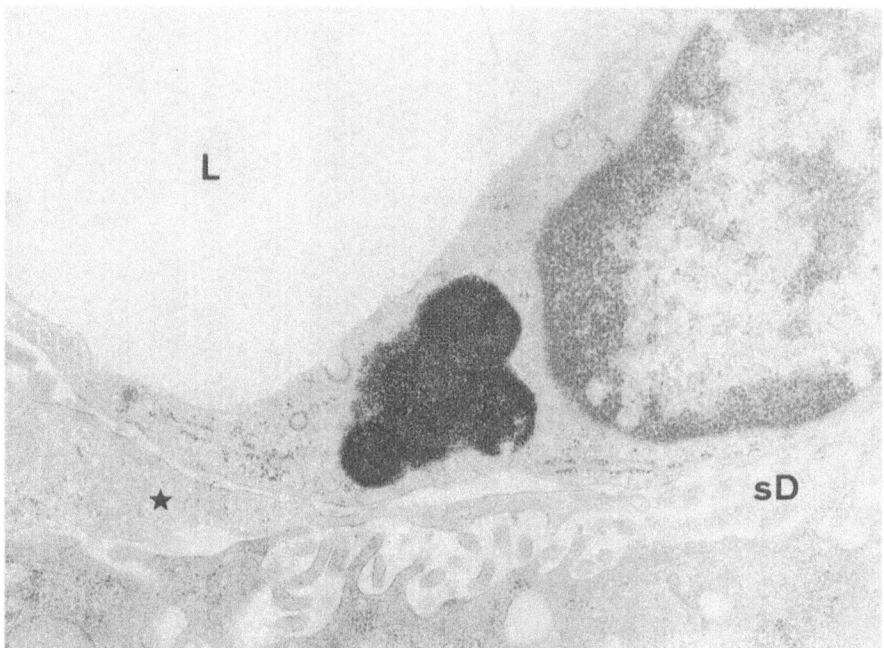

FIG. 8. TEM micrograph of an endothelial cell in rat liver, one month after the i.v. injection of particles, as in Figs. 5–7. At longer time intervals, lysosomes in endothelial cells form residual bodies, in which rounded aggregates of particles, with a diameter comparable to that of lysosomes, cohere to form a conglomerate. It is thought that these conglomerates are present for a very long time because of the indigestible nature of the particles. The space of Disse (*sD*) and a fat-storing cell process (*asterisk*) are seen. L, lumen of the sinusoid. (×72 000)

stances, digestion has been demonstrated after 1 h [107]. So far, little evidence exists on the possibilities to modulate the endocytotic capacity of endothelial cells, although it has been reported that IL-1 transiently enhances endocytosis by endothelial cells [128]. Is endothelial endocytosis a steady-state process with a fixed timetable?

Sometimes endothelial cells seem to function as preprocessing units for parenchymal cells, as in the case of lipoproteins, leading to the hydrolyzation and release of cholesterol, subsequently transported to parenchymal cells, where it is converted into bile acids [10]. Transferrin is desialylated by endothelial cells and also is transferred to parenchymal cells [135]. Endothelial cells possess membrane-bound lipase that has phospholipase and triacylglycerol hydrolase activity and metabolizes intermediate density lipoprotein (IDL) and high density liproprotein (HDL) [6]. Also, the specific receptor and uptake activity of endothelial cells might bring them in some cases in competition with Kupffer cells, for instance when glucocerebrosidase is administered i.v. to treat Gaucher's disease, in which case endothelial cells take up 60% of the injected compound, whereas the Kupffer cells suffer from the enzyme deficiency and take up less than 10% [18].

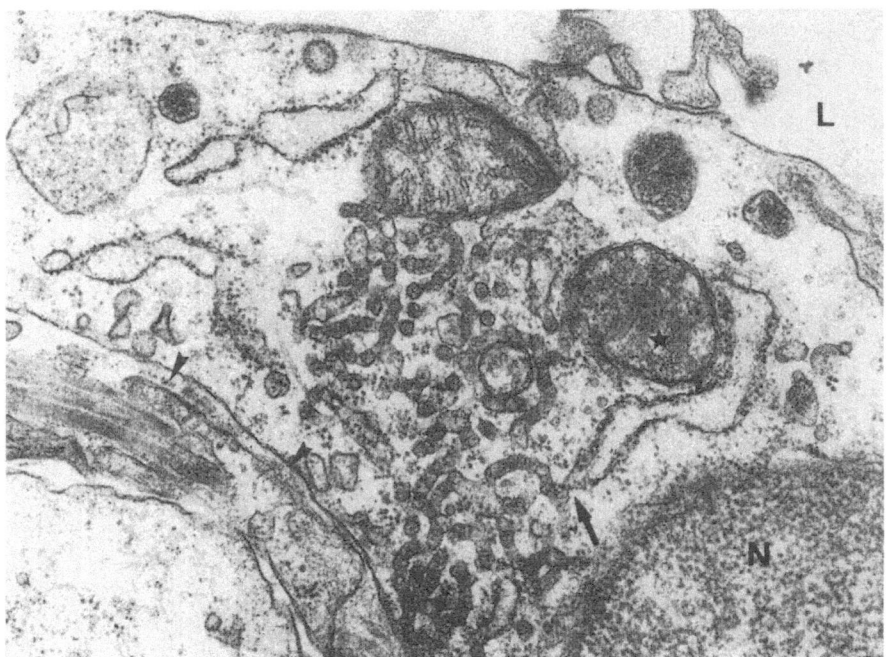

FIG. 9. TEM micrograph of an endothelial cell of rat liver, showing the presence of a tubular network of smooth endoplasmic reticulum. The tubules of smooth endoplasmic reticulum are continuous with cisternae of the rough endoplasmic reticulum (*arrow*). Other structures are a part of the nucleus (*N*), mitochondria (showing cristae parallel to the surface of the section [*asterisk*]). In the space of Disse, a bundle of collagen fibrils and a fragment of a basal lamina can be seen (*arrowheads*). *L*, lumen of the sinusoid. (×25 000)

Organelles, as found in all other cells, are present in endothelial cells. The nucleus bulges into the lumen of the sinusoid, which contributes to interaction with red and white blood cells passing by [231]. These cells may be temporarily retarded or stopped in their flow through the sinusoid. Other organelles include mitochondria, a Golgi apparatus, rough endoplasmic reticulum, and smooth endoplasmic reticulum, forming a peculiar tubular network (Fig. 9), centrioles, and a well developed cytoskeleton, consisting of microtubuli and microfilaments. Within the nucleus, a nucleolus and sometimes a sphaeridium [222] are to be recognized. Peroxisomes, Weibel-Palade bodies, or secretion granules are not found in rat sinusoidal endothelial cells; endothelial cells in other species, however, might show the presence of Weibel-Palade granules.

## Preparation of Endothelial Cells

Endothelial cells seem to be vulnerable cells, a fact which becomes obvious during preparation for electron microscopy (EM) [221] and during procedures for liver transplantation [66, 165]. Endothelial cells are apparently sensitive to ischemia and elevated pressure. Preparation for EM should preferably be performed by perfusion fixation with an osmotically balanced fixative, containing 1%–2% glutaraldehyde at physiological pressure (12 cmH$_2$O) at room temperature for 1 min through the portal vein, starting within seconds after laparotomy and cannulating the portal vein [229]. This seems obligatory to preserve the fine structure of the endothelial lining, such as intact fenestrae and sieve plates [221, 229, 230]. With retarded perfusion, or immersion fixation, the endothelial lining will develop large, irregular gaps. The endothelial cytoskeleton probably is destabilized and fenestrae fuse and create gaps.

Endothelial cells can be isolated by collagenase perfusion of the liver, isopycnic sedimentation in a two-step Percoll gradient, and selective adherence. The obtained purity and viability reaches 95% [23], whereas the yield is about 2.4 × 10$^6$ cells/g rat liver. Endothelial cells in culture display their normal morphologic and functional characteristics, such as fenestrae and pinocytotic vesicles. They also respond to agents such as alcohol by increasing fenestrae diameter, and serotonin by decreasing fenestrae diameter [23, 25, 33, 197]. The distribution and clustering of fenestrae in sieve plates seems to become diffuse in some isolated cell preparations [42]. Endothelial cells cultured on type I collagen gels formed a cobblestone layer on the surface of the gel. Cells cultured on laminin-containing type I collagen gels invaded the gel and exhibited tube formation with a low number of fenestrae. Endothelial cells cultured on Matrigel had many fenestrae and formed tubes (10 μm) [185]. All this indicates that extracellular matrix components are also determining the phenotype of endothelial cells.

## Fenestrae

An obvious function of endothelial cells seems to be sieving, in particular, sieving of the fluids exchanged between the sinusoidal lumen and the space of Disse [86]. Fenestrae have been visualized after perfusion fixation of livers with TEM and SEM and without chemical fixation in freeze-etch preparations of fresh liver tissue [221]. Recently, we were able to visualize fenestrae by atomic force microscopy (AFM) in cultured endothelial cells, briefly fixed and still in fluid [25]. Attempts to visualize fenestrae in living endothelial cells by AFM were only very occasionally successful, because these endothelial cells were found to be very vulnerable and soft compared with a number of other cell types [25]. This is an amazing experience, because one might expect sinusoidal endothelial cells to be quite strong to be able to resist the continuous friction with red and white blood cells. Filtering of fluids by the endothelial lining sets restrictions on the passage of lipoproteins, but may also restrict passage of other droplets and particles such as viruses and infecting agents. Lipoproteins concern chylomicrons and their remnants, transported from the lumen to the space of Disse, and very low-density lipoproteins (VLDL) from the space of Disse to the sinusoidal lumen. Chylomicrons have sizes equal to and larger than fenestrae, whereas remnants and VLDL have sizes equal to and smaller than fenestrae.

The most accurate measurements of fenestrae diameter have been performed with TEM preparations; SEM specimens shrink during preparation and change their measures by about 30%. Endothelial fenestrae in plastic-embedded sections measure 150–175 nm in TEM, and occur at a frequency of 9–13 per $\mu m^2$ in SEM and occupy 6%–8% of the total endothelial surface (i.e., porosity) in SEM preparations [230]. In SEM preparations, fenestrae diameter decreases from 111 nm to 105 nm on a periportal-to-pericentral gradient, whereas the number varies from 9 to 13 per $\mu m^2$ in the same

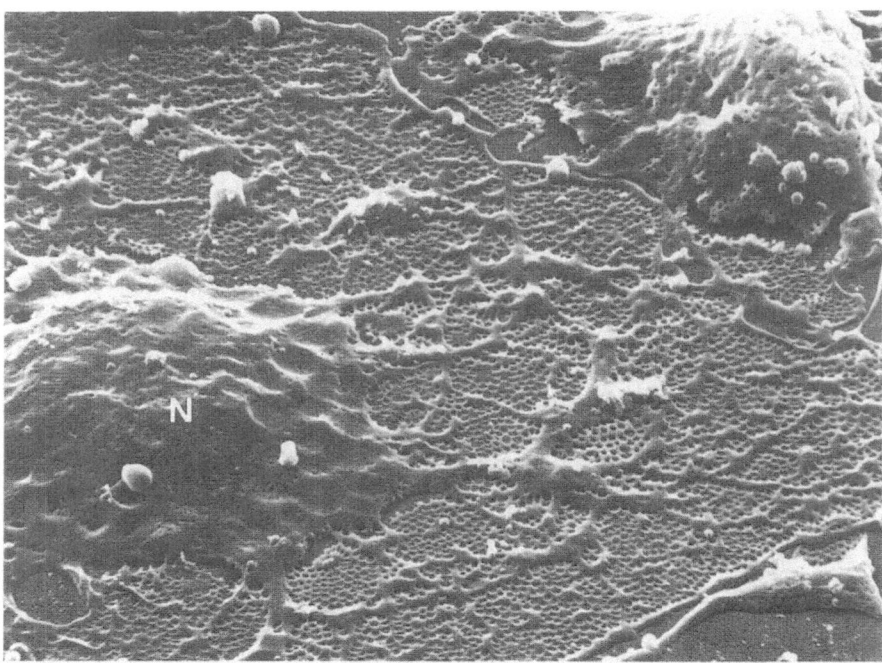

Fig. 10. SEM micrograph of an endothelial cell treated with latrunculin A, showing a substantially increased number of fenestrae. Cytoplasmic arms divide flat fields containing numerous fenestrae. The bulging area contains the nucleus (N) and shows many coated pits. (×10 000)

direction, thereby increasing the porosity from 6% to 8% [230]. It is not well understood why a higher porosity is seen in the centrolobular areas, because the level of metabolic activities in this area seems to be lower. The diameter of fenestrae can be influenced by agents such as serotonin, $CCl_4$, alcohol, nicotine, pantethine, and pressure [23, 25, 33, 62, 63, 86, 227].

Detergent-extracted whole mounts (Fig. 10) of slightly fixed, isolated endothelial cells studied with TEM, showed that fenestrae are delineated by a filamentous, fenestrae-associated cytoskeleton ring with a thickness of 16 nm (Fig. 11), whereas sieve plates are surrounded and delineated by a ring-like orientation of microtubuli

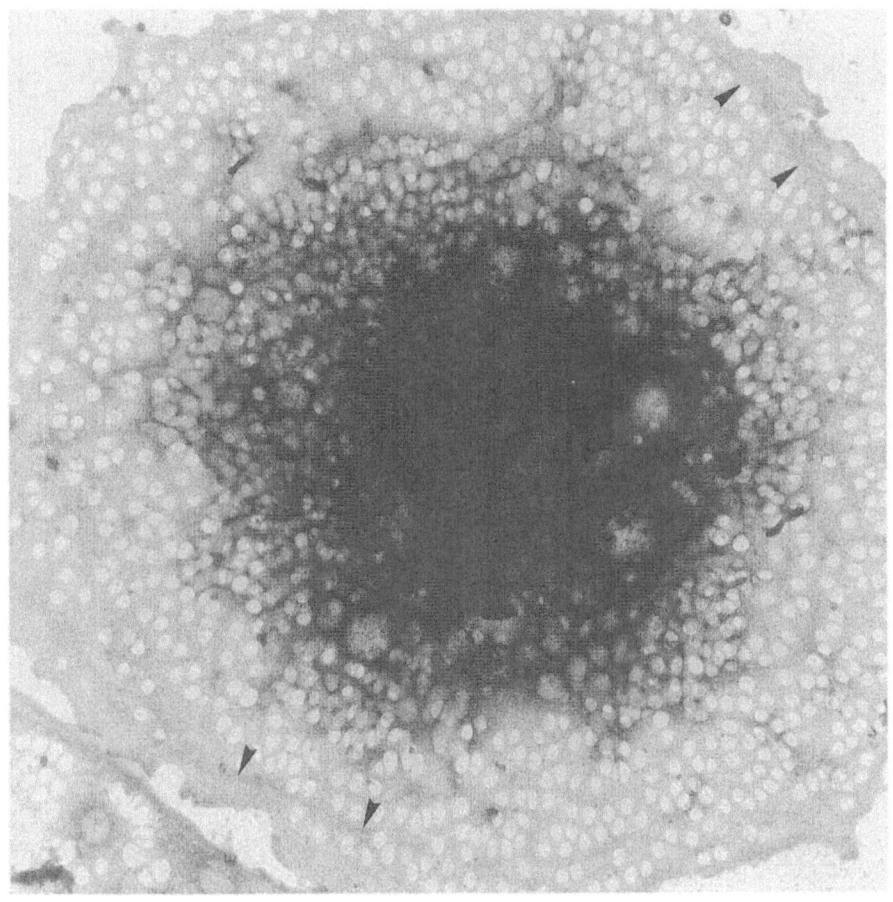

FIG. 11. TEM micrograph of a whole mount of a control (untreated) endothelial cell after isolation, purification, and culture for a short period on a formvar-coated EM grid. Numerous fenestrae are seen, many of which are arranged in rows or sieve plates. Bundles of microfilaments fix the rows of fenestrae (*arrowheads*) in the peripheral cytoplasm. The central dark area contains the nucleus, the contours of which are not shown. (×2125)

[24]. Ethanol enlarged the diameter of these rings, whereas serotonin reduced it [24]. The rings become thinner in relaxation and thicker when contracted. The fenestrae-associated cytoskeleton ring therefore seems to act as a supporting structure and "muscle" around fenestrae. Because the fenestrae-associated cytoskeleton ring opens and closes like fenestrae in response to ethanol and serotonin treatment, it is suggested that the fenestrae-associated cytoskeletal ring is composed of a contractile protein, most probably regulating the size-changes of the fenestrae. With regard to fenestrae contraction, myosin and actin might be involved, as it has been demonstrated that activation of myosin light chain kinase and protein kinase C occurs in response to serotonin [8]. This contraction is associated with a rapid influx of $Ca^{2+}$, which is dependent on extracellular $Ca^{2+}$ [27, 71].

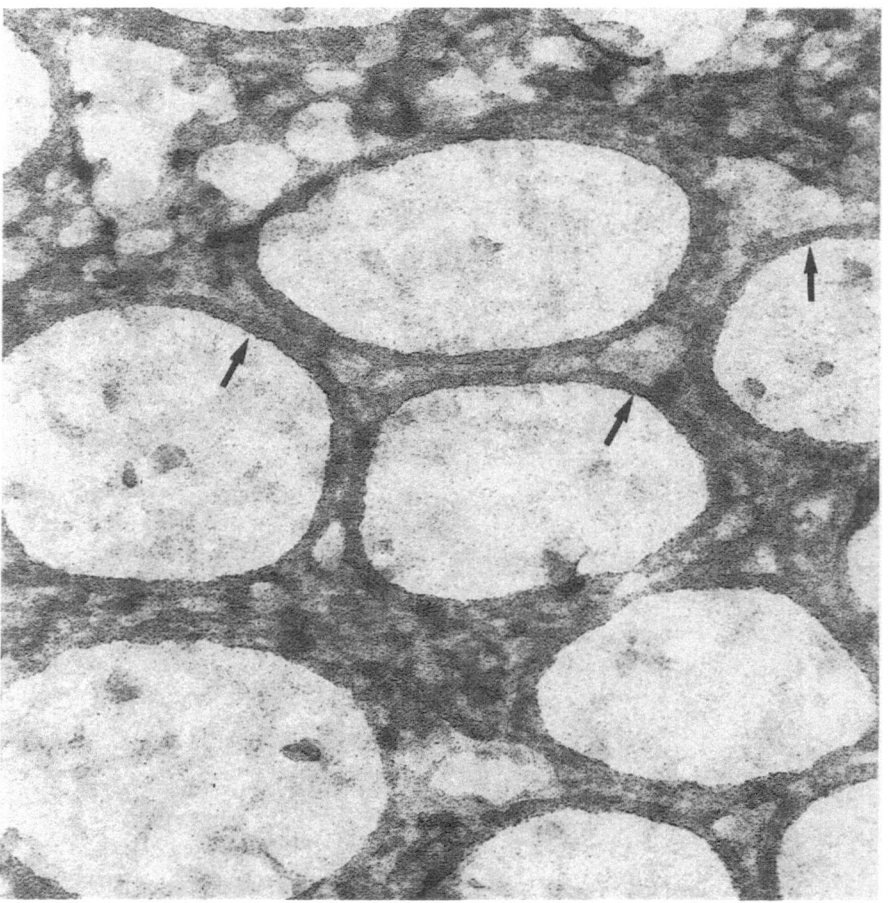

FIG. 12. TEM micrograph of a whole mount of an in vitro-cultured endothelial cell, showing the fenestrae-associated cytoskeleton rings (*arrows*) and branching and connecting filaments in the extracted cytoplasm. ($\times 270\,000$)

An intriguing phenomenon occurs when endothelial cells are treated with agents that interfere with the actin cytoskeleton. A number of these substances, such as cytochalasin B, latrunculin A (Fig. 12), misakinolide and jasplakinolide were tested with endothelial cells in vitro. These substances have different specific reaction mechanisms with actin monomers or filaments, but share their ability to disturb the actin cytoskeleton. They all induce, within half an hour, a doubling of the number of fenestrae, each provided with a (newly formed?) fenestrae-associated cytoskeleton ring [24, 26]. Latrunculin A seems to be one of the most powerful agents, because its effect was obtained at concentrations about 100 times lower than cytochalasin B [26]. Apparently, the cytoskeleton determines the numerical dynamics of fenestrae [26].

# Sieving

The fenestrated lining blocks the passage of particles such as chylomicrons and their remnants [45, 143, 237]. In unweaned baby rats, numerous chylomicrons were seen in the space of Disse [143]. The average size of fenestrae in these baby rats, as studied by TEM, was 130 nm with a maximum of 250 nm, and the values for remnants within the space of Disse were 120 nm (average) and 250 nm (maximum). When adult rats were fed corn oil, fenestrae were found to have an average size of 185 nm, with a maximum of 400 nm, whereas remnants within the space of Disse were 160 nm (average) and 450 nm (maximum) [45]. Larger chylomicrons were found in the portal blood. These data clearly prove the sieving effect of endothelial fenestrae. In addition, lecithin-coated polystyrene beads measuring 140 nm were observed within the space of Disse and in the parenchymal cells [102].

There are two important physiological consequences connected to the selective admission of lipoproteins to the space of Disse, both of which concern their cholesterol and vitamin A content. During circulation, chylomicrons selectively lose most of their triglycerides in the tissues, thereby becoming relatively enriched in cholesterol and cholesterol esters, in the meantime forming remnants with a smaller diameter, allowing their entrance into the space of Disse [65, 230]. The influx of cholesterol in parenchymal cells is therefore determined by the size and frequency of fenestrae and by parenchymal cell surface receptors for remnants. Furthermore, the uptake of cholesterol inhibits the de novo synthesis of cholesterol in parenchymal cells and contributes to both the production of bile acids and the synthesis of lipoproteins (VLDL). It is known that chronic alcohol abuse influences the diameter and frequency of fenestrae, at the same time affecting the metabolism of lipoproteins and vitamin A [65]. A short-time effect of alcohol is an increase in the diameter of fenestrae, allowing larger chylomicrons to transport their contents to the parenchymal cells, thereby contributing to the development of fatty liver [33]. Chronic alcohol abuse defenestrates the endothelial lining [86], resulting in hyperlipidemia [36] and inhibition of the transport of cholesterol and vitamin A to parenchymal and fat-storing cells. This phenomenon will turn sinusoids into capillaries with a continuous endothelial lining and a basal lamina.

A second important consequence of the selective admission of lipoproteins is the transport of vitamin A to the parenchymal and fat-storing cells [20, 85]. Vitamin A determines the differentiation or activation of fat-storing cells, and when the influx of retinoids is interrupted, fat-storing cells develop into activated myofibroblasts, synthesizing enormous amounts of extracellular matrix, causing fibrosis. The fenestrae are therefore thought to play an important role in the balance and distribution of lipids, cholesterol, and vitamin A, and are thought to play a major role in the development of liver cirrhosis.

It is known that rabbits have smaller fenestrae than rats [237], which might explain why rabbits are more sensitive to atherosclerosis, supposing they have equally sized circulating lipoprotein particles. Smaller fenestrae cause cholesterol-rich remnants to circulate longer before they are taken up by the liver. Partial (66%) hepatectomy induces a 10-fold increase in porosity of the endothelial lining and induces a 20-fold increase of fat-droplet volume in parenchymal cells [141]. Endotoxin (lipopolysaccharide, LPS) administration also decreased fenestration and accentuated the alcohol alterations [176]. Nicotine narrows the fenestrae [62], which might contribute to coronary disease, because of the effect on the distribution of cholesterol.

## Sinusoids, Forced Sieving, and Endothelial Massage

The word "sinusoid" seems to be composed of the Latin word *sinus* (a hollow) and the ancient Greek word *eidos* (form) [131]. The development of adult-type sinusoids is initiated at the 10th week of gestation and is completed by 20 weeks [39]. The rat liver sinusoid is a quite narrow type of capillary, with a diameter in the range of 5 to 7 μm [230] or 7 to 10 μm [15], depending on the method of measurement. The sinusoidal lumen occupies about 11% of the tissue volume, whereas the space of Disse takes about 5% of the tissue volume [21]. Narrow and tortuous sinusoids are found in the periportal area, whereas the sinusoids in the centrolobular region are wider and are arranged in a more parallel way. In SEM preparations, the wall of a small portal vein branch shows very few connections to sinusoids, whereas the wall of a central vein seems perforated with connections to sinusoids. In central veins, we sometimes observe a central bar occluding the outlet orifice of a sinusoid.

White blood cells often exceed the size of a sinusoid [230], resulting in regular, mechanical interaction between blood cells and the sinusoidal wall, causing retardation of flow or even plugging, as can be seen by in vivo microscopy (IVM). The occurrence of this type of interaction resulted in the postulation of two hypotheses: *endothelial massage* and *forced sieving*, which might occur together [230]. These hypotheses result from measurements of sinusoids and blood cells, together with IVM observations, indicating that red and white blood cells are in fact too big for sinusoids and therefore interact with the endothelial lining (Fig. 13) [230]. The hypotheses are considered to explain the driving forces behind the exchange of particles and fluids between the sinusoidal lumen and the space of Disse. Forced sieving promotes the transport of lipoprotein particles into the space of Disse, whereas endothelial massage supports the refreshing, mixing, and transporting of fluids contained within the space of Disse [230].

Forced sieving starts from the observation that blood flow in hepatic sinusoids consists of a slowly moving row of single red blood cells, separated by small volumes of plasma. By IVM, it is seen that red blood cells easily deform and constantly adapt to the size and shape of the sinusoid while flowing, thereby filling the lumen and occluding the separated volumes of plasma. Lipoproteins in these shifting fluid

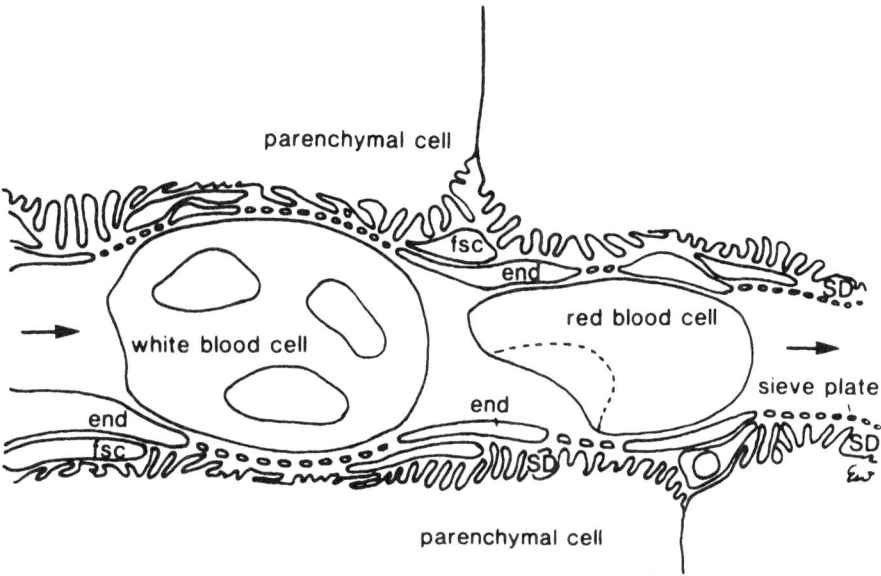

FIG. 13. Schematic explanation of the behavior of red and white blood cells within the hepatic sinusoid. Red blood cells are soft and pliable and therefore adapt their size and shape to the endothelial lining while flowing through a sinusoid. White blood cells are provided with a nucleus and a cytoskeleton, which make the cells less easy to deform and lets them regularly plug or interrupt flow while passing through the sinusoid. This behavior leads to two hypotheses, thought to be important for liver physiology, i.e., forced sieving and endothelial massage. See the text for further explanation. *Fsc*, fat-storing cell; *end*, endothelium; *SD*, space of Disse

compartments are vibrating in Brownian motion and will frequently be limited (one-sidedly) in their random movements by red blood cells. This interference is thought to enhance the chances of particles escaping through fenestrae into the space of Disse, especially when they are stuck in the limited zone of shear and friction forces between the red cell membrane and the surface of endothelial cells [230]. It is supposed that the particles roll between red blood cells and the endothelial cells surface, until they pass into fenestrae and disappear into the space of Disse. It is not unthinkable that these lipoprotein particles function as lubricating ball bearings during the passage of blood cells, keeping them at the same time at a little distance from the endothelial cell membrane to avoid membrane-to-membrane wear and shear.

Endothelial massage results mainly from the interaction of white blood cells (WBC) with the endothelial wall. WBC have a nucleus and cytoskeleton, which makes them relatively stiff as compared to the very flexible red blood cells. In IVM it is seen that WBC regularly plug periportal sinusoids, where they interrupt or retard blood flow. The size of WBC in IVM has an average value of 8.5 μm with a maximum of 12–13 μm for monocytes and polymorphs (PMN), whereas sinusoids measure between 6 and 7 μm in IVM [230]. Therefore, WBC have quite an impact on the endothelial lining, which they are supposed to compress together with the space of Disse. Compression of the space of Disse seems easy, because the microvilli on top of the parenchymal cells do not contain bundles of actin microfilaments and are not supposed to be rigid, like microvilli of the brush border of intestinal epithelial cells. WBC, however, have a shape and rigidity of their own, unlike red blood cells, and do not easily adapt to the size and shape of the sinusoid. Therefore, they get stuck in narrow, periportal sinusoids and impress a part of the endothelial lining and the space of Disse, depending on their shape and position in that particular sinusoid. Impression of the space of Disse causes displacement of fluids, which escape through the nearby fenestrae. It is also observed by IVM that this situation is solved by unplugging, during which the WBC change their shape or attach to the lining and move away from the spot. After this, the endothelial lining and the space of Disse will resume their normal shape and fresh fluids will enter the space of Disse.

Flow resistance decreases from periportal to centrolobular areas. The narrow diameter and the tortuous path of sinusoids and resistance factors appear to contribute to the slow velocity in the periportal area [115]. Owing to the narrowness and the tortuosity of the periportal sinusoids, the interaction with WBC is greatest in the periportal region [228], and by that interaction they contribute to the metabolism in the periportal region.

## Receptors

A number of substances are taken up by receptor-mediated endocytosis of endothelial cells: transferrin, ceruloplasmin, transcobalamine II, glucosaminoglucans, modified HDL and LDL, formaldehyde-treated serum albumin (FSA), liver lipase, collagen, remnant Apo E, VLDL, horseradish peroxidase, hyaluronic acid, chondroitin sulfate, lysosomal hydrolases, invertase, amylase A, asialo-orosomucoid, and ovalbumin [43, 55, 162, 163, 188].

Human sinusoidal endothelial cells, but not vascular endothelium, possess CD32/Fc receptors but there seems to be no direct evidence for antigen presentation by these cells [182, 208]. The monoclonal antibody 2E1 against the Fc receptor II reacts with sinusoidal endothelial cells except in the periportal area [142]. Fc receptors, found along the sinusoidal endothelial cells, decrease after GalN injury [94]. Circulating immune complexes were found to be ingested by Kupffer cells and endothelial cells according to the Fc receptor distribution [2, 94, 117]. In Kupffer cell-depleted or -defective rats, i.v. injected soluble aggregates of IgG, IgA, or IgM and immunocomplexes were cleared by Fc-receptor-mediated endocytosis in endothelial cells [22, 35, 195]. Endothelial cells can take up serum immunoglobulin, and its excessive storage results in the formation of cytoplasmic inclusions that are easily recognized in light microscopical preparations and which immunostain strongly with anti-immunoglobulin (Ig)G, IgA, and IgM antibodies and disappear by corticosteroid therapy [96].

The CD14 molecule, the receptor for lipopolysaccharide (LPS)-binding protein, is present on normal human liver sinusoidal endothelial cells but not on vascular endothelium [145, 182]. This LPS-binding protein receptor and the receptor III for the Fc fragment of IgG show heterogeneous distribution within the liver lobule and are not, or are barely, expressed in periportal areas [183].

The scavenger receptor is concentrated on hepatic endothelial cells and mediates an ultrarapid clearance of certain substances by endothelial cells. As an example, 80% of the $NH_2$-terminal propeptide of type I procollagen [133] disappeared with a plasma half-life of 0.6 min. Other substances taken up by the scavenger receptor are: acetylated-LDL [108, 212], formaldehyde-treated albumin [99], collagen [127], glycation end products of bovine serum albumin (BSA) [192], and acetaldehyde-modified proteins [207]. Polyinosinic acid is being used in these experiments as an inhibitor for the scavenger receptor [99]. Uptake of acetylated-LDL by endothelial cells is highly specific and can be used, in its fluorescent-labeled form, to recognize endothelial cells in the tissue or in mixed cultures.

The mannose receptor rapidly clears substances such as mannose-terminated ovalbumin [105, 196], mannosylated albumin [107], N-acetyl galactosamine [175], ricin [123], the C-terminal propeptide of type I procollagen [189], and tissue-type plasminogen activator [184]. Coated vesicles are clearly involved in receptor-mediated endocytosis, as becomes evident by treating the cells with 150 mM sucrose, which inhibits endocytosis in endothelial cells through coated pits, at the same time inhibiting receptor-mediated uptake of ricin by mannose receptors [123]. IL-1 and tumor necrosis factor (TNF-)$\alpha$ increase the uptake mediated by the endothelial mannose receptor [9, 127]. In contrast to the mannose-specific uptake of a number of substances by endothelial cells, it seems that uptake by parenchymal cells and Kupffer cells is mainly galactose-specific. There seem to be more mannose receptors on endothelial cells than on Kupffer cells.

It was found that part of the endocytotic capacity of endothelial cells is directed to retroendocytosis. This process is based on incomplete dissociation of ligands from receptors before receptor recycling to the cell surface [124] and involves partial processing of ingested molecules instead of a total digestion within lysosomes. Endocytosed ricin, which inhibits protein synthesis in endothelial cells, is recycled to the cell surface by retroendocytosis [123]. The rate of retroendocytosis was about four times higher in endothelial cells than in parenchymal cells. Binding to the scavenger receptor, however, decreases retroendocytosis.

The uptake of hyaluronan by endothelial cells is receptor-mediated [64]. The clearance of hyaluronic acid appears to be a useful test for liver endothelial cell function [46, 89, 191]. Uptake of hyaluronan by endothelial cells is inhibited by antibodies against a 100 kDa cell surface protein [60] and by heparin, which is competing for the receptor [46]. The endothelial hyaluronan receptor consists of two polypeptides (166 and 175 kDa) forming an oligomeric structure [239–241]. In addition, rat liver endothelial cells express $Ca^{2+}$-dependent hyaluronan-binding activity, distinct from the $Ca^{2+}$-independent hyaluronan receptor [240]. The clearance of hyaluronic acid, or abundance of the substance in perfusion fluids or circulating blood, seems to correlate well with endothelial damage after cold ischemia for liver preservation and/or warm reperfusion injury for liver transplantation [91, 186, 202, 242]. The effects of LPS on the clearance or abundance of hyaluronan in circulation are less clear. Some authors report enhancement of hyaluronan uptake [64]; others state that Kupffer cell activation by LPS results in suppression of hyaluronan uptake by sinusoidal endothelial cells [47]. Elevated plasma levels of hyaluronan in septicemia could not be attributed to a change in receptors on endothelial cells [64].

Other receptors, reported to occur on hepatic endothelial cells, are receptors for estradiol [137], estrogen [213], thromboxane A2 [90], IL-1 [3], ceruloplasmin [157], transferrin [158], flt-1 and KDR/flk-1 [140], and vascular endothelial growth factor [238]. Besides specific uptake of certain classes of molecules, endothelial cells have the capacity to endocytose all kinds of small particles up to the size of 0.1 μm [226]. The binding and endocytosis of much larger particles by endothelial cells, i.e., apoptotic bodies, was reported to also involve carbohydrate-specific receptors [50].

We might conclude, regarding the enormous and variate capacity of endothelial cells for endocytosis, that these cells have the task of protecting the circulation from components of the extracellular matrix, e.g. secreted by fat-storing cells into the space of Disse. Collagen is well known to be an inducer of platelet aggregation, and the presence of such products in the sinusoidal lumen might disturb liver blood flow. The clearance of (denaturated) collagen, propeptides, and hyaluronic acid by endothelial cells seems to be meaningful, regarding the capacity of (activated) fat-storing cells to produce components of the extracellular matrix. The endothelial cells, therefore, have a meaningful and strategic position between the space of Disse, containing the fat-storing cells, and the sinusoidal lumen.

## Adhesion Molecules

In normal liver, the selectins endothelial leucocyte adhesion molecule-1 (ELAM-1) and CD62 are present on portal and central vein endothelial cells [201]. Sinusoidal endothelial cells of normal liver do not stain for selectins, platelet endothelial cell adhesion molecule-1 (PECAM-1) and CD34, as they can be detected on other microvascular endothelia [183]. In addition, portal and central vein endothelial cells possess a basal lamina but lack fenestrae. These data illustrate the fact that sinusoidal endothelial cells differ from other endothelial cells within the liver and differ from endothelial cells in other organs and tissues of the body, both in structure and in immunophenotype.

Different lectin-FITC complexes have been used to demonstrate the presence of glucose, mannose, galactose, N-acetyl-neuraminic acid, and N-acetyl-glucosamine reactive sites on endothelial cells, especially in the periportal area [14]. Endothelial cells in normal liver possess a number of adhesion molecules, such as intercellular adhesion molecule-1 (ICAM-1) [56, 130, 149, 153, 182, 183], ICAM-2 [183], two integrins chains, $\alpha1,\beta1$ and $\alpha5,\beta1$ [38], CD4 [182, 183], CD36 [183], lymphocyte/leucocyte function associated-1 (LFA-1) and very late antigen-4 (VLA-4) [70], and vascular adhesion protein-1 (VAP-1) [132]. Selectins are not present in normal conditions [56], but are induced after LPS [56]. Also ICAM-1 is enhanced after administration of LPS, TNF-$\alpha$, IL-1, or IL-6 [56, 116, 130, 149, 153]. Interestingly, ICAM-1 on rat liver endothelial cells was found to be identical to the hyaluronan receptor [130].

It is thought that adhesion molecules or their increase after activation plays a role in the attachment of Kupffer cells [182, 183] and pit cells. It has been determined that CD2 and CD11a/CD18 (LFA-1) on pit cells play an important role in their recruitment to the liver [120]. Adhesion molecules are important for cells visiting the liver, such as lymphocytes (LFA-1 and VLA-4) or leukocytes in general [16, 74, 216]. In particular, the upregulation of adhesion factors for PMN and their subsequent activation might, together with the result of the activation of sinusoidal cells, be harmful to the tissue and cause acute liver injury [116, 139, 154, 216]. Vascular cell adhesion molecule-1 (VCAM-1) expression on endothelial cells is thought to be diagnostic for graft inflammation [41].

## Cytokines

The release of cytokines and other biologically active substances by endothelial cells has been investigated quite intensively during the past years. Endothelial cells synthesize endothelin-1 (ET-1), the most powerful vasoconstrictor of the hepatic vasculature [69]. ET-1 and also ET-3 induce constriction of sinusoids [15, 95, 244]. ET-1 also increases the sinusoidal pressure gradient and resistance [244]. Constriction occurs after the binding of ET to the ETB receptor [95]. ET receptors are present on fat-storing cells [103], making it logical to conclude and observe that sinusoidal constriction is based on the contraction of fat-storing cells [16, 69, 244]. LPS causes an increase in ET-1 mRNA in endothelial cells [53]. Endothelin release by endothelial cells in culture was not enhanced by LPS, but it was increased by TGF-$\beta$ and Kupffer cell conditioned medium, especially when Kupffer cells were activated by LPS [169]. In cirrhotic liver, activated fat-storing cells are major sites of ET-1 synthesis [159].

Nitroprusside, a NO donor, neutralizes the action induced by ET-1 [244]. NO, a vasodilator, is produced by parenchymal cells and endothelial cells [245]. NO increases liver flow, whereas NO synthase inhibitor decreases liver flow [245]. IL-1 $\beta$ induces NO synthesis in endothelial cells in culture. Endothelial cell endocytosis seems to be decreased by NO, whereas inhibition of NO synthesis up-regulates endocytosis [128]. Other products of endothelial cells include: IL-1 and IL-6 [59], platelet activating factor (PAF) [138], prostaglandin E2 (PGE$_2$) [82], and hepatocyte growth factor (HGF) [148].

## Effects of Endotoxin (LPS)

Endotoxin reduces the porosity of the endothelium to 40% by decreasing the diameter and number of fenestrae [51]. It is clear that administration of LPS, which is specifically taken up by Kupffer cells in normal intact liver, will cause indirect effects on endothelial cells. Cells cultured in the presence of LPS do not show toxic damage except when Kupffer cells are involved. This means that LPS toxicity is caused by products secreted by Kupffer cells after the uptake and activation by LPS. It is therefore very important to distinguish between direct and indirect effects of LPS, in other words, whether LPS has been administered in the presence or absence of Kupffer cells. In fact, endothelial cell damage is produced by LPS-induced release of TNF-$\alpha$ and super-oxide anions by activated Kupffer cells [139]. In spite of these indirect effects, normal human liver sinusoidal endothelial cells possess CD14 (LPS receptor) [145, 182].

In response to LPS, endothelial cells are reported to produce IL-6 [110], IL-1 [138], PAF [138], PGF$_1$-$\alpha$, PGE$_2$, thromboxane B2 [168], reactive oxygen species [4], and no reactive oxygen [161], and to induce inducible nitric oxide synthase (iNOS)

[172]. LPS is reported to increase $H_2O_2$-detoxifying capacity [194], G6PDH [193], intracellular $Ca^{2+}$ [161], adhesion for PMN [56, 57, 134, 139], endothelin-1 mRNA [53], and decrease the clearance of hyaluronan in vivo [64] or in situ, but not in vitro with purified endothelial cells [47], showing the effect of the presence of Kupffer cells. LPS reduced the number of thromboxane A2 binding sites on endothelial cells [90].

Some LPS effects are counteracted by IL-10, produced by Kupffer cells, which down-regulates IL-6 release [110]. $PGE_1$ decreases IL-1 production [138]. Alcohol elevates plasma levels of LPS, which activates Kupffer cells, having an impact on endothelial cells, as summarized above [48]. In a model of sepsis, i.e., polymicrobial sepsis evoked by cecal ligation and puncture, endothelial cell dysfunction occurred only late during the hypodynamic stage of sepsis [220]. Glucose utilization by the liver of fasted rats is predominantly due to sinusoidal cells. LPS enhanced the rate of glucose utilization by endothelial cells by a factor of 2.7 [134].

# Endothelial Cells in Liver Disease

As a result of pathological conditions, endothelial cells can change into continuous endothelial cells, i.e., lose their fenestrae, and start the formation of a basal lamina, a process called capillarization. The adhesion molecules of endothelial cells change during capillarization [38]. Capillarization occurs during fibrosis [7, 51, 129]. Cirrhotic, capillarized endothelial cells display PECAM-1 and laminin receptors $\alpha6,\beta1$ and $\alpha2,\beta1$ [38]. Also, during the development of hepatocellular carcinoma, capillarization was observed and included loss of staining for CD4, CD14, and/or CD32 [145], development of a continuous basement membrane [88], staining of cell surface glycoproteins by *Ulex europaeus* lectin [79, 83], appearance of CD34 [40, 122], and appearance of factor VIII-related antigen, laminin, and PAL-E [83]. In chronic liver diseases, capillarization of sinusoids was found to be accompanied by the appearance of factor VIII-related antigen and UEA-1 positive staining [211]. Factor VIII-related antigen is not an accurate marker of normal endothelial cells [119]. Capillarization also occurs in experimental liver injury when induced by thioacetamide treatment, where the development of a basement membrane, detection of laminin, and factor VIII were observed whereas fenestrae and anti-CD44 staining decreased [155, 203]. Capillarization seems to imply decreased parenchymal cell uptake [129], because the transport through fenestrae is blocked and replaced by transport through the wall of a continuous capillary.

The role of endothelial cells in different disease processes including liver fibrosis seems to be quite passive, i.e., the cells might become involved in the process of capillarization, but active participation in the synthesis of extracellular matrix products seems to be the task of activated fat-storing cells. Isolated sinusoidal endothelial cells of normal rat liver express mRNA for collagen types III and IV, as well as laminin [125]. Others find only small amounts of collagen type IV $\alpha I$ mRNA [72]. In cirrhotic liver, compared to normal liver, endothelial cells exhibit as much as five times the collagen type I mRNA whereas mRNA for type IV collagen and laminin decreased up to 50% [125]. Endothelial dysfunction occurs during hemorrhage [219]. Sera of patients with autoimmune hepatitis (AIH) type 1 appeared to contain an antibody against hepatic sinusoidal endothelial cells. Culture of rat liver sinusoidal endothelial cells in the presence of IgG from this serum reduced the number of viable cells [78]. A CD4$^+$ T-cell line (LnC2) displayed selective cytotoxicity against endothelial cells in the presence of concanavaline A in vitro, and the endothelial cell monolayer was rapidly destroyed [109].

Because of the limited porosity (<10%) of the endothelial cells, this sieve might contribute to the protection of the parenchymal cells against infectious agents circulating in the blood [106]. A viral particle with a diameter in the order of 45 nm, will probably not get the chance to directly contact parenchymal cells. The presence of defensive cells, such as the Kupffer cells, might contribute to the protective effect. Keller [104] demonstrated an antiviral activity in cocultures of endothelial and parenchymal cells after a stimulus with LPS, which induces the release of IL-1 and interferon from endothelial cells. On the other hand, endothelial cells were found to be permissive for mouse hepatitis virus 3, at the same time showing a decrease in the number of fenestrae which could not be reversed by cytochalasin B [199].

Feline immunodeficiency virus (FIV), as a model for human immunodeficiency virus(HIV), did not change the number of fenestrae upon infection. However, the infection of endothelial cells contributed to the progression of the infection [200]. HIV was found to infect human liver endothelial cells [198]. When human liver endothelial cells were infected with HIV in vitro, they showed the formation of syncytia and the budding of new viral particles, indicating the production of new viruses [198]. This infection by HIV is probably mediated by CD4 surface antigens on these endothelial cells, as were shown to be present by immunogold-TEM [145, 181, 198]. Cell membranes of Kupffer cells and endothelial cells were both labeled with three different Ab against CD4, indicating that both cell types constitute targets for HIV [181]. Treatment with anti-CD4 antibody abolishes the infection of endothelial cells in vitro [198], whereas morphine increases the reproduction of HIV [179]. It is concluded that endothelial cells might constitute a target and a reservoir for HIV [73].

# Endothelial Cells in Liver Transplantation

Preparing the liver for transplantation includes perfusion of a preserving fluid, lowering of the temperature, stagnant flow during preservation, and reperfusion with warm oxygenated blood when connecting the liver to the donor circulation. From clinical and fundamental studies, it is apparent that each of these steps includes a potential danger to the tissue. Many observations point to the endothelial cells as being very sensitive in this procedure, possibly leading to essential and lethal deficiency during the post-transplantational period.

Preservation is dependent on the composition of the preserving fluid [32, 150]. Additions to the preserving fluid were found to avoid endothelial cell injury, such as immunoerythrocytes [164], KCN [165], lowering of the pH [29], and gaseous oxygen persufflation [136]. Low oxygen levels cause a decrease in endothelial cell mitochondrial membrane potential [67], a decrease in intracellular sodium concentration [166], iron-dependent generation of reactive oxygen species, and subsequent lipid peroxidation [5, 167]. Endothelial cells are much more susceptible to reactive oxygen species than parenchymal cells, probably because they lack detoxifying enzymes [77]. In TEM, disruption of endothelial cells has been observed [152, 156]. Even after 48–96 h of cold storage, parenchymal cells seem to be intact and surviving [118].

Warm oxygenated reperfusion apparently damages endothelial cells [30, 32, 66, 165]. Only endothelial cells undergo this reoxygenation injury, because Kupffer cells and parenchymal cells seem to be less sensitive [144, 173]. In severe cases, reperfusion injury leads to complete de-endothelialization and the formation of blebs by parenchymal cells. When reperfusion conditions were simulated with cultured endothelial cells, 30% of the cells were injured [167]. The activity of xanthine oxidase, a cytoplasmic marker enzyme for endothelial cells, is increased after hypoxia, in parallel with a decrease in cell viability. [77]. Neutrophils and Kupffer cells in the tissue might contribute to the damage by releasing $O_2^-$ [98]. Creatine kinase-BB and soluble thrombomodulin in blood seem to be additional parameters to evaluate endothelial cell damage in liver transplantation [34]. Hepatic rejection, which is intensified in recipients sensitized to their donor liver by preliminary skin grafts, is mediated by antibody deposition, systemic activation of the complement cascade, and severe destruction of the endothelial cells [37].

## Endothelial Cells in Liver Cancer

The subject of endothelial cells and cancer can be divided into three parts:

1. reaction of endothelial cells during the development of a primary liver tumor, such as hepatocellular carcinoma
2. tumors which develop from endothelial cells
3. reactions between endothelial cells and immigrating hematogenic tumor cells, metastasizing to the liver from an extrahepatic origin

Sinusoids in early hepatocellular adenoma and carcinoma were found to be comparable to normal liver. In later stages of hepatocellular carcinoma with progressive de-differentiation of the tumor cells, capillarization of the sinusoids occurs. Other sinusoidal cells undergo changes as well: fat-storing cells lose their lipid droplets and Kupffer cells and pit cells seem to disappear from the sinusoids [79, 80, 88, 187].

Reports on tumor formation in different types of sinusoidal cells are rare, but mostly concern endothelial cells. Different causes are given for the transformation of endothelial cells into (benign) hemangioendothelioma and (malignant) angiosarcoma [13]. The recognition of sinusoidal cells is difficult in the light microscope, because of their small size in comparison with parenchymal cells. Morphological methods for characterizing the cells should therefore use either EM or immunocytochemical staining [1]. Cases of epithelioid hemangioendothelioma have been described [12, 17, 49, 58, 68, 87, 180] and were found to be immunoreactive for factor VIII-related antigen [12, 17, 49], BNH9, and vimentin [12] and to demonstrate Weibel-Palade bodies (dense granules, positive for factor VIII) [17, 180]. This disease seems to develop after oral contraceptives of 4–7 years' duration [49]. Hemangio-endotheliomas were induced in rat livers after a 12-week treatment with quinoline

[81]. Angiosarcoma is a malignant endothelial cell tumor progressing to tumorous vascular masses [11, 61, 75, 146, 147], showing peculiar vasculature of the tumors and capillarization of sinusoids with several layers of basement membrane [11]. Angiosarcoma development could possibly be related to the use of arsenic [170], long-term androgen therapy [11], vinyl chloride [61], or Thorotrast and arsenic [160]. Hepatic angiosarcomas could be induced by 1,2-dimethylhydrazine dihydrochloride in experimental animals with 100% incidence [177]. Isolated liver endothelial cells of rats given diethylnitrosamine developed angiosarcomas after transplantion into young rats [121]. Hepatic angiosarcoma was also found in a relatively large number of patients, up to 40 years after intravenous injection with Thorotrast, a preparation stored in endothelial cells [222] and used to increase X-ray contrast, but containing $\alpha$-emitting thorium dioxide [1, 100, 114, 126, 206].

The interactions between invading tumor cells and liver endothelial cells have been studied with different models using colon carcinoma, lymphoma and melanoma cell lines, eventually with different metastatic capacity.

The ability of colorectal tumor cells to colonize the liver depends on their adhesion and response to endothelial cells [178]. Surface glycoproteins and adhesion receptors on endothelial cells determine the success of seeding to the liver tissue. Colon carcinoma cell lines with high levels of cell surface sialyl Le(x) colonized to the liver of nude mice more efficiently than cells with low levels [97]. H-59 carcinoma cells adhered only slightly to E-selectin molecules of endothelial cells, which could be augmented by activating these cells with rTNF-$\alpha$ [28]. Adherence to the sinusoidal endothelium seems to be more important than mechanical trapping in narrow (i.e., periportal) sinusoids [101].

When lymphoma cells invade the liver, adhesion to endothelial cells is mediated by sialyl Le(x), a ligand for ELAM-1 [243]. NO production by endothelial cells retards the growth of these cells [171, 210], whereas pre-immunization against lymphoma cells led to the induction of NO production by endothelial cells and inhibition of metastasis [171]. SCID mice, which lack the production of NO by endothelial cells in response to contact with lymphoma cells, showed progressive metastasis [171]. Furthermore, endothelial cell-conditioned medium contains migration-stimulating activity for lymphoma cells [76].

As important as NO seems to be in the defense of the liver against lymphoma invasion, in the case of melanoma the focus is on IL-1. IL-1 is present on the cell surface of melanoma cells [3]. When IL-1 is added to cultured cells, the adherence to endothelial cells is also enhanced [4]. This adherence can be neutralized by antibodies against IL-1 [3], by antibodies against the IL-1 receptor on endothelial cells [214], by IL-1 receptor antagonists [215], or by antibodies against VCAM-1, which reacts to VLA-4 expressed on melanoma cells [4]. IL-1 also induces $H_2O_2$-production in endothelial cells, thereby contributing to cytotoxicity [3, 4]. IL-1 or LPS treatment of intact mice also enhances hepatic metastasis of melanoma cells [215]. This treatment correlates with enhanced adherence of melanoma cells to endothelial cells, probably because of increased mannose-receptor activity and the presence of growth factors secreted by endothelial cells [215]. These research data inspired the authors of this work to make the important suggestion to treat patients at risk for hepatic metastasis of melanoma with IL-R antagonist [215].

## Genetic Manipulation of Endothelial Cells

Genetic manipulation and therapeutic intervention, such as inserting a gene for enzyme replacement in endothelial cells, could be accomplished by infusing a recombinant replication-deficient adenovirus vector expressing human hepatic lipase in lipase-deficient mice [6]. The human hepatic lipase was immuno-localized on both lumenal and sublumenal surfaces of endothelial cells and on parenchymal cell microvilli in the space of Disse in transgenic rabbits, showing the same location as in the human liver [174]. ISIS-3082, a phosphorothioate antisense oligodeoxynucleotide specific for ICAM-1, was i.v. injected, and the majority of this material was cleared by endothelial cells within half an hour by the scavenger receptor, after which digestion in lysosomes could be demonstrated [19].

## Conclusion

The study of hepatic sinusoidal endothelial cells has made clear that this unique type of endothelial cell is characterized by a combination of specialized structures and functions. Hepatic endothelial cells are fenestrated and filter lipoprotein particles in the fluids exchanged between the blood and the space of Disse. They are therefore involved in the distribution of lipoprotein components, such as cholesterol and vitamin A. Endothelial massage and forced sieving sustain liver physiology by refreshing the fluids in the space of Disse and promoting the transport of particles into the space of Disse. The cells have a strongly developed endocytotic apparatus, consisting of bristle-coated micropinocytotic vesicles and macropinocytotic vacuoles, taking up material which is further transported to vacuoles of increasing density and to lysosomes. Sinusoidal endothelial cells possess a specific set of cell surface receptors and adhesion molecules. Endothelial cells secrete a limited amount of cytokines, but are in their turn sensitive to cytokines secreted by Kupffer cells after their activation by endotoxin. Liver transplantation seems to be hampered by endothelial cell injury, caused by the combination of cold ischemia and warm reperfusion. Capillarization of sinusoids includes the loss of fenestrae and the formation of a basal lamina, and occurs in experimental injury, fibrosis, hepatocellular carcinoma, and other (chronic) liver diseases. Endothelial cells are involved in liver metastasis of melanoma cells, colon carcinoma cells, and lymphoma, by attaching to adhesion molecules on these cells. Endothelial cells of the hepatic sinusoid form, together with Kupffer cells, pit cells, fat-storing cells, and parenchymal cells, a special histological unit or functional unit in the tissue, which constitutes and contributes a large part of the specific functions of the liver.

*Acknowledgements.* The authors wish to thank Ann De Dobbeleer, Marijke Baekeland, Chris Derom, and Carine Seynaeve for their administrative and technical support. Our work was financially supported by the Belgian Science Foundation FWO (Vlaanderen), grants 3.00053.92, 3.00050.95, G0038.96, and 1.5.411.98, and the Research Council of the Free University of Brussels (VUB), grants 195.332.1310, 196.322.0140, and OZR230.

# References

1. Abe M, Wakasa H (1987) Thorotrast-induced hepatic angiosarcoma with 39 years latency. A pathologic and immunohistochemical study. Acta Pathol Jpn 37:1653–1660

2. Ahmed SS, Muro H, Nishimura M, et al. (1995) Fc receptors in liver sinusoidal endothelial cells in NZB/W F1 lupus mice: a histological analysis using soluble immunoglobulin G-immune complexes and a monoclonal antibody (2.4G2). Hepatology 22:316–324

3. Anasagasti MJ, Alvarez A, Avivi C, et al. (1996) Interleukin-1-mediated H2O2 production by hepatic sinusoidal endothelium in response to B16 melanoma cell adhesion. J Cell Physiol 167:314–323

4. Anasagasti MJ, Alvarez A, Martin JJ, et al. (1997) Sinusoidal endothelium release of hydrogen peroxide enhances very late antigen-4-mediated melanoma cell adherence and tumor cytotoxicity during interleukin-1 promotion of hepatic melanoma metastasis in mice. Hepatology 25:840–846

5. Angermuller S, Schunk M, Kusterer K (1995) Alteration of xanthine oxidase activity in sinusoidal endothelial cells and morphological changes of Kupffer cells in hypoxic and reoxygenated rat liver. Hepatology 21:1594–1601

6. Applebaum-Bowden D, Kobayashi J, Kashyap VS, et al. (1996) Hepatic lipase gene therapy in hepatic lipase-deficient mice. Adenovirus-mediated replacement of a lipolytic enzyme to the vascular endothelium. J Clin Invest 97:799–805

7. Arai M, Mochida S, Ohno A, et al. (1993) Sinusoidal endothelial cell damage by activated macrophages in rat liver necrosis. Gastroenterology 104:1466–1471

8. Arias IM (1990) The biology of hepatic endothelial cell fenestrae. Prog Liver Dis 9:11–26

9. Asumendi A, Alvarez A, Martinez I, et al. (1996) Hepatic sinusoidal Ec heterogeneity with respect to mannose receptor activity is interleukin-1 dependent. Hepatology 23:1521–1529

10. Bakkeren HF, Kuipers F, Vonk RJ, et al. (1990) Evidence for reverse cholesterol transport in vivo from liver endothelial cells to parenchymal cells and bile by high-density lipoprotein. Biochem J 268:685–691

11. Balazs M (1991) Primary hepatocellular tumours during long-term androgenic steroid therapy. A light and electron microscopic study of 11 cases with emphasis on microvasculature of the tumours. Acta Morphol Hung 39:201–216

12. Bancel B, Patricot LM, Caillon P, et al. (1993) Hepatic epithelioid hemangioendothelioma. A case with liver transplantation. Review of the literature. Ann Pathol 13:23–28

13. Bannasch P, Zerban H (1986) Pathogenesis of primary liver tumors induced by chemicals. Recent Res Canc Res 100:1–15

14. Barbera-Guillem E, Rocha M, Alvarez A, et al. (1991) Differences in the lectin-binding patterns of the periportal and perivenous endothelial domains in the liver sinusoids. Hepatology 14:131–139

15. Bauer M, Zhang JX, Bauer I, et al. (1994) Endothelin-1 as a regulator of hepatic microcirculation: sublobular distribution of effects and impact on hepatocellular secretory function. Shock 1:457–465

16. Bauer C, Marzi I, Bauer M, et al. (1995) Interleukin-1 receptor antagonist attenuates leukocyte-endothelial interactions in the liver after hemorrhagic shock in the rat. Crit Care Med 23:1099–1105

17. Bellmunt J, Allende E, Navarro M, et al. (1989) Epithelioid hemangioendothelioma of the liver with myocardial metastases. Jpn J Clin Oncol 19:153–158

18. Bijsterbosch MK, Donker W, van de Bilt H, et al. (1996) Quantitative analysis of the targeting of mannose-terminal glucocerebrosidase. Predominant uptake by liver

endothelial cells. Eur J Biochem 237:344–349

19. Bijsterbosch MK, Manoharan M, Rump ET, et al. (1997) In vivo fate of pho-sphorothioate antisense oligodeoxynucleotides: predominant uptake by scavenger receptors on endothelial liver cells. Nucleic Acids Res 25:3290–3296

20. Blomhoff R, Helgerud P, Rasmussen M, et al. (1982) In vivo uptake of chylomicron [3H]retinyl ester by rat liver: evidence for retinol transfer from parenchymal to nonparenchymal cells. Proc Natl Acad Sci USA 79:7326–7330

21. Blouin A, Bolender RP, Weibel ER (1977) Distribution of organelles and membranes between hepatocytes and nonhepatocytes in rat liver parenchyma. J Cell Biol 72:441–455

22. Bogers WM, Stad RK, Janssen DJ, et al. (1991) Kupffer cell depletion in vivo results in preferential elimination of IgG aggregates and immune complexes via specific Fc receptors on rat liver endothelial cells. Clin Exp Immunol 86:328–333

23. Braet F, de Zanger RB, Sasaoki T, et al. (1994) Assessment of a method of isolation, purification, and cultivation of rat liver sinusoidal endothelial cells. Lab Invest 70:944–952

24. Braet F, de Zanger RB, Baekeland M, et al. (1995) Structure and dynamics of the fenestrae-associated cytoskeleton of rat liver sinusoidal endothelial cells. Hepatology 21:180–189

25. Braet FCP, Kalle WHJ, de Zanger RB, et al. (1996) Comparative atomic force and scanning electron microscopy: an investigation on fenestrated endothelial cells in vitro. J Microsc 181:10–17

26. Braet F, de Zanger RB, Jans D, et al. (1996) Microfilament-disrupting agent latrunculin A induces and increased number of fenestrae in rat liver sinusoidal endothelial cells: comparison with cytochalasin B. Hepatology 24:627–635

27. Brauneis U, Gatmaitan Z, Arias IM (1992) Serotonin stimulates a $Ca^{2+}$ permeant nonspecific cation channel in hepatic endothelial cells. Biochem Biophys Res Commun 186:1560–1566

28. Brodt P, Fallavollita L, Bresalier RS, et al. (1997) Liver endothelial E-selectin mediates carcinoma cell adhesion and promotes liver metastasis. Int J Cancer 71:612–619

29. Bronk SF, Gores GJ (1991) Acidosis protects against lethal oxidative injury of liver sinusoidal endothelial cells. Hepatology 14:150–157

30. Caldwell-Kenkel JC, Currin RT, Tanaka Y, et al. (1991) Kupffer cell activation and endothelial cell damage after storage of rat livers—Effects of reperfusion. Hepatology 13:83–95

31. Cardier JE, Barbera-Guillem E (1997) Extramedullary hematopoiesis in the adult mouse liver is associated with specific hepatic sinusoidal endothelial cells. Hepatology 26:165–175

32. Carles J, Fawaz R, Hamoudi NE, et al. (1994) Preservation of human liver grafts in UW solution—Ultrastructural evidence for endothelial and Kupffer cell activation during cold ischemia and after ischemia-reperfusion. Liver 14:50–56

33. Charels K, de Zanger RB, Van Bossuyt H, et al. (1986) Influence of acute alcohol administration on endothelial fenestrae of rat livers: an in vivo and in vitro scanning electron microscopic study. In: Kirn A, Knook DL, Wisse E (eds) Cells of the Hepatic Sinusoid, vol 1. The Kupffer Cell Foundation, Rijswijk, The Netherlands, pp 497–502

34. Chazouilleres O, Vaubourdolle M, Robert A, et al. (1996) Serum levels of endothelial injury markers creatine kinase-BB and soluble thrombomodulin during human liver transplantation. Liver 16:237–240

35. Chroneos ZC, Baynes JW, Thorpe SR (1995) Identification of liver endothelial cells as the primary site of IgM catabolism in the rat. Arch Biochem Biophys 319:63–73

36. Clark SA, Cook HB, Oxner RBG, et al. (1988) Defenestration of hepatic sinusoids as a cause of hyperlipoproteinaemia in alcoholics. The Lancet 26:1225–1227

37. Colletti LM, Johnson KJ, Kunkel RG, et al. (1994) Mechanisms of hyperacute rejection in porcine liver transplantation. Antibody-mediated endothelial injury. Transplantation 57:1357–1363

38. Couvelard A, Scoazec JY, Feldmann G (1993) Expression of cell-cell and cell-matrix adhesion proteins by sinusoidal endothelial cells in the normal and cirrhotic human liver. Am J Pathol 143:738–752

39. Couvelard A, Scoazec JY, Dauge MC, et al. (1996) Structural and functional differentiation of sinusoidal endothelial cells during liver organogenesis in humans. Blood 87:4568–4580

40. Cui S, Hano H, Sakata A, et al. (1996) Enhanced CD34 expression of sinusoid-like vascular endothelial cells in hepatocellular carcinoma. Pathol Int 46:751–756

41. Dahmen U, Bergese SD, Qian S, et al. (1995) Patterns of inflammatory vascular endothelial changes in murine liver grafts. Transplantation 60:577–584

42. David H, Kassner G, Krause W, et al. (1990) Ultrastructure and quantitative composition of isolated endothelial cells of rat liver. Exp Pathol 39:95–101

43. De Leeuw AM, Praaning-Van Dalen DP, Brouwer A, et al. (1989) Endocytosis in liver sinusoidal endothelial cells. In: Wisse E, Knook DL, Decker K (eds) Cells of the Hepatic Sinusoid. Vol 2, Kupffer Cell Foundation, Rijswijk, The Netherlands, pp 94–99

44. De Rijke YB, Biessen EA, Vogelezang CJ, et al. (1994) Binding characteristics of scavenger receptors on liver Ec and Kc for modified low-density lipoproteins. Biochem J 304:69–73

45. de Zanger RB, Wisse E (1982) The filtration effect of rat liver fenestrated sinusoidal endothelium on the passage of (remnant) chylomicrons to the space of Disse. In: Knook DL, Wisse E (eds) Sinusoidal Liver Cells. Elsevier, Amsterdam, pp 69–77

46. Deaciuc IV, Bagby GJ, Lang CH, et al. (1993) Hyaluronic acid uptake by the isolated, perfused rat liver—An index of hepatic sinusoidal endothelial cell function. Hepatology 17:266–272

47. Deaciuc IV, Bagby GJ, Niesman MR, et al. (1994) Modulation of hepatic sinusoidal endothelial cell function by Kupffer cells: an example of intercellular communication in the liver. Hepatology 19:464–470

48. Deaciuc IV, Spitzer JJ (1996) Hepatic sinusoidal endothelial cell in alcoholemia and endotoxemia. Alcohol Clin Exp Res 20:607–614

49. Dean PJ, Haggitt RC, O'Hara CJ (1985) Malignant epithelioid hemangioendothelioma of the liver in young women. Am J Surg Pathol 9:695–704

50. Dini L, Lentini A, Diez GD, et al. (1995) Phagocytosis of apoptotic bodies by liver endothelial cells. J Cell Sci 108:967–973

51. Dobbs BR, Rogers GW, Xing HY, et al. (1994) Endotoxin-induced defenestration of the hepatic sinusoidal endothelium: a factor in the pathogenesis of cirrhosis. Liver 14:230–233

52. Duijvestijn AM, Van Goor H, Klatter F, et al. (1992) Antibodies defining rat endothelial cells: RECA-1, a pan-endothelial cell-specific antibody. Lab Invest 66:459

53. Eakes AT, Howard KM, Miller JE, et al. (1997) Endothelin-1 production by hepatic endothelial cells: characterization and augmentation by endotoxin exposure. Am J Physiol 272:G605–G611

54. Earnest DL, Sim WW, Kirkpatrick DM, et al. (1989) Effects of ethanol and acetaldehyde on Kupffer cell function. In: Wisse E, Knook DL, Decker K (eds) Cells of the Hepatic Sinusoid. Vol 2, Kupffer Cell Foundation, Rijswijk, The Netherlands, pp 325–330

55. Eskild W, Henriksen T, Skretting G, et al. (1987) Endocytosis of acetylated low-density lipoprotein, endothelial cell-modified low-density lipoprotein and formaldehyde-treated serum albumin by rat liver endothelial cells. Evidence of uptake via a common receptor. Scand J Gastroenterol 22:1263–1269

56. Essani NA, McGuire GM, Manning AM, et al. (1995) Differential induction of mRNA for ICAM-1 and selectins in hepatocytes, Kupffer cells and endothelial cells during

endotoxemia. Biochem Biophys Res Commun 211:74–82
57. Essani NA, McGuire GM, Manning AM, et al. (1996) Endotoxin-induced activation of the nuclear transcription factor kappa B and expression of E-selectin messenger RNA in hepatocytes, Kupffer cells, and endothelial cells in vivo. J Immunol 156:2956–2963
58. Fedeli G, Certo M, Cannizzaro O, et al. (1991) Epithelioid hemangioendothelioma of the liver: report of two cases. Ital J Gastroenterol 23:261–263
59. Feder LS, Todaro JA, Laskin DL (1993) Characterization of interleukin-1 and interleukin-6 production by hepatic endothelial cells and macrophages. J Leukocyte Biol 53:126–132
60. Forsberg N, Gustafson S (1991) Characterization and purification of the hyaluronan-receptor on liver endothelial cells. Biochim Biophys Acta 1078:12–18
61. Fortwengler HP, Jones D, Espinosa E, et al. (1981) Evidence for endothelial cell origin of vinyl chloride-induced hepatic angiosarcoma. Gastroenterology 80:1415–1419
62. Fraser R, Clark SA, Day WA, et al. (1988) Nicotine decreases the porosity of the rat liver sieve: a possible mechanism for hypercholesteroleamia. Br J Exp Pathol 69:345–350
63. Fraser R, Clark SA, Bowler LM, et al. (1989) The opposite effects of nicotine and pantethine on the porosity of the liver sieve and lipoprotein metabolism. In: Wisse E, Knook DL, Decker K (eds) Cells of the Hepatic Sinusoid. Vol 2, Kupffer Cell Foundation, Rijswijk, The Netherlands, pp 335–339
64. Fraser JRE, Pertoft H, Alston Smith J, et al. (1991) Uptake of hyaluronan in hepatic endothelial cells is not directly affected by endotoxin and associated cytokines. Exp Cell Res 197:8–11
65. Fraser R, Dobbs BR, Rogers GW (1995) Lipoproteins and the liver sieve: the role of the fenestrated sinusoidal endothelium in lipoprotein metabolism, atherosclerosis, and cirrhosis. Hepatology 21:863–874
66. Fratte S, Gendrault JL, Steffan AM, et al. (1991) Comparative ultrastructural study of rat livers preserved in Euro-Collins or University-of-Wisconsin solution. Hepatology 13:1173–1180
67. Fujii Y, Johnson ME, Gores GJ (1994) Mitochondrial dysfunction during anoxia/reoxygenation injury of liver sinusoidal endothelial cells. Hepatology 20:177–185
68. Fukayama M, Nihei Z, Takizawa T, et al. (1984) Malignant epithelioid hemangioendothelioma of the liver, spreading through the hepatic veins. Virchows Arch [A] 404:275–287
69. Gandhi CR, Sproat LA, Subbotin VM (1996) Increased hepatic endothelin-1 levels and endothelin receptor density in cirrhotic rats. Life Sci 58:55–62
70. Garciabarcina M, Lukomska B, Gawron W, et al. (1995) Expression of cell adhesion molecules on liver-associated lymphocytes and their ligands on sinusoidal lining cells in patients with benign or malignant liver disease. Am J Pathol 146:1406–1413
71. Gatmaitan Z, Varticovski L, Ling L, et al. (1996) Studies on fenestral contraction in rat liver endothelial cells in culture. Am J Pathol 148:2027–2041
72. Geerts A, Greenwel P, Cunningham M, et al. (1993) Identification of connective tissue gene transcripts in freshly isolated parenchymal, endothelial, Kupffer and fat-storing cells by Northern hybridization analysis. J Hepatol 19:148–158
73. Gendrault JL, Steffan AM, Schmitt MP, et al. (1991) Interaction of cultured human Kupffer cells with HIV-infected CEM Cells—An electron microscopic study. Pathobiology 59:223–226
74. Gome DE, Gorczynski RM, Cohen Z, et al. (1994) Hepatic regulation of lymphocyte adhesion to, and activation on, syngeneic endothelial monolayers. Immunology 83:58–64
75. Goodman ZD (1984) Histologic diagnosis of hepatic tumors. Ann Clin Lab Sci 14:169–178
76. Hamada J, Cavanaugh PG, Miki K, et al. (1993) A paracrine migration-stimulating factor for metastatic tumor cells secreted by mouse hepatic sinusoidal endothelial

cells—Identification as complement component C3b. Cancer Res 53:4418–4423

77. Hamer I, Wattiaux R, Wattiaux-De Coninck S (1995) Deleterious effects of xanthine oxidase on rat liver endothelial cells after ischemia/reperfusion. Biochim Biophys Acta 1269:145–152

78. Han K, Hashimoto N, Ikeda Y, et al. (1995) Occurrence of antibody against rat hepatic sinusoidal endothelial cells in sera of patients with autoimmune hepatitis. Dig Dis Sci 40:1213–1220

79. Haratake J, Scheuer PJ (1990) An immunohistochemical and ultrastructural study of the sinusoids of hepatocellular carcinoma. Cancer 65:1985–1993

80. Haratake J, Hisaoka M, Yamamoto O, et al. (1992) An ultrastructural comparison of sinusoids in hepatocellular carcinoma, adenomatous hyperplasia, and fetal liver. Arch Pathol Lab Med 116:67–70

81. Hasegawa R, Furukawa F, Toyoda K, et al. (1989) Sequential analysis of quinoline-induced hepatic hemangioendothelioma development in rats. Carcinogenesis 10:711–716

82. Hashimoto N, Watanabe T, Shiratori Y, et al. (1995) Prostanoid secretion by rat hepatic sinusoidal endothelial cells and its regulation by exogenous adenosine triphosphate. Hepatology 21:1713–1718

83. Hattori M, Fukuda Y, Imoto M, et al. (1991) Histochemical properties of vascular and sinusoidal endothelial cells in liver diseases. Gastroenterol Jpn 26:336–343

84. Hellevik T, Bondevik A, Smedsrød B (1996) Intracellular fate of endocytosed collagen in rat liver endothelial cells. Exp Cell Res 223:39–49

85. Hendriks HFJ, Elhanany E, Brouwer A, et al. (1988) Uptake and processing of 3H retinoids in rat liver studied by electron microscopy autoradiography. Hepatology 8:276–285

86. Horn T, Christoffersen P, Henriksen JH (1987) Alcoholic liver injury: defenestration in noncirrhotic livers—A scanning electron microscopy study. Hepatology 7:77–82

87. Ichida T, Kojima T, Shibata M, et al. (1981) Fine structure of malignant hemangioendothelioma of the liver. J Clin Elect Microsc 14:5–6

88. Ichida T, Hata K, Yamada S, et al. (1990) Subcellular abnormalities of liver sinusoidal lesions in human hepatocellular carcinoma. J Submicrosc Cytol Pathol 22:221–229

89. Imamura H, Sutto F, Brault A, et al. (1995) Role of Kupffer cells in cold ischemia/reperfusion injury of rat liver. Gastroenterology 109:189–197

90. Ishiguro S, Arii S, Monden K, et al. (1994) Identification of the thromboxane A2 receptor in hepatic sinusoidal endothelial cells and its role in endotoxin-induced liver injury in rats. Hepatology 20:1281–1286

91. Itasaka H, Suehiro T, Wakiyama S, et al. (1995) Significance of hyaluronic acid for evaluation of hepatic endothelial cell damage after cold preservation/reperfusion. J Surg Res 59:589–595

92. Ito T, Nemoto M (1952) Uber die Kupfferschen Sternzellen und die Fettspeicherungszellen (fat-storing cells) in der Blutkapillarwand der menschlichen Leber. Okajimas Folia Anat Jpn 24:243–258

93. Ito T, Shibasaki S (1968) Electron microscopic study on the hepatic sinusoidal wall and the fat-storing cells in the normal human liver. Arch Histol Jpn 29:137–192

94. Ito I, Muro H, Kosugi I, et al. (1990) Alterations in Fc receptor activity in sinusoidal endothelial cells and Kupffer cells during D-galactosamine (Galn)-induced liver injury in rats. Virchows Arch [B] 58:417–425

95. Ito Y, Katori M, Majima M, et al. (1996) Constriction of mouse hepatic venules and sinusoids by endothelins through ETB receptor subtype. Int J Microcirc Clin Exp 16:250–258

96. Iwamura S, Enzan H, Saibara T, et al. (1995) Hepatic sinusoidal endothelial cells can store and metabolize serum immunoglobulin. Hepatology 22:1456–1461

97. Izumi Y, Taniuchi Y, Tsuji T, et al. (1995) Characterization of human colon carcinoma variant cells selected for sialyl Lex carbohydrate antigen: liver colonization and

adhesion to vascular endothelial cells. Exp Cell Res 216:215–221

98. Jaeschke H, Bautista AP, Spolarics Z, et al. (1992) Superoxide generation by neutrophils and Kupffer cells during in vivo reperfusion after hepatic ischemia in rats. J Leukocyte Biol 52:377–382

99. Jansen RW, Molema G, Harms G, et al. (1991) Formaldehyde treated albumin contains monomeric and polymeric forms that are differently cleared by endothelial and Kupffer cells of the liver: evidence for scavenger receptor heterogeneity. Biochem Biophys Res Commun 180:23–32

100. Jennings RC, Priestley SE (1978) Haemangioendothelioma (Kupffer cell angiosarcoma), myelofibrosis, splenic atrophy, and myeloma paraproteinaemia after parenteral thorotrast administration. J Clin Pathol 31:1125–1132

101. Kan ZX, Ivancev K, Lunderquist A, et al. (1995) In vivo microscopy of hepatic metastases: dynamic observation of tumor cell invasion and interaction with Kupffer cells. Hepatology 21:487–494

102. Kanai M, Murata Y, Mabuchi Y, et al. (1996) In vivo uptake of lecithin-coated polystyrene beads by rat hepatocytes and sinusoidal endothelial cells. Anat Rec 244:175–181

103. Kawada N, Kuroki T, Kobayashi K, et al. (1995) Action of endothelins on hepatic stellate cells. J Gastroenterol 30:731–738

104. Keller F, Schmidt S, Nonnenmacher H, et al. (1989) Inflammatory and non-specific immunological functions induced in murine endothelial liver cells by in vitro treatment with LPS. In: Wisse E, Knook DL, Decker K (eds) Cells of the Hepatic Sinusoid. Vol 2, Kupffer Cell Foundation, Rijswijk, The Netherlands, pp 308–313

105. Kindberg GM, Magnusson S, Berg T, et al. (1990) Receptor-mediated endocytosis of ovalbumin by two carbohydrate-specific receptors in rat liver cells. The intracellular transport of ovalbumin to lysosomes is faster in liver endothelial cells than in parenchymal cells. Biochem J 270:197–203

106. Kirn A, Steffan AM, Anton M, et al. (1978) Phagocytic properties displayed by mouse hepatocytes after virus induced damage of the sinusoidal lining. Biomedicine 29:25–28

107. Kjeken R, Brech A, Løvdal T, et al. (1995) Involvement of early and late lysosomes in the degradation of mannosylated ligands by rat liver endothelial cells. Exp Cell Res 216:290–298

108. Kleinherenbrink-Stins MF, van de Boom JH, Schouten D, et al. (1991) Visualization of the interaction of native and modified lipoproteins with parenchymal, endothelial and Kupffer cells from human liver. Hepatology 14:79–90

109. Knolle PA, Gerken G, Loser E, et al. (1996) Role of sinusoidal endothelial cells of the liver in concanavalin A-induced hepatic injury in mice. Hepatology 24:824–829

110. Knolle PA, Loser E, Protzer U, et al. (1997) Regulation of endotoxin-induced IL-6 production in liver sinusoidal endothelial cells and Kupffer cells by IL-10. Clin Exp Immunol 107:555–561

111. Knook DL, Sleyster EC (1976) Separation of Kupffer and endothelial cells of the rat liver by centrifugal elutriation. Exp Cell Res 99:444–449

112. Knook DL, Blansjaar N, Sleyster EC (1977) Isolation and characterization of Kupffer and endothelial cells from the rat liver. Exp Cell Res 109:317–329

113. Knook DL, Sleyster EC (1980) Isolated parenchymal, Kupffer and endothelial rat liver cells characterized by their lysosomal enzyme content. Biochem Biophys Res Commun 96:250–257

114. Kojiro M, Nakashima T, Ito Y, et al. (1985) Thorium dioxide-related angiosarcoma of the liver. Pathomorphologic study of 29 autopsy cases. Arch Pathol Lab Med 109:853–857

115. Komatsu H, Koo A, Guth PH (1990) Leukocyte flow dynamics in the rat liver microcirculation. Microvasc Res 40:1–13

116. Komatsu Y, Shiratori Y, Kawase T, et al. (1994) Role of polymorphonuclear leukocytes in galactosamine hepatitis: mechanism of adherence to hepatic

endothelial cells. Hepatology 20:1548-1556

117. Kosugi I, Muro H, Shirasawa H, et al. (1992) Endocytosis of soluble IgG immune complex and its transport to lysosomes in hepatic sinusoidal endothelial cells. J Hepatol 16:106-114

118. Lemasters JJ, Caldwell-Kenkel JC, Currin RT, et al. (1989) Endothelial cell killing and activation of Kupffer cells following reperfusion of rat liver stored in Euro-Collins solution. In: Wisse E, Knook DL, Decker K (eds) Cells of the Hepatic Sinusoid. Vol 2, Kupffer Cell Foundation, Rijswijk, The Netherlands, pp 277-281

119. Lenzi R, Alpini G, Liu MH, et al. (1990) von Willebrand factor antigen is not an accurate marker of rat and guinea pig liver endothelial cells. Liver 10:372-379

120. Luo D, Vanderkerken K, Bouwens L, et al. (1996) The role of adhesion molecules in the recruitment of hepatic natural killer cells (pit cells) in rat liver. Hepatology 24:1475-1480

121. Luquette MH, Kimball PM, Pretlow TP, et al. (1985) Vascular sarcomas (probably angiosarcomas) transplanted from suspensions of liver cells from diethy-lnitrosamine-treated rats. Lab Invest 53:546-555

122. Maeda T, Adachi E, Kajiyama K, et al. (1995) CD34 expression in endothelial cells of small hepatocellular carcinoma: its correlation with tumour progression and angiographic findings. J Gastroenterol Hepatol 10:650-654

123. Magnusson S, Berg T, Turpin E, et al. (1991) Interactions of ricin with sinusoidal endothelial rat liver cells. Different involvement of two distinct carbohydrate-specific mechanisms in surface binding and internalization. Biochem J 277:855-861

124. Magnusson S, Faerevik I, Berg T (1992) Characterization of retroendocytosis in rat liver parenchymal cells and sinusoidal endothelial cells. Biochem J 287:241-246

125. Maher JJ, McGuire RF (1990) Extracellular matrix gene expression increases preferentially in rat lipocytes and sinusoidal endothelial cells during hepatic fibrosis in vivo. J Clin Invest 86:1641-1648

126. Manning JT, Ordonez NG, Barton JH (1983) Endothelial cell origin of thorium oxide-induced angiosarcoma of liver. Arch Pathol Lab Med 107:456-458

127. Martinez I, Sveinbjornsson B, Vidal-Vanaclocha F, et al. (1995) Differential cytokine-mediated modulation of endocytosis in rat liver endothelial cells. Biochem Biophys Res Commun 212:235-241

128. Martinez I, Sveinbjornsson B, Smedsrød B (1996) Nitric oxide down-regulates endocytosis in rat liver endothelial cells. Biochem Biophys Res Commun 222:688-693

129. Martinez Hernandez A, Martinez J (1991) The role of capillarization in hepatic failure—studies in carbon tetrachloride-induced cirrhosis. Hepatology 14:864-874

130. McCourt PAG, Ek B, Forsberg N, et al. (1994) Intercellular adhesion molecule-1 is a cell surface receptor for hyaluronan. J Biol Chem 269:30081-30084

131. McCuskey RS (1998) Personal communication.

132. McNab G, Reeves JL, Salmi M, et al. (1996) Vascular adhesion protein 1 mediates binding of T cells to human hepatic endothelium. Gastroenterology 110:522-528

133. Melkko J, Hellevik T, Risteli L, et al. (1994) Clearance of NH2-terminal propeptides of types I and III procollagen is a physiological function of the scavenger receptor in liver endothelial cells. J Exp Med 179:405-412

134. Meszaros K, Bojta J, Bautista AP, et al. (1991) Glucose utilization by Kupffer cells, endothelial cells, and granulocytes in endotoxemic rat liver. Am J Physiol 260:G7-12

135. Mihas AA, Tavassoli M (1991) The effect of ethanol on the uptake, binding, and desialylation of transferrin by rat liver endothelium: implications in the pathogenesis of alcohol-associated hepatic siderosis. Am J Med Sci 301:299-304

136. Minor T, Isselhard W, Klauke H (1996) Reduction in nonparenchymal cell injury and

vascular endothelial dysfunction after cold preservation of the liver by gaseous oxygen. Transpl Int 9 Suppl 1:S425–S428

137. Mizoguchi Y, Ichikawa Y, Kobayashi K, et al. (1991) Effect of sho-saiko-to (TJ-9, Japanese herbal medicine) on estradiol receptors in the cytosol of hepatic sinusoidal endothelial cells. Osaka City Med J 37:79–87

138. Mizoguchi Y, Ichikawa Y, Kioka K, et al. (1991) Effects of arachidonic acid metabolites and interleukin-1 on platelet activating factor production by hepatic sinusoidal endothelial cells from mice. J Gastroenterol Hepatol 6:283–288

139. Mochida S, Ohno A, Arai M, et al. (1995) Role of adhesion between activated macrophages and endothelial cells in the development of two types of massive hepatic necrosis in rats. J Gastroenterol Hepatol 10 Suppl 1:S38–S42

140. Mochida S, Ishikawa K, Inao M, et al. (1996) Increased expressions of vascular endothelial growth factor and its receptors, flt-1 and KDR/flk-1, in regenerating rat liver. Biochem Biophys Res Commun 226:176–179

141. Morsiani E, Mazzoni M, Aleotti A, et al. (1995) Increased sinusoidal wall permeability and liver fatty change after two-thirds hepatectomy: an ultrastructural study in the rat. Hepatology 21:539–544

142. Muro H, Shirasawa H, Kosugi I, et al. (1993) Defect of Fc receptors and phenotypical changes in sinusoidal endothelial cells in human liver cirrhosis. Am J Pathol 143:105–120

143. Naito M, Wisse E (1978) Filtrating effect of endothelial fenestrations on chylomicron transport in the neonatal rat liver. Cell Tissue Res 190:371–382

144. Nakagami M, Morimoto T, Mitsuyoshi A, et al. (1996) Difference in onset of warm ischemia and reperfusion injury between parenchymal and endothelial cells of the liver. Evaluation by purine nucleoside phosphorylase and hyaluronic acid. J Surg Res 62:118–124

145. Nakamura S, Muro H, Suzuki S, et al. (1997) Immunohistochemical studies on endothelial cell phenotype in hepatocellular carcinoma. Hepatology 26:407–415

146. Nguyen GK, McHattie JD, Jeannot A (1982) Cytomorphologic aspects of hepatic angiosarcoma. Fine needle aspiration biopsy of a case. Acta Cytol 26:527–531

147. Noguchi M, Upton MP, Hirohashi S, et al. (1987) A case of epithelioid hemangioendothelioma of the liver. Jpn J Clin Oncol 17:275–284

148. Noji S, Tashiro K, Koyama E, et al. (1990) Expression of hepatocyte growth factor gene in endothelial and Kupffer cells of damaged rat livers, as revealed by in situ hybridization. Biochem Biophys Res Commun 173:42–47

149. Ohira H, Ueno T, Shakado S, et al. (1994) Cultured rat hepatic sinusoidal endothelial cells express intercellular adhesion molecule-1 (ICAM-1) by tumor necrosis factor-alpha or interleukin-1 alpha stimulation. J Hepatol 20:729–734

150. Ohkohchi N, Sakurada M, Koyamada M, et al. (1994) The importance of prevention of sinusoidal endothelial cell injury during cold preservation of liver graft. Tohoku J Exp Med 174:317–331

151. Ohmura T, Enomoto K, Satoh H, et al. (1993) Establishment of a novel monoclonal antibody, SE-1, which specifically reacts with rat hepatic sinusoidal endothelial cells. J Histochem Cytochem 41:1253–1257

152. Ohno A, Mochida S, Arai M, et al. (1994) Fat-storing cell abnormalities associated with endothelial cell damage after cold ischemic storage of rat liver in UW solution. Dig Dis Sci 39:861–865

153. Ohteki T, Okamoto S, Nakamura M, et al. (1993) Elevated production of interleukin-6 by hepatic MNC correlates with ICAM-1 expression on the hepatic sinusoidal endothelial cells in autoimmune MRL/lpr mice. Immunol Lett 36:145–152

154. Ohtsuka M, Miyazaki M, Kondo Y, et al. (1997) Neutrophil-mediated sinusoidal endothelial cell injury after extensive hepatectomy in cholestatic rats. Hepatology 25:636–641

155. Okanoue T, Mori T, Sakamoto S, et al. (1995) Role of sinusoidal endothelial cells in

liver disease. J Gastroenterol Hepatol 10 Suppl 1:S35–S37

156. Okouchi Y, Sasaki K, Tamaki T (1994) Ultrastructural changes in hepatocytes, sinusoidal endothelial cells and macrophages in hypothermic preservation of the rat liver with University of Wisconsin solution. Virchows Arch 424:477–484

157. Omoto E, Tavassoli M (1990) Purification and partial characterization of ceruloplasmin receptors from rat liver endothelium. Arch Biochem Biophys 282:34–38

158. Omoto E, Minguell JJ, Tavassoli M (1990) Proteoglycan synthesis by cultured liver endothelium: the role of membrane-associated heparan sulfate in transferrin binding. Exp Cell Res 187:85–89

159. Pinzani M, Milani S, De Franco R, et al. (1996) Endothelin 1 is overexpressed in human cirrhotic liver and exerts multiple effects on activated hepatic stellate cells. Gastroenterology 110:534–548

160. Popper H, et al. (1978) Development of hepatic angiosarcoma in man induced by vinyl chloride, thorotrast and arsenic: comparison with cases of unknown etiology. Am J Pathol 92:2

161. Portoles MT, Arahuetes RM, Pagani R (1994) Intracellular calcium alterations and free radical formation evaluated by flow cytometry in endotoxin-treated rat liver Kupffer and endothelial cells. Eur J Cell Biol 65:200–205

162. Praaning-Van Dalen DP, Knook DL (1982) Quantitative determination of in vivo endocytosis by rat liver Kupffer and endothelial cells facilitated by an improved cell isolation method. FEBS Lett 141:229–232

163. Praaning-Van Dalen DP, De Leeuw AM, Brouwer A, et al. (1987) Rat liver endothelial cells have a greater capacity than Kupffer cells to endocytose N-Acetylglucosamine- and Mannose-terminated glycoproteins. Hepatology 7:672–679

164. Rao PN, Walsh TR, Makowka L, et al. (1990) Inhibition of free radical generation and improved survival by protection of the hepatic microvascular endothelium by targeted erythrocytes in orthotopic rat liver transplantation. Transplantation 49:1055–1059

165. Rauen U, Hanssen M, Lauchart W, et al. (1993) Energy-dependent injury to cultured sinusoidal endothelial cells of the rat liver in UW solution. Transplantation 55:469–473

166. Rauen U, Kirsch M, Reuters I, et al. (1997) Rapid decrease in cellular sodium and chloride content during cold incubation of cultured liver endothelial cells and hepatocytes. Biochem J 322 :693–699

167. Rauen U, Elling B, de Groot H (1997) Injury to cultured liver endothelial cells after cold preservation: mediation by reactive oxygen species that are released independently of the known trigger hypoxia/reoxygenation. Free Radic Biol Med 23:392–400

168. Rieder H, Ramadori G, Allmann KH, et al. (1990) Prostanoid release of cultured liver sinusoidal endothelial cells in response to endotoxin and tumor necrosis factor. Comparison with umbilical vein endothelial cells. J Hepatol 11:359–366

169. Rieder H, Ramadori G, Meyer zum Büschenfelde KH (1991) Sinusoidal endothelial liver cells in vitro release endothelin—augmentation by transforming growth factor beta and Kupffer cell-conditioned media. Klin Wochenschr 69:387–391

170. Roat JW, Wald A, Mendelow H, et al. (1982) Hepatic angiosarcoma associated with short-term arsenic ingestion. Am J Med 73:933–936

171. Rocha M, Kruger A, Van Rooijen N, et al. (1995) Liver endothelial cells participate in T-cell-dependent host resistance to lymphoma metastasis by production of nitric oxide in vivo. Int J Cancer 63:405–411

172. Rockey DC, Chung JJ (1996) Regulation of inducible nitric oxide synthase in hepatic sinusoidal endothelial cells. Am J Physiol 271:G260–G267

173. Samarasinghe DA, Farrell GC (1996) The central role of sinusoidal endothelial cells in hepatic hypoxia-reoxygenation injury in the rat. Hepatology 24:1230–1237

174. Sanan DA, Fan J, Bensadoun A, et al. (1997) Hepatic lipase is abundant on both hepatocyte and endothelial cell surfaces in the liver. J Lipid Res 38:1002–1013

175. Sano A, Taylor ME, Leaning MS, et al. (1990) Uptake and processing of glycoproteins by isolated rat hepatic endothelial and Kupffer cells. J Hepatol 10:211–216

176. Sarphie TG, Deaciuc IV, Spitzer JJ, et al. (1995) Liver sinusoid during chronic alcohol consumption in the rat: an electron microscopic study. Alcohol Clin Exp Res 19:291–298
177. Sato N, Kaku T, Dempo K, et al. (1984) The relationship of colonic carcinogenesis and hepatic vascular tumors induced by subcutaneously injected-1,2-dimethylhydrazine dihydrochloride in specific pathogen free mice. Cancer Letters 24:313–320
178. Sawada H, Wakabayashi H, Nawa A, et al. (1996) Differential motility stimulation but not growth stimulation or adhesion of metastatic human colorectal carcinoma cells by target organ-derived liver sinusoidal endothelial cells. Clin Exp Metastasis 14:308–313
179. Schweitzer C, Keller F, Schmitt MP, et al. (1991) Morphine stimulates HIV replication in primary cultures of human Kupffer cells. Res Virol 142:189–195
180. Scoazec JY, Degott C, Reynes M, et al. (1989) Epithelioid hemangioendothelioma of the liver: an ultrastructural study. Hum Pathol 20:673–681
181. Scoazec JY, Feldmann G (1990) Both macrophages and endothelial cells of the human hepatic sinusoid express the CD4 molecule, a receptor for the human immunodeficiency virus. Hepatology 12:505–510
182. Scoazec JY, Feldmann G (1991) In situ immunophenotyping study of endothelial cells of the human hepatic sinusoid: results and functional implications. Hepatology 14:789–797
183. Scoazec JY, Racine L, Couvelard A, et al. (1994) Endothelial cell heterogeneity in the normal human liver acinus: in situ immunohistochemical demonstration. Liver 14:113–123
184. Seydel W, Stang E, Roos N, et al. (1991) Endocytosis of the recombinant tissue plasminogen activator alteplase by hepatic endothelial cells. Arzneimittelforsch 41:182–186
185. Shakado S, Sakisaka S, Noguchi K, et al. (1995) Effects of extracellular matrices on tube formation of cultured rat hepatic sinusoidal endothelial cells. Hepatology 22:969–973
186. Shimizu H, He W, Guo P, et al. (1994) Serum hyaluronate in the assessment of liver endothelial cell function after orthotopic liver transplantation in the rat. Hepatology 20:1323–1329
187. Shoji Y, Kaneda K, Wake K, et al. (1994) Light and electron microscopic analysis of liver sinusoids during hepatocarcinogenesis with 2-acetylaminofluorene in rats. Jpn J Cancer Res 85:491–498
188. Smedsrød B (1989) Endocytosis of collagen and procollagen peptide in liver endothelial cells. In: Wisse E, Knook DL, Decker K (eds) Cells of the Hepatic Sinusoid. Vol 2, Kupffer Cell Foundation, Rijswijk, The Netherlands, pp 69–73
189. Smedsrød B, Melkko J, Risteli L, et al. (1990) Circulating C-terminal propeptide of type-I procollagen is cleared mainly via the mannose receptor in liver endothelial cells. Biochem J 271:345–350
190. Smedsrød B, De Bleser PJ, Braet F, et al. (1994) Cell biology of liver endothelial and Kupffer cells. Gut 35:1509–1516
191. Smedsrød B (1995) Non-invasive means to study the functional status of sinusoidal liver endothelial cells. J Gastroenterol Hepatol 10 Suppl 1:S81–S83
192. Smedsrød B, Melkko J, Araki N, et al. (1997) Advanced glycation end products are eliminated by scavenger-receptor-mediated endocytosis in hepatic sinusoidal Kupffer and endothelial cells. Biochem J 322:567–573
193. Spolarics Z, Navarro L (1994) Endotoxin stimulates the expression of glucose-6-phosphate dehydrogenase in Kupffer and hepatic endothelial cells. J Leukocyte Biol 56:453–457
194. Spolarics Z, Stein DS, Garcia ZC (1996) Endotoxin stimulates hydrogen peroxide detoxifying activity in rat hepatic endothelial cells. Hepatology 24:691–696
195. Stad RK, Bogers WM, van Es LA, et al. (1995) The involvement of Kupffer cells and liver endothelial cells in the clearance of large sized soluble IgA aggregates in rats.

Adv Exp Med Biol 371B:1053–1055

196. Stang E, Kindberg GM, Berg T, et al. (1990) Endocytosis mediated by the mannose receptor in liver endothelial cells. An immunocytochemical study. Eur J Cell Biol 52:67–76

197. Steffan AM, Gendrault JL, Kirn A (1987) Increase in the number of fenestrae in mouse endothelial liver cells by altering the cytoskeleton with cytochalasin B. Hepatology 7:1230–1238

198. Steffan AM, Lafon ME, Gendrault JL, et al. (1992) Primary cultures of endothelial cells from the human liver sinusoid are permissive for human immunodeficiency virus type-1. Proc Natl Acad Sci USA USA 89:1582–1586

199. Steffan AM, Pereira CA, Bingen A, et al. (1995) Mouse hepatitis virus type 3 infection provokes a decrease in the number of sinusoidal endothelial cell fenestrae both in vivo and in vitro. Hepatology 22:395–401

200. Steffan AM, Lafon ME, Gendrault JL, et al. (1996) Productive infection of primary cultures of endothelial cells from the cat liver sinusoid with the feline immunodeficiency virus. Hepatology 23:964–970

201. Steinhoff G, Behrend M, Schrader B, et al. (1993) Expression patterns of leukocyte adhesion ligand molecules on human liver endothelia—lack of ELAM-1 and CD62 inducibility on sinusoidal endothelia and distinct distribution of VCAM-1, ICAM-1, ICAM-2, and LFA-3. Am J Pathol 142:481–488

202. Sutto F, Brault A, Lepage R, et al. (1994) Metabolism of hyaluronic acid by liver endothelial cells: effect of ischemia-reperfusion in the isolated perfused rat liver. J Hepatol 20:611–616

203. Tamaki S, Ueno T, Torimura T, et al. (1996) Evaluation of hyaluronic acid binding ability of hepatic sinusoidal endothelial cells in rats with liver cirrhosis. Gastroenterology 111:1049–1057

204. Tanikawa K (1988) The pathology of the liver: an ultrastructural approach. In: Motta PM (ed) Biopathology of the liver. pp 131–147

205. Tanikawa K, Sata M, Kumashiro R, et al. (1989) Kupffer cell function in cholestasis. In: Wisse E, Knook DL, Decker K (eds) Cells of the Hepatic Sinusoid. Vol 2, Kupffer Cell Foundation, Rijswijk, The Netherlands, pp 288–293

206. Tateno H, Hosoda S, Yamada S, et al. (1984) Proliferative lesions in thorotrast-deposited livers pertaining to the development of primary cancers. Gan No Rinsho 30:23–34

207. Thiele GM, Miller JA, Klassen LW, et al. (1996) Long-term ethanol administration alters the degradation of acetaldehyde adducts by liver endothelial cells. Hepatology 24:643–648

208. Tomita M, Yamamoto K, Kobashi H, et al. (1994) Immunohistochemical phenotyping of liver macrophages in normal and diseased human liver. Hepatology 20:317–325

209. Ueno M, Oda M, Funatsu K, et al. (1989) Endotoxemia and endotoxin excretion into bile in carbon tetrachloride-induced liver cirrhosis, impairment of Kupffer cell functions. In: Wisse E, Knook DL, Decker K (eds) Cells of the Hepatic Sinusoid. Vol 2, Kupffer Cell Foundation, Rijswijk, The Netherlands, pp 293–297

210. Umansky V, Rocha M, Schirrmacher V (1996) Liver endothelial cells: participation in host response to lymphoma metastasis. Cancer Metastasis Rev 15:273–279

211. Urashima S, Tsutsumi M, Nakase K, et al. (1993) Studies on capillarization of the hepatic sinusoids in alcoholic liver disease. Alcohol Alcohol 28:77–84

212. van Berkel TJ, De Rijke YB, Kruijt JK (1991) Different fate in vivo of oxidatively modified low density lipoprotein and acetylated low density lipoprotein in rats. Recognition by various scavenger receptors on Kupffer and endothelial liver cells. J Biol Chem 266:2282–2289

213. Vickers AE, Lucier GW (1996) Estrogen receptor levels and occupancy in hepatic sinusoidal endothelial and Kupffer cells are enhanced by initiation

with diethylnitrosamine and promotion with 17alpha-ethinylestradiol in rats. Carcinogenesis 17:1235–1242

214. Vidal-Vanaclocha F, Amezaga C, Asumendi A, et al. (1994) Interleukin-1 receptor blockade reduces the number and size of murine B16 melanoma hepatic metastases. Cancer Res 54:2667–2672

215. Vidal-Vanaclocha F, Alvarez A, Asumendi A, et al. (1996) Interleukin 1 (IL-1)-dependent melanoma hepatic metastasis in vivo; increased endothelial adherence by IL-1-induced mannose receptors and growth factor production in vitro. J Natl Cancer Inst 88:198–205

216. Vollmar B, Senkel A, Menger MD (1995) In vivo evidence that intercellular adhesion molecule-1 does not mediate endotoxin-induced hepatic leukocyte-endothelial cell interaction. J Hepatol 23:613–616

217. Wake K (1971) Sternzellen in the liver: perisinusoidal cells with special reference to storage of vitamin A. Am J Anat 132:429–461

218. Wake K (1980) Perisinusoidal stellate cells (fat-storing cells, interstitial cells, lipocytes), their related structure in and around the liver sinusoids, and vitamin A-storing cells in extrahepatic organs. Int Rev Cytol 66:303–353

219. Wang P, Ba ZF, Biondo A, et al. (1996) Liver endothelial cell dysfunction occurs early following hemorrhagic shock and persists despite crystalloid resuscitation. J Surg Res 63:241–247

220. Wang P, Ba ZF, Chaudry IH (1997) Liver endothelial cell function is depressed only during hypodynamic sepsis. J Surg Res 68:38–43

221. Wisse E (1970) An electron microscopic study of the fenestrated endothelial lining of rat liver sinusoids. J Ultrastruct Res 31:125–150

222. Wisse E (1972) An ultrastructural characterization of the endothelial cell in the rat liver sinusoid under normal and various experimental conditions, as a contribution to the distinction between endothelial and Kupffer cells. J Ultrastruct Res 38:528–562

223. Wisse E (1974) Kupffer cell reactions in rat liver under various conditions as observed in the electron microscope. J Ultrastruct Res 46:499–520

224. Wisse E (1974) Observations on the fine structure and peroxidase cytochemistry of normal rat liver Kupffer cells. J Ultrastruct Res 46:393–426

225. Wisse E, Van't Noordende JM, Van Der Meulen J, et al. (1976) The pit cell: description of a new type of cell occurring in rat liver and peripheral blood. Cell Tissue Res 173:423–435

226. Wisse E (1977) Ultrastructure and function of Kupffer cells and other sinusoidal cells in the liver. In: Wisse E, Knook DL (eds) Kupffer cells and Other Liver Sinusoidal Cells. Elsevier, Amsterdam, pp 33–60

227. Wisse E, Van Dierendonck JH, de Zanger RB, et al. (1980) On the role of the liver endothelial filter in the transport of particulate fat (chylomicrons and their remnants) to parenchymal cells and the influence of certain hormones on the endothelial fenestrae. In: Popper H, Bianchi L, Gudat F, et al. (eds) Communications of Liver Cells, Falk Symposium 27. MTP Press, pp 195–200

228. Wisse E, de Zanger RB, Jacobs R, et al. (1983) Scanning electron microscope observations on the structure of portal veins, sinusoids and central veins in rat liver. Scanning Electron Microsc III:1441–1452

229. Wisse E, De Wilde A, de Zanger RB (1984) Perfusion fixation of human and rat liver tissue for light and electron microscopy. In: Popper H, Bianchi L, Gudat F, et al. (eds) Science of Biological Specimen Preparation. Vol 1, SEM, AMF O'Hare, Chicago, pp 31–38

230. Wisse E, de Zanger RB, Charels K, et al. (1985) The liver sieve: considerations concerning the structure and function of endothelial fenestrae, the sinusoidal wall and the space of Disse. Hepatology 5:683–692

231. Wisse E, McCuskey RS (1986) On the application and possibilities of in vivo

microscopy in liver research. In: Popper H, Bianchi L, Gudat F, et al. (eds) Science of Biological Specimen Preparation. SEM, AMF O'Hare, Chicago, pp 79–84

232. Wisse E, Doucet D, Van Bossuyt H (1991) A TEM study on the uptake of AMI 25 by sinusoidal liver cells. In: Wisse E, Knook DL, McCuskey RS (eds) Cells of the Hepatic Sinusoid. Vol 3, The Kupffer Cell Foundation, Rijswijk, The Netherlands, pp 534–539

233. Wisse E, Vanderkerken K, Crabbé E, et al. (1995) The role of pit cells in the defense of the liver against metastasizing tumor cells. In: Wisse E, Knook DL, Wake K (eds) Cells of the Hepatic Sinusoid. Vol 5, The Kupffer Cell Foundation, Leiden, The Netherlands, pp 90–95

234. Wisse E, Braet F, Luo D, et al. (1996) Structure and function of sinusoidal lining cells in the liver. Toxicol Pathol 24:100–111

235. Wisse E, Luo D, Vermijlen D, et al. (1997) On the function of pit cells, the liver-specific natural killer cells. Sem Liver Dis 17:265–286

236. Wisse E, Braet F, Luo D, et al. (1997) On the tumoricide function of pit cells, the NK cells of the liver. In: Vidal-Vanaclocha F (ed) Functional heterogeneity of the liver tissue. Medical Intelligence Unit, R.G. Landes, Austin, pp 207–235

237. Wright PL, Smith KF, Day WA, et al. (1983) Small liver fenestrae may explain the susceptibility of rabbits to atherosclerosis. Arteriosclerosis 3:344–348

238. Yamane A, Seetharam L, Yamaguchi S, et al. (1994) A new communication system between hepatocytes and sinusoidal endothelial cells in liver through vascular endothelial growth factor and Flt tyrosine kinase receptor family (Flt-1 and KDR/Flk-1). Oncogene 9:2683–2690

239. Yannariello-Brown J, Frost SJ, Weigel PH (1992) Identification of the Ca2+-independent endocytic hyaluronan receptor in rat liver sinusoidal endothelial cells using a photoaffinity cross-linking reagent. J Biol Chem 267:20451–20456

240. Yannariello-Brown J (1996) Identification and characterization of a divalent cation-dependent glycosaminoglycan-binding protein from rat liver endothelium. Glycobiology 6:111–119

241. Yannariello-Brown J, Zhou B, Weigel PH (1997) Identification of a 175 kDa protein as the ligand-binding subunit of the rat liver sinusoidal endothelial cell hyaluronan receptor. Glycobiology 7:15–21

242. Yokoi Y, Nakamura S, Muro H, et al. (1994) Functional abnormalities of sinusoidal endothelial cells in rats with acute liver rejection. Transplantation 57:27–31

243. Yoneda J, Saiki I, Kobayashi H, et al. (1994) Inhibitory effect of recombinant fibronectin polypeptides on the adhesion of liver-metastatic lymphoma cells to hepatic sinusoidal Ec and tumor invasion. Jpn J Cancer Res 85:723–734

244. Zhang JX, Pegoli W, Clemens MG (1994) Endothelin-1 induces direct constriction of hepatic sinusoids. Am J Physiol 266:G624–G632

245. Zhang B, Borderie D, Sogni P, et al. (1997) NO-mediated vasodilation in the rat liver. Role of hepatocytes and liver endothelial cells. J Hepatol 26:1348–1355

246. Zimmermann KW (1923) Z Anat Entwicklungsgesch 68:29–109

# Hepatic Stellate Cells

KENJIRO WAKE

*Summary.* In 1876, von Kupffer discovered star-shaped cells in the hepatic lobules using the gold chloride method, and called them "Sternzellen" (stellate cells). In 1898, however, he misconstrued these cells as phagocytic cells. The original stellate cells were rediscovered in 1971. These cells are located perisinusoidally, and extend several long branching cytoplasmic processes onto the abluminal surface of the endothelial cells. These cytoplasmic processes are studded with numerous thorn-like microprojections which make contact with the hepatocytes. The space of Disse in the mammalian liver is the space between the endothelial cell–stellate cell complex and the hepatocytes. The postnatal growth of the stellate cells of the rat continues up to at least week 5. The morphology of cultured stellate cells is variable depending on the culture conditions. In electron micrographs, hepatic stellate cells are seen to have two types of lipid droplets: membrane-bounded (Type I) and nonmembrane-bounded (Type II). In the lamprey, *Lampetra japonica*, abundant vitamin A is stored not only in the hepatic stellate cells, but also in fibroblast-like cells in various aplanchnic organs. Vitamin A storage is mainly restricted to the hepatic stellate cells in all mammalian species. The low-vitamin-A territory in the hepatic lobule is in the centrilobular zones and along the bridging line between the central vein and the central vein in the neighboring lobule. These areas are compatible with sites of fibrosis and septum formations in hepatic cirrhosis.

*Key words.* Liver, Stellate cell, Vitamin A, Fibrosis, Hepatocyte

## Historical Account

The original paper [1] in which von Kupffer first described the Sternzellen (stellate cells) has been cited in subsequent studies of sinusoidal cells in the liver. Nevertheless, some misconceptions about stellate cells have survived. Kupffer's first paper on these

Department of Anatomy, School of Medicine, Tokyo Medical and Dental University, 1-5-45 Yushima, Bunkyo-ku, Tokyo 113-0033, Japan
Present address: Liver Research Unit, Minophagen Pharmaceutical Co. Ltd., No. 3 Tomizawa Bldg. 4F, 3-2-7 Yotsuya, Shinjuku-ku, Tokyo 160-0004, Japan

FIG. 1. Rothe's drawing of the "Sternzellen der Leber" (*sz*, hepatic stellate cells) of a rat in 1882. *b*, Gitterfaser; *c*, capillary (sinusoid); *vc*, central vein; *vp*, portal vein

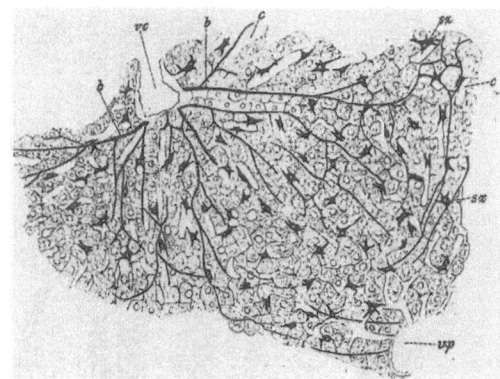

cells reported the existence of perisinusoidal cells in the liver [1, 2]. These cells were shown by the gold chloride method. We now know that this method is the specific demonstration method for vitamin-A-containing lipid droplets [3]. Rothe (1882) [4] confirmed the presence of stellate cells in various mammalian livers using the same gold chloride method (Fig. 1). A further observation by him [4] showed that there were some inclusion bodies in the cytoplasm of the stellate cells. He thought that these bodies were small nuclei of the stellate cells. About 90 years later, however, these bodies were found to be lipid droplets containing vitamin A [5].

In later papers on the stellate cells, Kupffer (1898, 1899) [6, 7] was concerned with intravenous (i.v.) injection of India ink into a rabbit in order to compare the phagocytic cells with the gold-reactive cells of the human liver. Unfortunately, he confused these two cell types and changed his initial opinion, concluding that his stellate cells were the special endothelial cells which incorporated the India ink. His new idea was widely accepted. As a result, Kupffer's stellate cells came to be referred to as phagocytic cells in the liver. It is important to notice, however, that this misinterpretation stimulated studies on vital staining [8, 9], followed by Aschoff's work on the "reticulo-endothelial system" in 1924 [10]. The distribution of vitamin A in the liver attracted research interest. Vitamin A autofluorescence was released from scattered cells in the hepatic lobules. Since, at that time, Kupffer cells (macrophages) were thought to be only one of the cell types scattered in the hepatic lobules, it was believed that vitamin A was stored in Kupffer cells in the liver [11–13]. However, cells located in the perisinusoidal space had been reported by several investigators using their own methods, and were named independently: Berkley's "granular cells" were found by the Golgi silver and picric acid silver methods [14], Zimmermann's "pericytes in the liver" by the Golgi silver method [15], Ito's "fat-storing cells" by the fat staining method [16], and Suzuki's "interstitial cells" by his silver method [17].

I reported that the perisinusoidal cells described above were the same cells as Kupffer's original stellate cells, which were rediscovered by the use of the gold chloride method (Fig. 2), and that vitamin A was stored not in Kupffer cells (macrophages) but in the perisinusoidal stellate cells [2, 5, 18]. In 1996, many researchers in the field of nonparenchymal liver cell biology and hepatic fibrosis

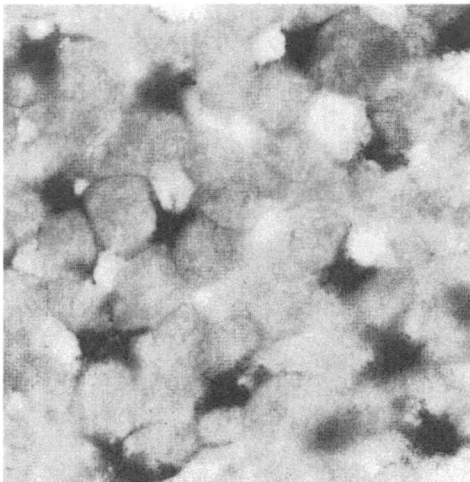

FIG. 2. Hepatic stellate cells of a rat demonstrated by Kupffer's gold chloride method. ×620

proposed that the term "hepatic stellate cell" should be used in referring to this cell type [19].

## Whole View and Size of Hepatic Stellate Cells

The three-dimensional structure of hepatic stellate cells has been investigated by Golgi's silver impregnation method and scanning electron microscopy [18, 20]. The Golgi method is the only suitable method for a whole-view demonstration of hepatic stellate cells (Fig. 3).

Stellate cells are made up of spindle-shaped or angular cell bodies and dendritic cytoplasmic processes. These cytoplasmic processes are one of the most characteristic

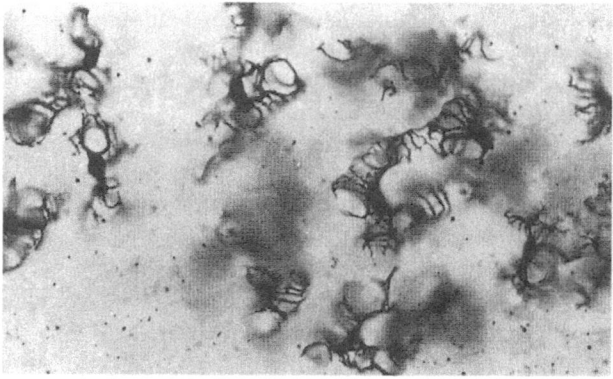

FIG. 3. Hepatic stellate cells of pig liver revealed by the rapid Golgi method. ×420

features of stellate cell morphology. The subendothelial processes protrude laterally or obliquely from the cell body along the sinusoidal wall, and surrounding the endothelial cells. Some of them run longitudinally and have numerous secondary branches which encircle the sinusoid at fairly regular intervals. An outstanding feature of the subendothelial processes is their thorny microprojections, also called "spines" [18, 20]. The intersinusoidal processes are another type of cytoplasmic process. These project from the cell body and follow a vertical course toward the nearby sinusoids through interhepatocellular space, penetrating hepatic cell cords as smooth, straight and thick processes.

A single stellate cell surrounds two or three, or sometimes more, nearby sinusoids. The total length of sinusoidal segments surrounded by a single stellate cell is approximately 60–140 μm in the rat liver [20].

The three-dimensional form and size of stellate cells differ significantly from zone to zone in the pig liver [21]. They are small in the periportal zone, and possess short, smoothly contoured subendothelial processes, which only occasionally exhibit branches and spines. In the intermediate zone they are larger and have better developed processes, bearing conspicuous secondary branching processes with numerous spines. In the centrilobular zone, these cells spread widely with several long, thick processes studded with long spines. According to Chen et al. [22], who were able to equalize the surface area to which these cells were attached, the spreading cells were not as likely to undergo apoptosis and therefore thrived compared with the more rounded cells. Consequently, the spreading stellate cells distributed in the centrilobular zone are thought to thrive better than those in the periportal zone. When hepatocytes are injured during pericentral necrosis following administration of $CCl_4$, it stimulates the proliferation of local stellate cells.

## Location of Stellate Cells and the Space of Disse

The subendothelial processes of stellate cells are closely associated with the upluminal surface of endothelial cells (Fig. 4). The smooth cytoplasmic membrane of the stellate cells adjoins the endothelial cells, and in mammalian species there is no collagen fibril between these cells but only a poorly developed basal lamina. Numerous spines extend from the edges of the subendothelial processes and are directed obliquely through the space of Disse away from the abluminal surface of the endothelial cells to make contact with the parenchymal cells [20]. Thus, these spines are called "hepatocyte-contacting processes" (HCP) [20, 23]. This geometrical relationship between stellate cells and parenchymal cells suggests that the hepatic stellate cells are different from the conventional pericytes of capillaries, because all of the cytoplasmic processes of the pericytes are in contact with the abluminal surface of the endothelial capillary cells.

The space between the liver sinusoids and the hepatocytes has traditionally been designated as the space of Disse (perisinusoidal space). However, now that the location of the stellate cells is known more accurately, the space of Disse should be defined as the space between the endothelial–stellate cell complex and the hepatocytes. This space is bridged by many HCP from the stellate cells and contains collagen bundles and occasional unmyelinated nerve fibers.

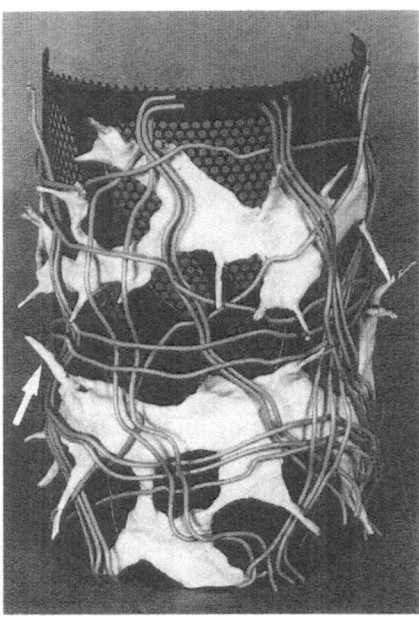

Fig. 4. A model of the sinuoidal wall in the liver. Two subendothlial processes of the stellate cell (*bright*) encircle the fenestrated endothelial cell (*dark*). Thorn-like micro-projections, or spines (*arrow*), extend from the lateral edges of the subendothelial processes. Collagen fibers (*grey*) form a network around the outer side of the endothelial cell–stellate cell complex

## Hepatocyte-Contacting Processes of Stellate Cells

Hepatocyte-contacting processes (HCP), or spines, are one of the most characteristic structures of stellate cells; they are found in the hepatic stellate cells of all vertebrates.

Scanning electron microscopy reveals that these minute projections face the microvillous facets of the hepatocytes and establish intercellular contacts between the stellate cells and the hepatocytes. Careful transmission electron microscopy reveals that the opposing cell membranes at these contact points, especially those of the hepatocytes, are reinforced by dense, submembranous material of a fine filamentous nature [20].

Gressner and Lahme [24] proposed the hypothesis that the loss of cell-to-cell contacts between stellate cells and hepatocytes might play an important role in the proliferation and transformation of stellate cells as a result of hepatocellular damage. To verify this hypothesis, they showed that the growth and fuctional activity of the stellate cells are suppressed by adding liver cell membranes.

The other possible functions of HCP are mechanical. When the endothelial lining is compressed by blood cells or the blood stream in the sinusoidal lumen, the underlying stellate cells and their HCP may play the role of a spring. At the same time, this movement accelerates the fluid exchange between the sinusoidal lumen and the space of Disse through endothelial fenestrations ("pumping mechanism") [20]. The mechanism involved is the contraction and relaxation of the stellate cells [20].

The arrangement of parenchymal cells with stellate cells is highly organized, and may offer new ideas for the design of an artificial liver (i.e., a device for supporting liver-failure patients awaiting a transplant).

# Development of Cytoplasmic Processes

Using the Golgi method, the postnatal development of the cytoplasmic processes of stellate cells has been clearly defined [23]. The stellate cells have not yet achieved their final form when the animal is born, and the cytoplasmic processes develop rapidly during the early postnatal stages. In 1-day-old rats, the cells are rather rounded with slim, scanty processes. Primary processes branch out from the cell body proximally and distally with an abundance of secondary processes extending toward the sinusoidal endothelial cells. Cell growth continues steadily up to at least week 5, when it is possible to identify the almost typical form of the stellate cell. The cellular outline has strikingly thorny edges at 5 weeks (Fig. 5).

As a consequence of lobular expansion, the radial sinusoids elongate. It seems natural to assume that the stellate cells which form an uninterrupted pericytic layer encasing each sinusoid from its periphery to its center would be similarly involved in this growing process.

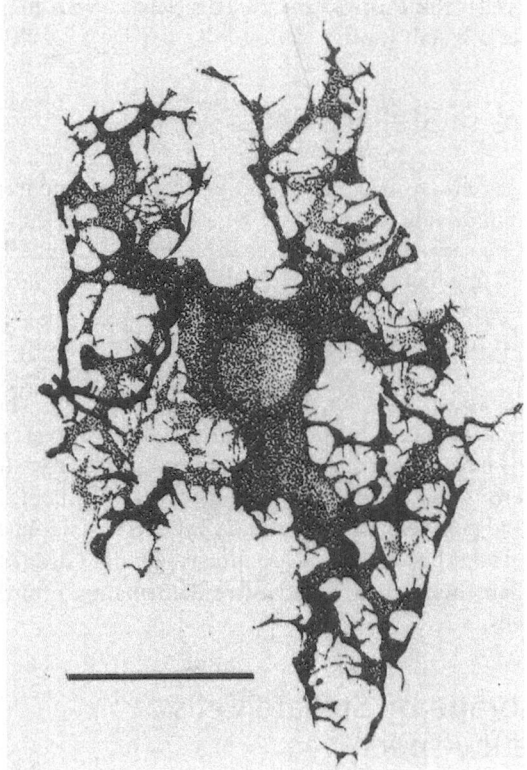

FIG. 5. Drawing depicting a total view of a stellate cell in rat liver at 5 weeks. This single cell surrounds an H-shaped section of the sinusoid with branching subendothelial processes. Rapid Golgi method. Bar = 20 μm

## Morphology of Stellate Cells in Vitro

Cultured stellate cells change their form continuously after seeding on plastic dishes [25]. They extend thin, fan-shaped membranous processes around the nuclei. As these membranous processes expand further, they change and become dendritic in appearance. Dendritic processes are characteristically studded with spines, 2–3 µm in length. Two days after seeding, the cells change their shape gradually from dendritic to membranous. Lipid droplets and cytoplasmic granules disperse toward the periphery of the cell. Characteristically, the cellular edge becomes smooth and looses its spines. Three to four days after seeding, the stellate cells look like fibroblasts. They show prominent stress fibers in the cytoplasm and the vitamin A–lipid droplets decrease in number.

When Kupffer cell-conditioned media (KCCM) is added to the culture medium of the stellate cells 2–3 days after seeding, the membranous processes change dramatically to dendritic ones [25]. Cytoplasmic processes become narrow and many spines appear. These changes are reversible; when the KCCM is removed, the dendritic stellate cells revert to being membranous. Similar rapid changes in stellate cell morphology occur after adding $PGE_2$ to the culture medium. Since $PGE_2$ is released from activated Kupffer cells, the form of the stellate cells in vivo might be under the influence of Kupffer cell activation.

## Fine Structure of Stellate Cells

The nuclei in stellate cells are oval or more or less elongated, and frequently indented by lipid droplets containing vitamin A . One or more nucleoli, and sometimes "spheridium," can be seen. The granular endoplasmic reticulum is well developed. The cisterns contain fine filamentous materials. The Golgi complex consists of well-developed lamellae associated with many vesicles, but large Golgi vacuoles are rarely seen. Since agranular reticulum and glycogen particles are also rarely seen, these cells may not participate in active glycogen metabolism. In the stellate cells of mammalian livers, multivesicular bodies are frequently seen in the cytoplasm. The most conspicuous feature of these stellate cells is the occurrence of lipid droplets in the cytoplasm. These lipid droplets have a high content of vitamin A, primarily stored in the form of retinyl esters. Two types of lipid droplets have been distinguished: membrane-bounded (Type I) and nonmembrane-bounded (Type II) [26]. Lipid droplets accumulate in the multivesicular bodies to develop into Type I lipid droplets. Microtubules, i.e., intermediate filaments of desmin and microfilaments, are prominent in the cytoplasm of stellate cells.

## Vitamin A Storage by Stellate Cells: A Phylogenetic Aspect

The liver is a major storage site of vitamin A in mammals (Fig. 6). Ninety-five per cent of the total vitamin A in rats is stored in the liver, and as much as 80% or more of the total vitamin A in the liver is present in the hepatic stellate cells [27]. Endothelial cells,

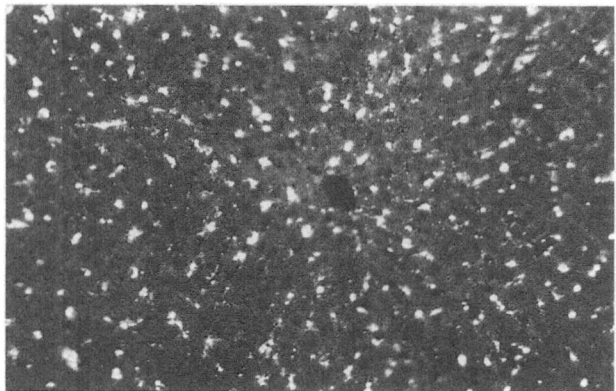

FIG. 6.  Vitamin A autofluorescence of stellate cells in rat liver. ×80

Kupffer cells, and fibroblast-like cells in the interlobular connective tissue contain negligible amounts of vitamin A.

In the lamprey, *Lampetra japonica*, vitamin A is stored not only in the liver, but also in all splanchnic organs [28–31]. In contrast, no vitamin A storage is observed in the somatic organs. In the liver of the lamprey, vitamin A is stored in the hepatic stellate cells as well as in fibroblast-like cells in the periportal, perivenular, and subcapsular connective tissue in the liver [29]. The individual fibroblast-like cells have fewer vitamin-A-containing lipid droplets than the hepatic stellate cells. Since the fibroblast-like cells are distributed close to each other, the quantity of stored vitamin A per cubic meter in the interlobular connective tissue seems to be much larger than that in the lobules. The cytological characteristics of the fibroblast-like cells in the liver and other splanchnic organs resemble those of the hepatic stellate cells.

From the distribution of vitamin A in the vertebrate body, it has been concluded that two different major mesenchymal cell systems exist: the first is the conventional fibroblast system of the somatic organs, and the second is the vitamin-A-storing cell system of the splanchnic organs. Among the latter cell populations, the hepatic stellate cells, which retain vitamin A during phylogenetic development, are the most typical. The remaining cell populations in the vitamin-A-storing system of mammalian species store much less vitamin A than the hepatic stellate cells in the physiological condition. However, after the administration of excess vitamin A to animals, these cell populations also store vitamin A moderately in the cytoplasm as lipid droplets.

## Intralobular Gradient of Vitamin A Storage

Stellate cells in the same liver contain variable amounts of vitamin A [21, 32]. This unhomogeneous storage by stellate cells depends on the intralobular position of the cells. The size of the lipid droplet is correlated approximately to the quantity of vitamin A stored in the individual stellate cells. The volume of the lipid droplets differs not only among zones along the sinusoidal axis, but also from region to region within a single zone [32]. The mean volume in the peripheral zone is small, increases by the middle zone, and then decreases gradually towards the central zone. Most stellate cells near the central vein contain no lipid droplets, and even when they are present, they are too small to be measured by light microscopy.

The heterogeneity of the stellate cells is also evidenced by subtle differences in desmin expression along the sinusoidal axis [21]. The desmin is strong in the periportal zone, and becomes weaker and disappears in the centrilobular zone. Ramm et al. [33] demonstrated that a vitamin-A-poor, desmin-negative stellate cell subpopulation produces as much collagen as a vitamin-A-replete, desmin-positive one after 7 days in culture.

Vitamin A storage capacity was significantly higher at sinusoids in the portal regions than at those in the midseptal regions, forming a decrescendo–crescendo profile between two adjacent portal tracts [32]. Along the periphery of the hepatic lobule, the inlet venules of the portal which was quantified revealed an occurrence rate of 60% at the periportal and 5% at the midseptal regions, which is closely compatible with the regional gradient of the vitamin A storage capacity. Thus, the vitamin-A-low territory in the hepatic lobule is located in the centrilobular zones and along the bridging line between the central vein and the central vein in the neighboring lobules (C–C bridging). This territory is compatible with sites of fibrogenetic propensity in hepatic fibrosis and cirrhosis [34].

## References

1. von Kupffer C (1876) Ueber Sternzellen der Leber. Briefliche Mitteilung an Prof. Waldyer. Arch Mikrosk Anat 12:353–358
2. Wake K (1980) Perisinusoidal stellate cells (fat-storing cells, interstitial cells, lipocytes), their related structure in and around the liver sinusoids, and vitamin A-storing cells in extrahepatic organs. Int Rev Cytol 66:303–353
3. Wake K, Motomatsu K, Senoo H, et al. (1986) Improved Kupffer's gold chloride method for the demonstration of the stellate cells storing retinol (vitamin A) in the liver and extrahepatic organs of vertebrates. Stain Technol 61:193–200
4. Rothe P (1882) Ueber die Sternzellen der Leber. Inaug-Dissertation, Munich University
5. Wake K (1971) "Sternzellen" in the liver: perisinusoidal cells with special reference to storage of vitamin A. Am J Anat 132:429–462
6. von Kupffer C (1898) Ueber Sternzellen der Leber. Verh anat Ges 12 Versammlung in Kiel, pp 80–86
7. von Kupffer C (1899) Ueber die sogenannten Sternzellen der Sugetheir leber Arch Mikrosk Anat 54:254–288
8. Ribbert H (1904) Die Ausscheidung intravenos injizierten gelosten Karmins in den Geweben. Allg Physiol 4:101–214
9. Kiyono K (1914) Die Vitale Karminspeicherung. Fischer, Jena
10. Aschoff L (1924) Das reticulo-endotheliale System. Erged Inn Med Kinderheilkd 26:1–118
11. Hirt A, and co-workers (1929) cited from Hirt A, Wimmer K (1940) Luminescenzmikroskopische Untersuchungen am lebenden Tier. Die Bedeutung des Retculoendothelialensystems und der Tragersubstanzen im Vitaminstoffwechsel. Klin Wochenschr 19:123–128
12. Querner F, Strum K (1934) Die paraplasmatische Fetteinschlusse der Leberzellen und der Leuchtstoff X. Zweite Mitteilung. Anat Anz 78:289–295

13. Popper H (1944) Distribution of vitamin A in tissue as revealed by fluorescence microscopy. Physiol Rev 24:205–224
14. Berkley HJ (1893) Studies in the histology of the liver. III. The perivascular cells of the rabbit's liver. Anat Anz 8:787–792
15. Zimmermann KW (1923) Der feinere Bau der Blutcapillaren. A f d ges Anat 63:29–109
16. Ito T (1951) Cytological studies on stellate cells of Kupffer and fat storing cells in the capillary wall of the human liver. Acta Anat Nippon 26:2
17. Suzuki K (1958) A silver impregnation method in histology (in Japanese). Takeda Pharmaceut Ind. Osaka, No. 310–320
18. Wake K (1988) Liver perivascular cells revealed by gold and silver impregnation methods and electron microscopy. In: Motta PM (ed) Biopathology of the liver. An ultrastructural approach. Kluwer, Dordrecht, pp 23–36
19. Ahern M, Hall P, Halliday J, et al. (1996) Hepatic stellate cell nomenclature [letter], Hepatology 23:193
20. Wake K (1995) Structure of the sinusoidal wall in the liver. In: Wisse E, Knook DL, Wake K (eds) Cells of the hepatic sinusoid, vol 5. Kupffer Cell Foundation, Leiden, pp 241–246
21. Wake K, Sato T (1993) Intralobular heterogeneity of perisinusoidal stellate cells in porcine liver. Cell Tissue Res 273:227–237
22. Chen CS, Mrksich M, Huang S, et al. (1997) Geometric control of cell life and death. Science 276:1425–1428
23. Wake K, Motomatsu K, Ekataksin W (1991) Postnatal development of the perisinusoidal stellate cells in the rat liver. In: Wisse E, Knook DL, McCuskey RS (eds) Cells of the hepatic sinusoid, vol 3. Kupffer Cell Foundation, Leiden, pp 269–275
24. Gressner AM, Lahme B (1991) Inhibitory actions of hepatocyte plasma membranes on proliferation, protein- and proteoglycan-synthesis of cultured rat fat storing cells. In: Wisse E, Knook DL, McCuskey RS (eds) Cells of the hepatic sinusoid, vol 3. Kupffer Cell Foundation, Leiden, pp 237–241
25. Wake K, Kishiye T, Yamamoto H, et al. (1993) Kupffer cells modulate the configuration of perisinusoidal stellate cells. In: Knook DL, Wisse E (eds) Cells of the hepatic sinusoid, vol 4. Kupffer Cell Foundation, Leiden, pp 157–160
26. Wake K (1974) Development of vitamin A-rich lipid droplets in multivesicular bodies of rat liver stellate cells. J Cell Biol 63:683–691
27. Blomhoff R, Wake K (1991) Perisinusoidal stellate cells of the liver: important roles in retinol metabolism and fibrosis. FASEB J 5:271–277
28. Wake K, Senoo H (1986) Morphological aspects of the differentiation of stellate cell line in the vertebrates. In: Kirn A, Knook DL, Wisse E (eds) Cells of the hepatic sinusoid, vol 1. Kupffer Cell Foundation, Rijswijk, pp 215–220
29. Wake K, Motomatsu K, Senoo H (1987) Stellate cells storing retinol in the liver of adult lamprey, *Lampetra japonica*. Cell Tissue Res 249:289–299
30. Wake K, Saato T, Ekataksin W, et al. (1989) Pillar cells in gill filaments of the lamprey, *Lampetra japonica*, store retinol. Biomed Res 10(Suppl 3):597–605
31. Bauer P, Wake K (1996) Mesangial cells of the lamprey, *Lampetra japonica*, store vitamin A. Arch Histol Cytol 59:71–78
32. Zou Z, Ekataksin W, Wake K (1998) Zonal and regional differences identified from precision mapping of vitamin A-storing lipid droplets of the hepatic stellate cells in pig liver: a novel concept of addressing the intralobular area of heterogeneity. Hepatology 27:1098–1108
33. Ramm GA, Britton RS, O'neill R, et al. (1995) Vitamin A-poor lipocytes: a novel desmin-negative lipocyte subpopulation, which can be activated to myofibroblasts. Am J Physiol 269(Gastrointest Liver Physiol 32):G532–G541
34. Bhunchet E, Wake K (1992) The role of mesenchymal cell populations in porcine serum-induced rat liver fibrosis. Hepatology 16:1452–1473

# Development, Differentiation, and Host Defense Function of Kupffer Cells

Makoto Naito[1], Go Hasegawa[1], Yusuke Ebe[1], and Masao Mitsuyama[2]

*Summary.* Kupffer cells are a proliferating resident macrophage population in the fetal and adult liver. Kupffer cells are derived from macrophage precursors, differentiating in the yolk sac and fetal liver in ontogeny. In macrophage colony-stimulating factor (M-CSF)-deficient (*op/op*) mice, the number of Kupffer cells is reduced and those which are present are characterized by immature morphology. The administration of M-CSF to *op/op* mice results in the immediate proliferation and maturation of Kupffer cells, indicating that M-CSF plays a pivotal role in the differentiation and proliferation of Kupffer cells. After depletion of Kupffer cells by the intravenous administration of liposome-entrapped dichloromethylene diphosphonate (lipo-MDP), small peroxidase-negative macrophages appear, proliferate, and differentiate into large peroxidase-positive Kupffer cells by 2 weeks. Macrophage precursors present in the liver proliferate after a lipo-MDP injection and differentiate into Kupffer cells. The enhanced M-CSF production in the liver after Kupffer cell depletion is thought to provide the microenvironment for Kupffer cell differentiation.

Kupffer cells play an important role in host defense mechanisms by trapping and killing various bacteria. In mice depleted of Kupffer cells, the size and number of zymosan-induced granulomas were smaller than in nontreated mice. When Kupffer-cell-depleted mice were infected with *Listeria monocytogenes*, there was a significant decrease in their natural resistance to this microbe. These findings imply that Kupffer cells are indispensable for antimicrobial protection by phagocytosis, bactericidal functions, and granuloma formation.

*Key words.* Kupffer cells, Monocytes, Differentiation, Macrophage colony-stimulating factor (M-CSF), Granulomas

## Introduction

Kupffer cells are resident macrophages in the hepatic sinusoid with various cytoplasmic apparatuses for brisk phagocytosis (Fig. 1). These cells are involved in various metabolic, immunologic, and host defense mechanisms. They are ultrastructurally

---

[1] Second Department of Pathology and [2] Department of Bacteriology, Niigata University School of Medicine, 757 Asahimachidori-Ichibancho, Niigata 951-8510, Japan

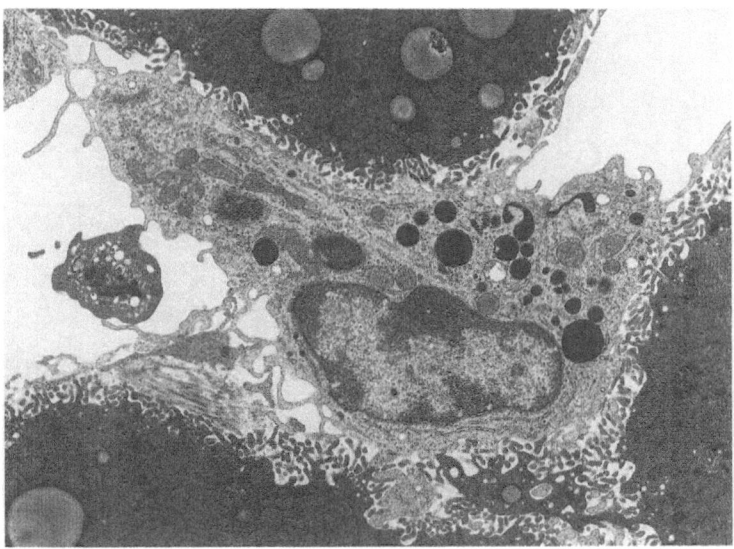

FIG. 1. A murine Kupffer cell situated in the hepatic sinusoid and equipped with well-developed lysosomes and microvilli. ×5000

characterized by abundant lysosomes, microvilli, filopodia, pseudopodia, worm-like structures, and pinocytic vesicles (Fig. 2). Kupffer cells show a localization pattern of endogenous peroxidase activity as resident macrophages [1] (Fig. 3). Since the discovery of these cells by von Kupffer [2], several different views have been presented on their origin. Based on the mononuclear phagocyte system (MPS) proposed by van Furth and colleagues [3, 4], Kupffer cells are a short-lived and nondividing population and are supplied by a monocyte influx to the liver. However, Kupffer cells are derived from primitive/fetal macrophages developing in the yolk sac and fetal liver in ontogeny [5]. In addition, the proliferation of Kupffer cells has been confirmed in adult liver under various experimental conditions [6–8] as well as in fetal liver. Osteopetrotic mice lacking macrophage colony-stimulating factor (M-CSF) activity have provided important insights regarding the role of M-CSF in Kupffer cell differentiation and function [9]. Liposomes containing dichloromethylene diphosphonate (lipo-MDP) have been used to deplete tissue macrophages [10] and have proven to be a useful tool for observing macrophage development and function. Using these models, we examined the differentiation pathways of Kupffer cells, with special reference to the biological significance of M-CSF. The biological significance of Kupffer cells in host defense mechanisms was also investigated.

## Kupffer Cell Development and Kinetics

Based on the concept of MPS [3, 4], tissue macrophages under a normal steady state are considered to be derived from blood monocytes. Monocytes leave the bone marrow after their production, enter the peripheral circulation, and circulate in the

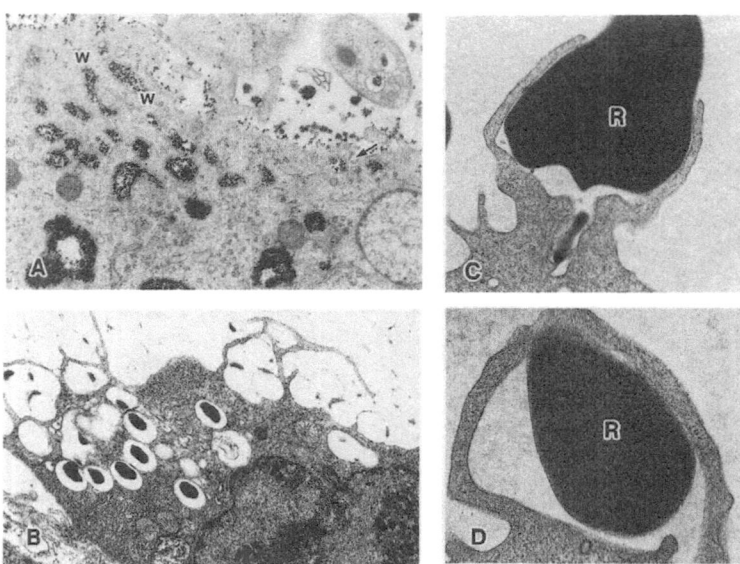

FIG. 2A–D. Various endocytic apparatuses of Kupffer cells. **A** Tiny thorotorast particles are incorporated by pinocytosis (*arrow*) and worm-like structures (*w*). ×20 000. **B** Latex particles of 0.8 μm in diameter are taken up by microvili and filopodia. ×10 000. **C, D** Red blood cells (*R*) are incorporated by extending pseudopodia. ×15 000

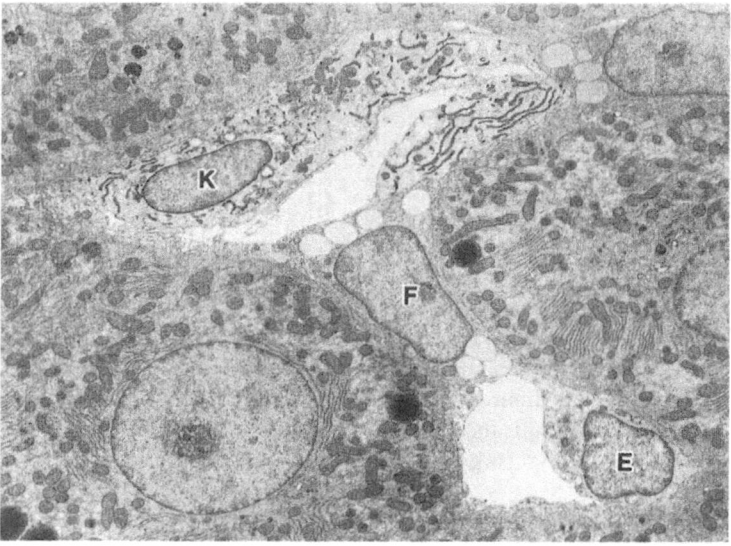

FIG. 3. Sinusoidal cells in the rat liver. Only Kupffer cells show the localization of peroxidase activity in the nuclear envelope and rough endoplasmic reticulum. *K*, Kupffer cell; *F*, fat-storing cell; *E*, endothelial cell. ×2000

blood stream. They migrate into tissues and differentiate into macrophages [3, 4]. However, immature macrophages (primitive macrophages) first develop in the yolk sac and then differentiate into peroxidase-negative fetal macrophages [5]. Primitive/ fetal macrophages in the yolk sac enter the blood stream and immigrate into the fetal liver. Fetal macrophages in the liver possess a high proliferative capacity and express macrophage antigens. They further develop the peroxidase activity of Kupffer cells with the lapse of gestational days [5]. In contrast, myelopoiesis and monocytopoiesis are poorly active in yolk sac hematopoiesis and in the early stages of hepatic hematopoiesis. Macrophage precursors also exist in the yolk sac and fetal liver in vivo and in vitro. During culturing of yolk sac cells and hepatic hematopoietic cells on a monolayer of the mouse stromal cell line ST2, primitive/fetal macrophage colonies developed before the formation of monocyte colonies [11], suggesting the existence of a direct pathway of differentiation from primitive macrophages into fetal macrophages during ontogeny.

In adult life, Kupffer cells have been thought to be nonproliferating cells in the terminal differentiation stage, and the lifespan of murine Kupffer cells was calculated to be 3.8 days [4]. However, conflicting data on the proliferation and lifespan of Kupffer cells have been presented. Kupffer cells show marked proliferative capacity after partial hepatectomy [6] or the administration of several macrophage stimulators [7]. In strontium-89-induced monocytopenic mice, Kupffer cells can be maintained for more than 6 weeks [8]. During the period of monocytopenia, the proliferation capacity of Kupffer cells increased. These findings indicate that Kupffer cells are a long-lived and slowly proliferating resident macrophage population.

## Kupffer Cell Differentiation in *op/op* Mice

Colony-stimulating factors largely define the role of the microenvironment for macrophage differentiation, phenotypes, and functions. Among these factors, M-CSF enhances the production of monocytes and their precursors, the chemotactic activity for monocyte/macrophages, the differentiation of monocytes into macrophages, macrophage proliferation, and endocytic and secretory functions. It has also been demonstrated that M-CSF and granulocyte/macrophage colony-stimulating factor (GM-CSF) play important roles in the proliferation of Kupffer cells [12].

Osteopetrotic (*op/op*) mice are an animal model of osteopetrosis; they develop osteosclerosis due to the complete absence of osteoclasts [13]. It has been found that *op/op* mice are defective in the production of functional M-CSF [9]. The impaired differentiation of monocytes into macrophages in these mutant mice results in severe deficiencies of blood monocytes, Kupffer cells, and other tissue macrophages [9, 14, 15]. In the mutant mice, the number of Kupffer cells is about 30% of that of their normal littermates, and their Kupffer cells are small, round (Fig. 4), and reveal no peroxidase activity [14, 16]. Because the GM-CSF levels in the mutant mice are within the normal range [17], the development and differentiation of such M-CSF-independent immature macrophages appear to be regulated by the effects of GM-CSF [14–18]. These results suggest the existence of a pathway of macrophage differentiation from granulocyte/macrophage colony-forming units (CFU-GM) or earlier macrophage precursors, bypassing the stage of monocytic cell series.

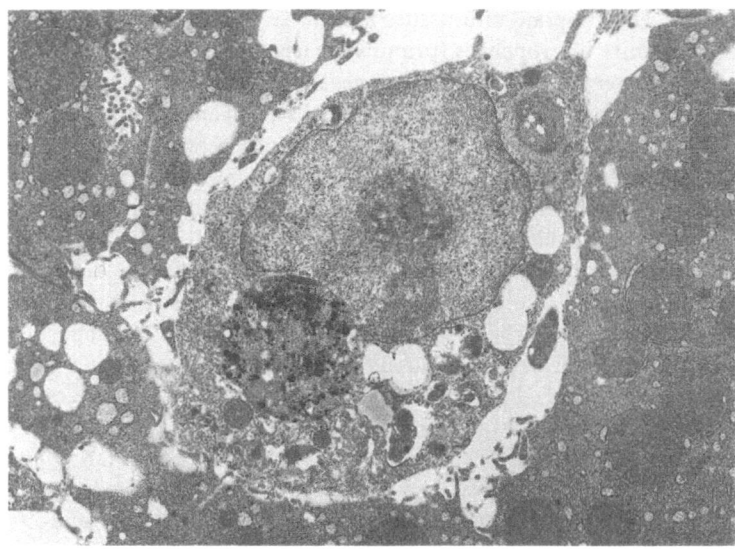

FIG. 4. Kupffer cell in an *op/op* mouse. The cell is small and round in shape and has poorly developed intracytoplasmic organelles. ×5000

The administration of M-CSF to *op/op* mice remarkably improves their osteosclerosis by the development and differentiation of osteoclasts [19, 20]. The number of Kupffer cells also rapidly increases before the influx of monocytes [21]. Kupffer cells develop peroxidase activity in the nuclear envelope and rough endoplasmic reticulum, as seen in resident macrophages [16]. These findings indicate that M-CSF is responsible for the differentiation of at least 70% of M-CSF-dependent Kupffer cells in the liver.

It was recently shown that dendritic cells differentiate and accumulate in the liver [22]. Dendritic cells are normally distributed in *op/op* mice, and they are considered to be a GM-CSF-dependent population [23]. However, the biological significance of hepatic dendritic cells has not been clarified. The relationship between Kupffer cells and dendritic cells may be an interesting subject to be investigated in further studies.

## Kupffer Cell Repopulation After Macrophage Depletion

Liposomes containing dichloromethylene diphosphonate (lipo-MDP) are ingested by macrophages and induce macrophage apoptosis [24]. At 5 days after the injection of lipo-MDP into mice, small peroxidase-negative macrophages appear. They increase in number and differentiate into large peroxidase-positive Kupffer cells. Repopulating macrophages actively proliferate and their number returns to the normal level by 2 weeks (Fig. 5) after injection. The M-CSF mRNA expression and the serum level of M-CSF were enhanced after the lipo-MDP injection [25]. These findings imply that the

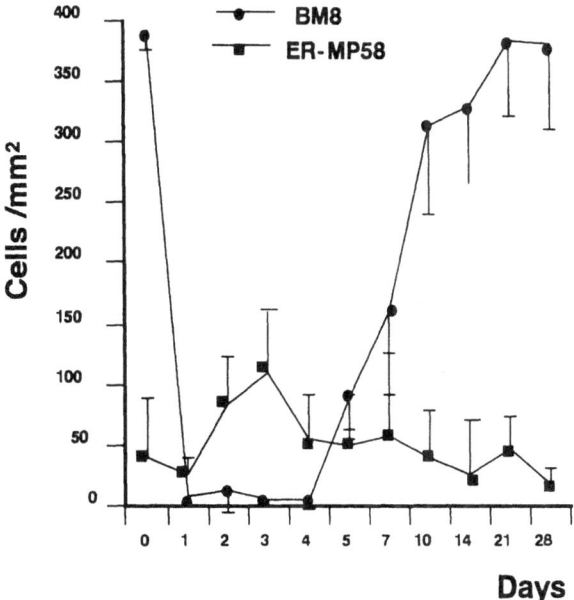

FIG. 5. Numbers of Kupffer cells (BM8-positive cells) and macrophage precursors (ER-MP58-positive cells) in a mouse liver after intravenous administration of lipo-MDP

local as well as the systemic production of M-CSF may provide a microenvironment for the differentiation and proliferation of Kupffer cells.

In the Kupffer-cell-depleted model, we have identified the existence of macrophage precursors in the liver. A monoclonal antibody (ER-MP58) [26] recognizes antigens on macrophage precursors from CFU-M to monocytes. The ER-MP58-positive precursors proliferated during the period of Kupffer cell depletion. The existence of hematopoietic stem cells in the adult liver has recently been suggested [25, 27]. In addition to the fetal period, extramedullary hematopoiesis is temporarily induced by various stimuli in the adult murine liver [7]. Since the production of M-CSF in the liver was enhanced during Kupffer cell depletion, it is suggested that locally produced M-CSF may induce the proliferation and differentiation not only of Kupffer cells, but also of their precursors.

## Role of Kupffer Cells in Host Defense Mechanisms

Kupffer cells phagocytize intravenously injected zymosan particles and accumulate together with monocytes and lymphocytes to form granulomas. Kupffer cells and monocyte-derived macrophages differentiate into epithelioid cells and multi-nucleated giant cells. The number and the size of the zymosan-induced granulomas were smaller in Kupffer-cell-depleted mice than in nontreated mice (Fig. 6). This finding is similar to that of glucan-induced granuloma formation in Kupffer-cell-deficient *op/op* mice [28]. Granulomas in the Kupffer-cell-depleted mice were formed along with the repopulation of Kupffer cells. These data suggest that preexisting

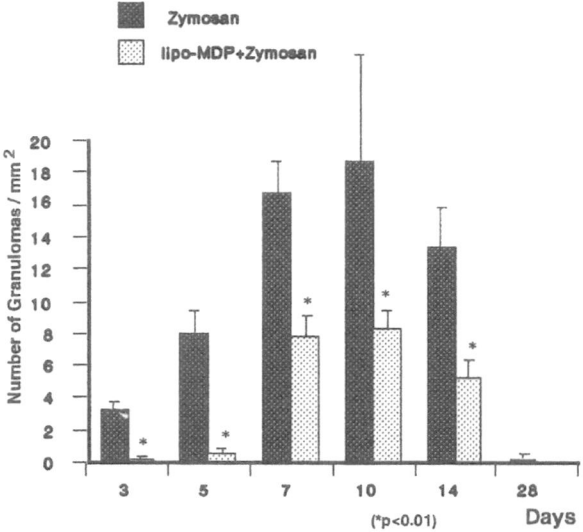

FIG. 6. Numbers of zymosan-induced granulomas in Kupffer-cell-depleted and control mice

Kupffer cells may provide an important microenvironment for macrophage differentiation and granuloma formation. The expressions of M-CSF, interleukin-1, monocyte chemoattractant protein-1, tumor necrosis factor-$\alpha$, and interferon-$\gamma$ mRNA were enhanced in the stage of granuloma formation in the control mouse liver, whereas they were suppressed in Kupffer-cell-depleted mice. The proliferation of macrophages after zymosan injection was parallel to the intensity of their M-CSF

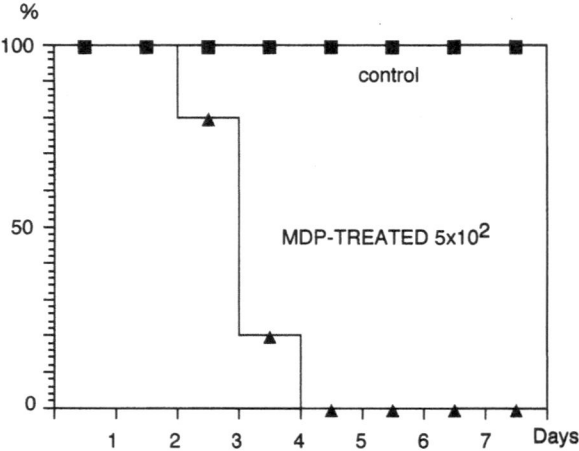

FIG. 7. Survival rates of Kupffer-cell-depleted mice and control mice after *Listeria* infection

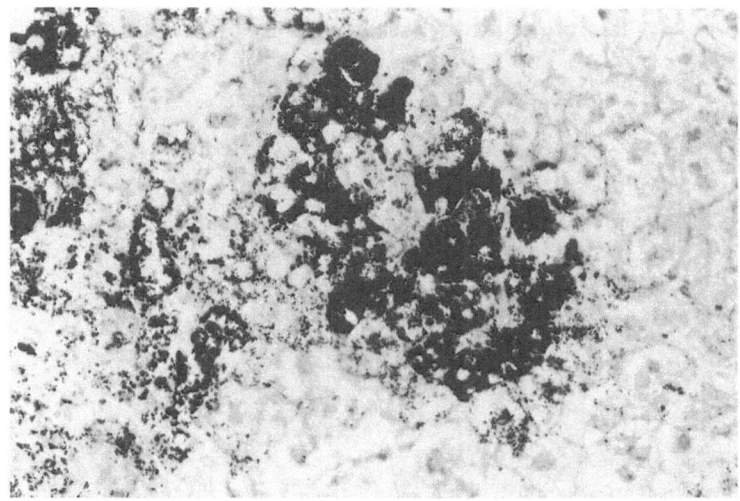

Fig. 8. The liver of a Kupffer-cell-depleted mouse at 3 days after *Listeria* infection. A large number of *Listeria* proliferated in the hepatocytes. ×400. Gram staining

expression [28]. These findings imply that Kupffer cells are indispensable for granuloma formation and the production of various cytokines.

*Listeria monocytogenes* is a gram-positive microorganism that causes amnionitis and acute exudative leptomeningitis. Focal abscesses can occur in any organ, including the lung, liver, spleen, and lymph nodes. In infections of longer duration, macrophages appear in large numbers and form granulomas. To assess the antimicrobial function of Kupffer-cells, we depleted Kupffer cells by the administration of lipo-MDP and injected *L. monocytogenes*. The natural resistance of the Kupffer cell-depleted mice to *L. monocytogenes* was significantly decreased. Mortality was increased from 0% in the control mice to 100% in the lipo-MDP-treated mice that were infected with $5 \times 10^2$ CFU doses (Fig. 7). Histologically, granulomas were not formed. *Listeria* bacilli were not detected in Kupffer cells, but were heavily accumulated in hepatocytes (Fig. 8). These findings clearly indicate that Kupffer cells are required for the expression of natural resistance against microbial infection.

## Conclusion

The differentiation pathways of Kupffer and related cells are shown in Fig. 9. Kupffer cells differentiate from precursor cells developing in the fetal hematopoietic organs in ontogeny. After birth, Kupffer cells may be derived from bone marrow and intrahepatic macrophage precursors. Locally produced M-CSF may be a key molecule for Kupffer cell differentiation and proliferation. In granulomatous inflammation, Kupffer cells play a critical role at the front line of host defense mechanisms against pathogens.

## Differentiation Pathway of Kupffer Cells

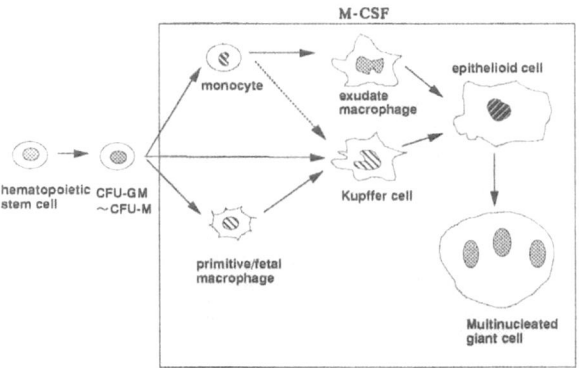

FIG. 9. Schematic representation of the development of Kupffer cells and related cells. *CFU-GM*, granulocyte/macrophage colony-forming unit; CFU-M, macrophage colony-forming unit

## *References*

1. Wisse E (1974) Observations on the fine structure and peroxidase cytochemistry of normal rat liver Kupffer cells. J Ultrastruct Res 46:393–426
2. Kupffer CV (1876) Über Sternzellen der Leber. Arch Mikrosk Anat 12:353–358
3. Furth R van, Cohn ZA, Hirsh JG, et al. (1972) The mononuclear phagocyte system: A new classification of macrophages, monocytes, and their precursors. Bull WHO 46:845–852
4. Furth R van (1989) Origin and turnover of monocytes and macrophages. Curr Top Pathol 79:125–147
5. Naito M, Hasegawa G, Takahashi K (1997) Development, differentiation, and maturation of Kupffer cells. Microsc Res Tech 39:350–364
6. Bouwens L, Knook DL, Wisse E (1986) Local proliferation and extrahepatic recruitment of liver macrophages (Kupffer cells) in partial-body irradiated rats. J Leukoc Biol 39:687–697
7. Deimann W, Fahimi D (1980) Induction of focal hemopoiesis in adult rat liver by glucan, a macrophage activator. A cytochemical and ultrastructural study. Lab Invest 42:217–224
8. Naito M, Takahashi K (1991) The role of Kupffer cells in glucan-induced granuloma formation in the liver of mice depleted of blood monocytes by administration of strontium-89. Lab Invest 64:664–674
9. Yoshida H, Hayashi S-I, Kunisada T, et al. (1990) The mutation "osteopetrosis" (op) is a mutation in the coding region of the macrophage colony stimulating factor (*Cfms*) gene. Nature 345:442–443
10. Rooijen NV, Kors N, Ende vdM, et al. (1990) Depletion and repopulation of macrophages in spleen and liver of rat after intravenous treatment with liposome-encapsulated dichloromethylene diphosphonate. Cell Tissue Res 260:215–222
11. Naito M, Takahashi K, Nishikawa S-I (1990) Development, differentiation, and maturation of macrophages in the fetal mouse liver. J Leukoc Biol 48:27–37
12. Hoedemakers RMJ, Scherphof GL, Daemaen T (1994) Proliferation of rat liver macrophages in vitro: Influence of hemopoietic growth factors. Hepatology 19:666–674

13. Marks SC (1982) Morphological evidence of reduced bone resorption in osteopetrotic (op) mice. Am J Anat 163:157–167
14. Naito M, Hayashi S-I, Yoshida H, et al. (1991) Abnormal differentiation of tissue macrophage populations in "osteopetrosis" (op) mice defective in the production of macrophage colony-stimulating factor. Am J Pathol 139:657–667
15. Wiktor-Jedrzejczak W, Ahmed A, Szczylik C, et al. (1982) Hematological characterization of congenital osteopetrosis in op/op mouse. Possible mechanism for abnormal macrophage differentiation. J Exp Med 156:1516–1527
16. Takahashi K, Naito M, Umeda S, et al. (1994) The role of macrophage colony-stimulating factor in hepatic glucan-induced granuloma formation in the osteopetrosis (op) mutant mouse defective in the production of macrophage colony-stimulating factor. Am J Pathol 144:1381–1392
17. Wiktor-Jedrzejczak W, Bartocci A, Ferrante AW Jr, et al. (1990) Total absence of colony-stimulating factor in the macrophage-deficient osteopetrotic (op/op) mouse. Proc Natl Acad Sci USA 87:4828–4832
18. Wiktor-Jedrzejczak W, Ansari AA, Sperl M, et al. (1992) Distinct in vivo functions of two macrophage subpopulations as evidenced by studies using macrophage-deficient op/op mouse. Eur J Immunol 22:1951–1954
19. Kodama H, Yamasaki A, Nose M, et al. (1991) Congenital osteoclast deficiency in osteopetrotic (op/op) mice is cured by injections of macrophage colony-stimulating factor. J Exp Med 173:269–272
20. Umeda S,Takahashi K, Naito M, et al. (1996) Neonatal changes of osteoclasts in osteopetrosis (op/op) mice defective in production of functional macrophage colony-stimulating factor (M-CSF) protein and effects of M-CSF on osteoclast development and differentiation. J Submicrosc Cytol Pathol 28:1–9
21. Umeda S, Takahashi K, Shultz LD, et al. (1996) Effects of macrophage colony-stimulating factor (M-CSF) on macrophages and related cell populations in osteopetrosis (op) mouse defective in production of functional M-CSF protein. Am J Pathol 149:559–574
22. Kudo S, Matsuno K, Ezaki T, et al. (1997) A novel migration pathway for rat dendritic cells from the blood: Hepatic sinusoids–lymph translocation. J Exp Med 185:777–784
23. Takahashi K, Naito M, Shultz LD, et al. (1993) Differentiation of dendritic cell populations in macrophage colony stimulating factor-deficient mice homozygous for the osteopetrosis (op) mutation. J Leukoc Biol 53:19–28
24. Naito M, Nagai H, Kawano S, et al. (1996) Liposome-encapsulated dichloromethylene diphosphonate induces macrophage apoptosis in vivo and in vitro. J Leukoc Biol 60:337–344
25. Yamamoto T, Naito M, Moriyama H, et al. (1996) Repopulation of murine Kupffer cells after intravenous administration of liposome-encapsulated dichloromethylene diphosphonate. Am J Pathol 149:1271–1286
26. Leenen PJM, Melis M, Slieker WAT, et al. (1990) Murine macrophage precursor characterization. II. Monoclonal antibodies against macrophage precursor antigens. Eur J Immunol 20:27–34
27. Hays EF, Hays DM, Golde DW (1978) Hemopoietic stem cells in mouse liver. Exp Hematol 6:18–27
28. Moriyama H, Yamamoto T, Takatsuka H, et al. (1997) Expression of macrophage colony stimulating factor and its receptor in hepatic granulomas of Kupffer cell-depleted mice. Am J Pathol 150:2047–2060

# Pit Cells as Liver-Associated Natural Killer Cells

Kenji Kaneda

*Summary.* Pit cells, the fourth type of hepatic sinusoidal cells, are liver-associated natural killer (NK) cells. They represent a morphologically and functionally modified form of peripheral blood NK cells. They are localized inside the lumen of the sinusoid, closely adhering to the endothelial cells and Kupffer cells, and often extending well-developed pseudopodia suggestive of migration along the sinusoidal wall. Multivesicular body-related dense granules and rod-cored vesicles are frequently found in the cytoplasm of pit cells and may be involved in the cytotoxicity against bound tumor cells. Pit cells increase in number after treatment with various biological response modifiers such as interleukin-2 and interleukin-12 via the local proliferation and influx of peripheral blood NK cells, resulting in the augmentation of liver-associated NK activity and a decrease in liver metastasis. They thus constitute the defense system of the liver together with Kupffer cells and extrathymic T cells, and profoundly contribute to the modulation of the development of liver diseases.

*Key words.* Pit cells, Natural killer cells, Rod-cored vesicles, Dense granules, Ultrastructure

## Introduction: An Overview of the Research on Hepatic Natural Killer Cells

Nowadays the liver is considered to be a major immune organ owing to the fact that a large number of immune-competent cells such as macrophages, natural killer (NK) cells, and extrathymic T cells populate the hepatic sinusoids. The research on hepatic NK cells followed two paths, which started independently in the middle of the 1970s (Table 1) [1–10]. In the field of immunology dealing with peripheral blood and splenic lymphocytes, spontaneous cytotoxicity or natural cytotoxicity against tumors was found to be present in the spleen of non-tumor-bearing mice in 1975 [1]. The morphological relevance of such NK-mediated cytotoxicity was then investigated, and it was found that large granular lymphocytes (LGLs) were responsible for this activity

Department of Anatomy, Osaka City University Medical School, 1-4-54 Asahimachi, Abeno-ku, Osaka 545, Japan

TABLE 1. Summarized history of the research on pit cells, NK cells, and related lymphocytes in the liver

| Years | Peripheral blood and spleen | Liver |
|---|---|---|
| 1975 | Natural killer activity in the spleen (Herberman et al. 1975 [1]) | Pit cells as the fourth sinusoidal cell (Wisse et al. 1976 [2]) |
| | Large granular lymphocytes and their morphological relevance to NK cells (Saksela et al. 1979 [3]) | |
| 1980 | Ultrastructure of peripheral blood NK cells (Grossi et al. 1982 [4]) | Rod-cored vesicles characteristic of pit cells (Kaneda et al. 1982 [5]) |
| | | Pit cells as NK cells (Kaneda et al. 1983 [6]) Liver-associated NK activity (Wiltrout et al. 1984 [7]) |
| 1985 | | NK activity of isolated pit cells (Bouwens et al. 1987 [8]) |
| 1990 | | Extrathymic T cells in the liver (Ohteki et al. 1990 [9]) |
| | | Pit cells as a differentiated form of NK cells (Vanderkerken et al. 1993 [10]) |

[3]. At the same time, in the field of histology of the liver, pit cells were first described in the rat liver in 1976 as the fourth type of sinusoidal cell, and were morphologically characterized by dense granules [2], although their function was unclear. In 1983, these two lines of research were joined by our study which demonstrated that pit cells were NK cells with the morphology of LGLs [6]. Wiltrout et al. [7, 11] showed that various biological response modifiers (BRMs) significantly augmented liver-associated NK activity and as a result suppressed liver metastasis, thus opening the possibilities of immunotherapy of liver metastasis with BRMs. Since then, much attention has been paid to the immunological function of the liver by basic and clinical researchers. This new aspect of the liver as an immune organ led to the finding of extrathymic T cells in the liver by Abo and co-workers in 1990 [9]. In researching the origin of pit cells, Bouwens et al. [8] and Vanderkerken et al. [10] compared the functional and morphological properties of pit cells with those of NK cells in other anatomical compartments, and suggested that peripheral blood NK cells might differentiate into liver-specific ones, or pit cells, in the microenvironment of the liver.

## Pit Cells as Liver-Associated LGLs

As revealed by electron microscopy, there is a difference in tissue distribution between LGLs (NK cells) and agranular lymphocytes (T and B cells) in rats [12]; the former cells exist abundantly in nonlymphoid organs such as the liver and lungs,

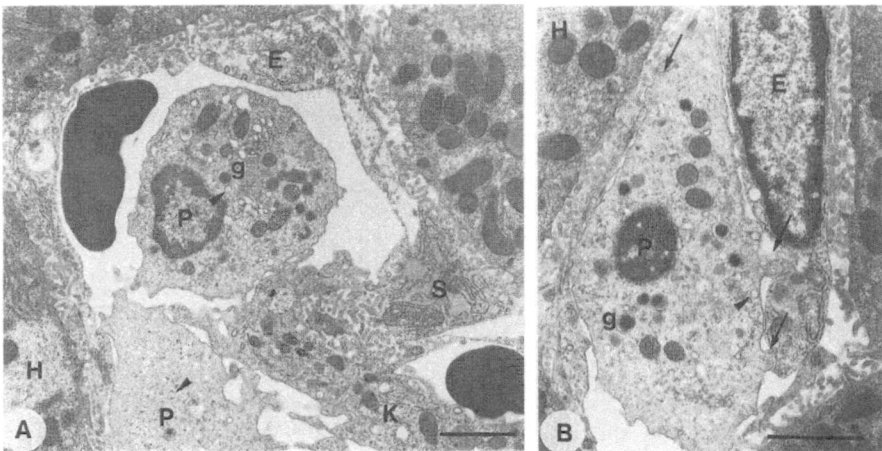

FIG. 1. **A** Sinusoidal cells of the rat liver. Kupffer cells (*K*) and pit cells (*P*) are located in the lumen of sinusoids, while stellate cells (*S*) exist in the space of Disse between hepatocytes (*H*) and endothelial cells (*E*). Pit cells contain dense granules (*g*) and rod-cored vesicles (*arrowheads*). Bar = 2 μm. **B** A pit cell (*P*) closely adheres to endothelial cells (*E*) extending small projections (*arrows*) toward the latter. They contain dense granules (*g*) and rod-cored vesicles (*arrowhead*). Bar = 2 μm

while the latter are abundant in lymphoid organs such as lymph nodes and the white pulp of the spleen. Such preferential localization of LGLs in the organs where metastasis frequently occurs may be related to the ability of NK cells to react promptly with tumor cells. The hepatic LGLs are termed pit cells, and are distinct from extrahepatic LGLs in both morphology and function, as described later.

Pit cells are located in the lumen of hepatic sinusoids, adhering to the Kupffer cells (Fig. 1A) and endothelial cells (Fig. 1B). They have spherical dense granules at one aspect of the nucleus [2, 13]. This feature is common among animal species including reptiles (iguana), birds (bantam), and mammals (rabbit, sheep, hamster, guinea pig, mouse, rat, human being), but there is a difference in the size and number of dense granules. The frequency of granules is much higher in rats than in mice and human beings.

Pit cells are likely to adhere more tightly to the sinusoidal walls than conventional lymphocytes, as is indicated by the morphometric data that the percentage of LGLs to total leukocytes in the hepatic sinusoid after intraportal perfusion with saline was 28.1%, which was much higher than that in the peripheral blood (0.8%), while the percentages of agranular lymphocytes in the liver and peripheral blood were 38.3% and 75.3%, respectively [14]. Such preferential localization of LGLs in the hepatic sinusoid may be related to the cytoplasmic processes which are extended, and often penetrate, the endothelial pores (Fig. 1B). On the other hand, when compared with the Kupffer cells, the pit cells attach to the sinusoidal endothelial cells less tightly, which allows the isolation of pit cells by high-pressure perfusion via the portal vein, as reported by Bouwens et al. [8].

Fig. 2. Cell organelles of pit cells in the rat liver. Spherical dense granules (*g*), multivesi-cular bodies (*m*), rod-cored vesicles (*arrowheads*), and empty 0.2 μm-vesicles (*arrows*) are characteristic of pit cells. Golgi apparatus (*go*) is well developed. Bar = 0.5 μm

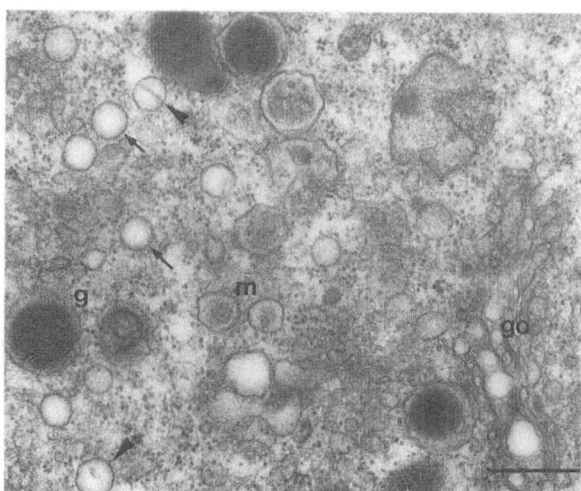

## Ultrastructural Characteristics of Pit Cells

Pit cells are ultrastructurally characterized by dense spherical granules and rod-cored vesicles (Fig. 2) [5, 13]. The dense granules are identified as azurophil granules by Giemsa stain. They are formed by the accumulation of a dense matrix in multivesicular bodies, a type of lysosome. Granules contain perforin and serine esterase as bio-active substances and acid phosphatase as lysosomal enzymes. Rod-cored vesicles are a unique structure of NK cells. They are approximately 0.2 μm in diameter and exhibit various profiles of rod-structures, i.e., a complete bridge over the diameter, a dot-appearance, etc., depending on the cutting plane of the vesicle. Empty vesicles of the same size as rod-cored vesicles are also found. Rod-cored vesicles and empty vesicles, collectively termed 0.2-μm-vesicles, are derived from the Golgi apparatus and are considered to be exocytosed.

## Ultrastructural and Functional Comparison of Pit Cells with Peripheral Blood and Splenic NK Cells

There are several differences in the function and ultrastructure of NK cells in the liver, peripheral blood, and spleen (Table 2) [15]. Liver NK cells, or pit cells, have various kinds of cytotoxicity, including lymphokine-activated killer (LAK) activity, and contain a large number of granules and rod-cored vesicles. Furthermore, pit cells themselves can be divided into two populations according to their density; pit cells with a high density resemble peripheral blood NK cells, while those with a low density possess the typical features of liver-specific NK cells. Vanderkerken et al. [10] considered that the former would be derived from peripheral blood NK cells and would differentiate into the latter after a certain period of time in the hepatic sinusoid. This

TABLE 2. Comparison of morphological and functional properties of LGLs by anatomical sites

|  | Liver | Peripheral blood | Spleen |
|---|---|---|---|
| Cell size | Large | Small | Small |
| Granules: Number | ++ | + | + |
|        Size | Small | Large | Small |
| 0.2-μm vesicles | ++ | +-++ | + |
| Rod-cored vesicles | ++ | + | + |
| Mitochondria | Large | Small | nd[a] |
| Expression of asialo GM1 | −/+ | + | + |
| NK activity | ++ | + | + |
| NC activity | + | + | + |
| LAK activity | + | − | nd |
| Adherence to endothelial cells | ++ | nd | + |

[a] nd, not examined.

interpretation has been confirmed by an experiment using rat natural killer (RNK) leukemia cells which have similar ultrastructural and fuctional properties as normal NK cells. RNK cells metastasized into the liver after intraperitoneal injection exhibited a larger number of rod-cored vesicles than those metastasized into the spleen (Fig. 3A,B), suggesting that the microenvironment of the liver may play a role in the differentiation of peripheral blood NK cells into liver-specific NK cells [16]. Pit cells are also capable of undergoing mitosis in the normal liver [2]. They are thus considered to be supplied by both local proliferation and influx from the peripheral blood in the normal state.

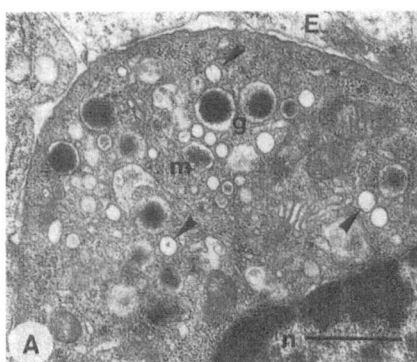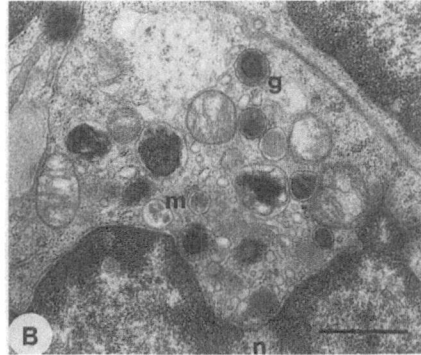

FIG. 3. Metastatic rat natural killer leukemia-0 (RNK-0) cells 3 months after intraperitoneal inoculation. **A** RNK-0 cells metastasized into the liver. There are many dense granules (*g*) and rod-cored vesicles (*arrowheads*) in the cytoplasm. *E*, sinusoidal endothelial cells; *n*, nucleus; *m*, multivesicular bodies. Bar = 1 μm. **B** RNK-0 cells metastasized into the spleen. There are fewer rod-cored vesicles than in RNK-0 cells in the liver. *g*, dense granules; *n*, nucleus; *m*, multivesicular bodies. Bar = 1 μm. (Photographed by Dr. Akiko Kojima, Osaka City University Medical School)

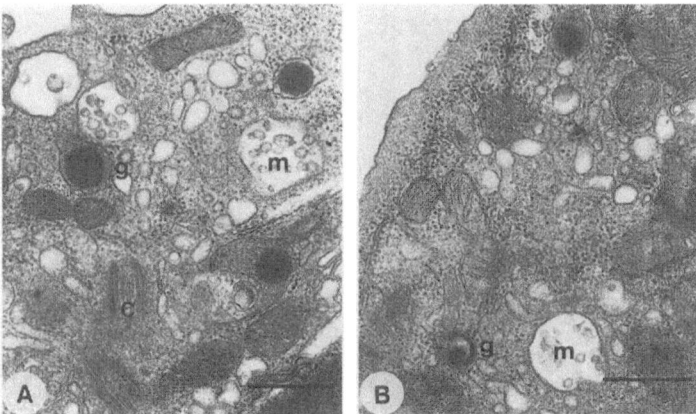

FIG. 4. Ultrastructural comparison between $CD3^-IL\text{-}2R\beta^+$ cells ($=$ NK cells; **A**) and $CD3^{intermediate+}IL\text{-}2R\beta^+$ cells ($=$ extrathymic T cells; **B**) obtained by cell sorting from the mouse liver. These two populations have a common feature of LGLs except in the size of dense granules ($g$). Granules of NK cells are larger than those of extrathymic T cells. $m$, multivesicular bodies; $c$, centrioles. **A, B**: bar $= 0.5\,\mu$m

## Pit Cells and Extrathymic T Cells in the Liver: Ultrastructural Comparison

In the mouse liver, as well as NK cells, there are a large number of extrathymic T cells which are phenotypically defined as $CD3^{intermediate+}IL\text{-}2R\beta^+$ cells or $NK1.1^+$ $TCR^{intermediate+}$ cells. These constitute the defense system of the liver against tumor metastasis and microbial infection, together with NK cells and Kupffer cells [17]. In the liver of human beings and rats, however, the presence of extrathymic T cells has not been clearly demonstrated, probably owing to the lack of appropriate antibodies to characterize them. In the human liver, as well as $CD3^-CD56^+$ cells ($=$ NK cells), there are many $CD3^+CD56^+$ cells [18] which may correspond to the extrathymic T cells of mouse liver.

As revealed by electron microscopy, $CD3^-IL\text{-}2R\beta^+$ cells ($=$ NK cells; Fig. 4A) and $CD3^{intermediate+}IL\text{-}2R\beta^+$ cells ($=$ extrathymic T cells; Fig. 4B) obtained by the cell sorting of mouse hepatic mononuclear cells show a common feature of LGLs, although the number and size of dense granules are smaller in the latter cells than in the former [19, 20].

## Tumor Cell Lysis by Pit Cells: Involvement of Dense Granules and the Fas–Fas Ligand System

Pit cells have natural killer-, natural cytotoxic (NC)-, and lymphokine-activated killer (LAK)-mediated cytotoxicities, by which they are capable of preventing liver metastasis of various kinds of tumors. Both in vivo and in vitro experiments have demon-

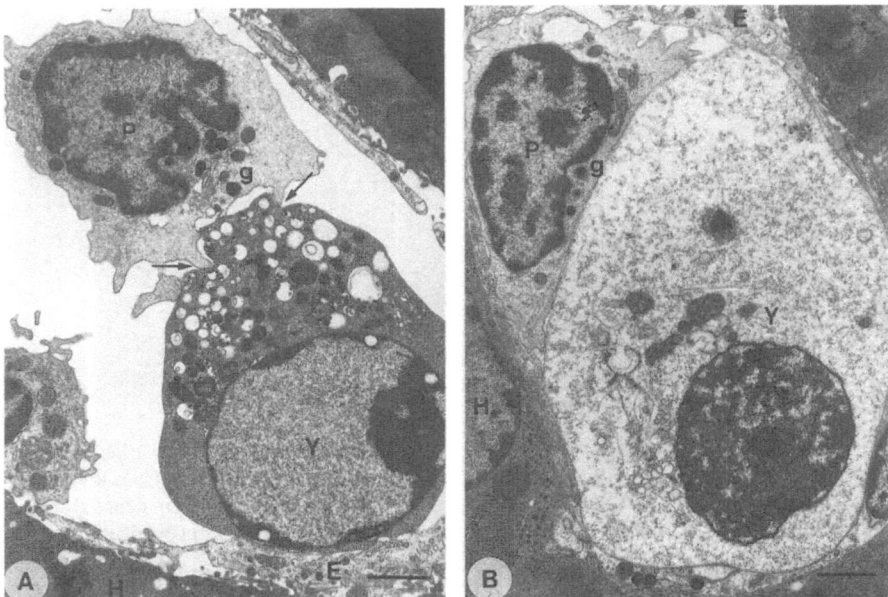

FIG. 5A,B.   In vivo tumor cell lysis by pit cells. Pit cell-Yac-1 cell conjugate is seen in the sinusoid 1 h after intraportal injection. **A** A pit cell (*P*) holds a Yac-1 cell (*Y*) with cytoplasmic projections (*arrows*). Dense granules (*g*) are oriented toward the target cell, which exhibits nuclear chromatin condensation and vacuolation of cell organelles. *E*, sinusoidal endothelial cells; *H*, hepatocytes. Bar = 2 μm. **B** A pit cell (*P*) adheres closely to a Yac-1 cell (*Y*), the cytoplasm of which becomes pale due to cytolysis. *g*, dense granules; *E*, endothelial cells; *H*, hepatocytes. Bar = 2 μm. (From [20], with permission of the Biomedical Research Foundation)

strated that pit cells are bound to target cells with their cell bodies and cytoplasmic processes, and then orient dense granules toward the target and ultimately induce apoptosis (Fig. 5A) or cell lysis (Fig. 5B) [21]. Although the mechanism by which pit cells exert cytotoxicity against tumor cells is not fully understood, there are two possibilities; one is perforin-induced osmotic disruption of cells, and another is Fas–Fas ligand system-mediated apoptosis. Dense granules of NK cells and LAK cells contain perforin and serine esterase, as has been demonstrated biochemically and immunohistochemically [22, 23]. Being exocytosed, perforin will make pores in the plasma membrane of bound target cells, resulting in the osmotic rupture of cells. However, no correlation has been found between the size of granules and cytolytic activity. For example, both LAK cells and granular metrial glandular cells (NK cell lineage in the uterus) have very large granules. The former cells exhibit strong cytotoxicity, whereas the latter display low NK activity. As for the involvement of the Fas–Fas ligand system in NK-mediated cytolyis, Tsutsui et al. [24] clearly showed this by using mouse hepatic NK cell clones which lacked the effective mechanism of perforin-mediated cytolysis in spite of a sufficient amount of perforin in the granules. These NK cell clones exerted cytotoxicity against an intact Fas-expressing tumor cell line A-1, but did not do so against a mutant Fas-expressing one F-10.

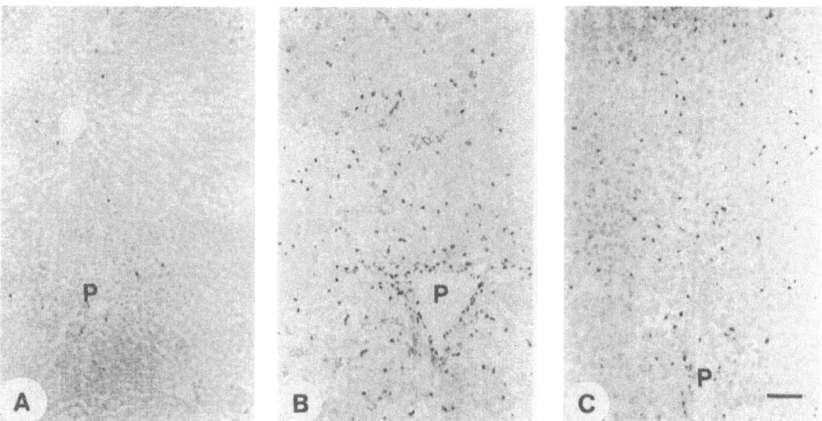

FIG. 6. Immunohistochemistry for mAb 3.2.3 (A) in normal, (B) IL-2-treated, and (C) IL-12-treated rat livers. MAb 3.2.3-positive cells, i.e., NK cells, significantly increase in number in both IL-2- and IL-12-treated livers. P, portal veins. Bar = 100 μm. (Photographed by Dr. Yun Sun Lee, Kinki University School of Medicine)

## Augmentation of Liver-Associated NK Activity by BRMs and Suppression of Liver Metastasis

By treatment with various BRMs such as OK-432 and poly IC:LC, liver-associated NK activity is more profoundly augmented than spleen-associated activity [7]. This augmentation is considered to result from an increased influx of peripheral blood NK cells into the liver [25]. Pit cells are also activated, as demonstrated by the increment of rod-cored vesicles and the enlargement of Golgi apparatus [26]. By treatment with IL-2 or IL-12 for five consecutive days, monoclonal antibody 3.2.3-positive NK cells significantly increased in number in the rat liver (Fig. 6). Experimental hepatic metastases of rat colon carcinoma RNC-H4 were concurrently reduced [27]. In mice, $NK1.1^+TCR^{intermediate+}$ cells or $NK1^+$ T cells are considered to be the effector cells in IL-12-induced immune responses and suppression of liver metastasis [28, 29].

## Liver NK Cells in a Tumor-Bearing State

In Japan, IL-2 is the only BRM that is under clinical trial for patients with hepatic tumors. For successful immunotherapy with IL-2, the dose and time schedule for administration is important because high-dose IL-2 often causes serious side-effects, especially in the tumor-bearing state. Intraperitoneal injection of IL-2 at a dose of $10^5$ IU twice daily for 3 days resulted in the death of MH134-hepatoma-bearing mice, while it had no lethal effect on non-tumor-bearing mice [30]. In a tumor-bearing state, the numbers of $CD3^-IL-2R\beta^+$ cells (= NK cells) and $CD3^{intermediate+}IL-$

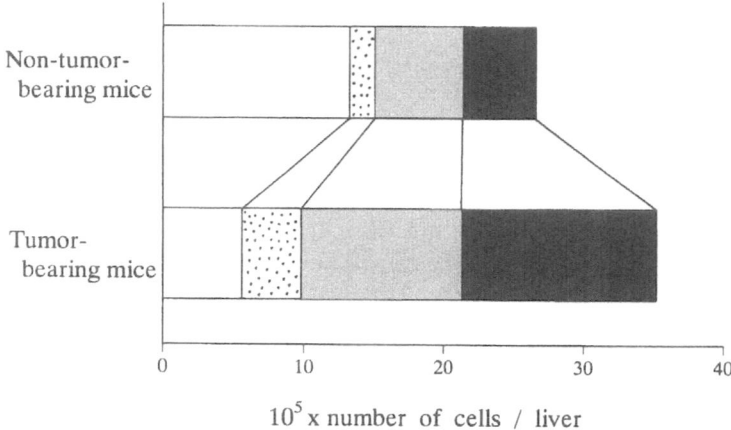

FIG. 7. Number of four lymphocyte subsets per liver in non-tumor-bearing and MH134-tumor-bearing mice 7 days after tumor implantation. *Black areas*, CD3⁻IL-2R$\beta^+$ cells (= NK cells); *shaded areas*, CD3$^{intermediate+}$IL-2R$\beta^+$ cells (= extrathymic T cells); *dotted areas*, CD3⁻IL-2R$\beta^-$ cells (= B cells etc.); *white areas*, CD3$^+$IL-2R$\beta^-$ cells (= conventional T cells). The former two lymphocyte subsets significantly increase in number in tumor-bearing mice. (Modified from the data in [30])

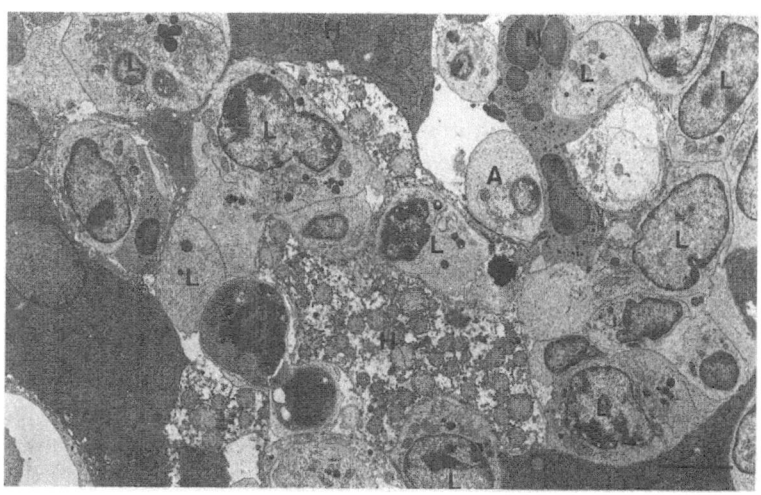

FIG. 8. Accumulation of large granular lymphocytes in the liver of MH134-tumor-bearing mice after treatment with high-dose IL-2 (6 × 10⁵ IU in 3 days). Large granular lymphocytes (*L*), agranular lymphocytes (*A*), and neutrophils (*N*) are accumulated in the space of Disse. *H*, hepatocytes. Bar = 5 μm

$2R\beta^+$ cells (= extrathymic T cells) per liver were much larger than those in a non-tumor-bearing state, while the number of $CD3^+IL\text{-}2R\beta^-$ cells (= thymic T cells) was smaller (Fig. 7) [30]. When high-dose IL-2 was given to tumor-bearing mice, LGLs including NK cells and extrathymic T cells underwent a population increase in the liver (Fig. 8) and lungs, leading to the functional disturbance of these organs.

# Biological Functions of Pit Cells Other than Anti-Tumor Activity

There have been few studies on the function of pit cells other than their anti-tumor activity. In general, NK cells are considered to have a wide variety of functions, including antiviral and antifungal activities, regulation of immune reactions, regulation of hemopoiesis, rejection of allografts, etc. Pit cells may have these functions as well. Recently, it has been demonstrated that hepatic NK cells are involved in the progress [31] or termination [32] of liver regeneration by suppressing or augmenting, respectively, NK-mediated cytotoxicity against immature hepatocytes.

## References

1. Herberman RB, Nunn ME, Lavrin DH (1975) Natural cytotoxic reactivity of mouse lymphoid cells against syngeneic and allogeneic tumors. I. Distribution of reactivity and specificity. Int J Cancer 16:216–229
2. Wisse E, van't Noordende JM, van der Meulen J, et al. (1976) The pit cell: Description of a new type of cell occuring in rat liver sinusoids and peripheral blood. Cell Tiss Res 173:423–435
3. Saksela E, Timonen T, Ranki A, et al. (1979) Morphological and functional characterization of isolated effector cells responsible for human natural killer activity to fetal fibroblasts and to cultured cell line targets. Immunol Rev 44:71–123
4. Grossi CE, Cadoni A, Zicca A, et al. (1982) Large granular lymphocytes in human peripheral blood: Ultrastructural and cytochemical characterization of the granules. Blood 59:277–283
5. Kaneda K, Wake K, Senoo H (1982) The "rod-cored vesicle": A new type of vesicle in the pit cells. In: Knook DL, Wisse E (eds) Sinusoidal liver cells. Elsevier, Amsterdam, pp 77–84
6. Kaneda K, Dan C, Wake K (1983) Pit cells as natural killer cells. Biomed Res 4:567–576
7. Wiltrout RH, Mathieson BJ, Talmadge JE, et al. (1984) Augmentation of organ-associated natural killer activity by biological response modifiers. Isolation and characterization of large granular lymphocytes from the liver. J Exp Med 160:1431–1449
8. Bouwens L, Remels L, Baekeland M, et al. (1987) Large granular lymphocytes or "pit cells" from rat liver: Isolation, ultrastructural characterization and natural killer activity. Eur J Immunol 17:37–42
9. Ohteki T, Seki S, Abo T, et al. (1990) Liver is a possible site for the proliferation of abnormal $CD3^+4^-8^-$ double-negative lymphocytes in autoimmune MRL–lpr/lpr mice. J Exp Med 172:7–12
10. Vanderkerken K, Bouwens L, de Neve W, et al. (1993) Origin and differentiation of hepatic natural killer cells (pit cells). Hepatology 18:919–925

11. Wiltrout RH, Herberman RB, Zhang S-R, et al. (1985) Role of organ-associated NK cells in decreased formation of experimental metastasis in lung and liver. J Immunol 134:4267–4275
12. Kaneda K, Wake K (1985) Pit cells in extrahepatic organs of the rat. Anat Rec 211:192–197
13. Kaneda K, Wake K (1983) Distribution and morphological characteristics of the pit cell of the rat. Cell Tiss Res 233:485–505
14. Kaneda K (1989) Liver-associated large granular lymphocytes: Morphological and functional aspects. Arch Histol Cytol 52:447–459
15. Kaneda K, Pilaro AM, Sayers TJ, et al. (1994) Quantitative analysis of rod-cored vesicles and dense granules of large granular lymphocytes in the liver, spleen, and peripheral blood of rats. Cell Tiss Res 276:187–195
16. Kaneda K, Sayers TJ, Wiltrout TA, et al. (1996) Rod-cored vesicles in large granular lymphocyte (LGL) leukemia cells of rats: Alterations induced following metastasis to the liver. Biomed Res 17:53–65
17. Abo T (1992) Extrathymic differentiation of T lymphocytes and its biological function. Biomed Res 13:1–39
18. Takii Y, Hashimoto S, Iiai T, et al. (1994) Increase in the proportion of granulated $CD56^+$ T cells in patients with malignancy. Clin Exp Immunol 97:522–527
19. Fujikura S, Watanabe H, Abo T, et al. (1995) Ultrastructural comparison of CD3-intermediate positive T cells and natural killer cells from the liver of mice. In: Wisse E, Knook DL, Wake K (eds) Cells of the hepatic sinusoid, vol 5. Kupffer Cell Foundation, Leiden, pp 156–157
20. Watanabe H, Miyaji C, Kawachi Y, et al. (1995) Relationship between intermediate TCR cells and $NK1.1^+$ T cells in various immune organs: $NK1.1^+$ T cells are present within a population of intermediate TCR cells. J Immunol 155:2972–2983
21. Kaneda K, Wake K (1990) Ultrastructural study of in vivo tumor lysis by liver-associated natural killer cells. Biomed Res 11:137–143
22. Burkhardt JK, Hester S, Lapham CK, et al. (1990) The lytic granules of natural killer cells are dual-function organelles combining secretory and pre-lysosomal compartments. J Cell Biol 111:2327–2340
23. Ojcius DM, Zheng LM, Sphicas EC, et al. (1991) Subcellular localization of perforin and serine esterase in lymphokine-activated killer cells and cytotoxic T cells by immunogold labeling. J Immunol 146:4427–4432
24. Tsutsui H, Nakanishi K, Matsui K, et al. (1996) IFN-$\gamma$-inducing factor up-regulates Fas ligand-mediated cytotoxic activity of murine natural killer cell clones. J Immunol 157:3967–3973
25. Wiltrout RH, Pilaro AM, Gruys ME, et al. (1989) Augmentation of mouse liver-associated NK activity by biological response modifiers occurs largely via rapid recruitment of LGL from the bone marrow. J Immunol 143:372–378
26. Dan C, Kaneda K, Wake K (1985) A striking increase in rod-cored vesicles in pit cells (natural killer cells) and augmentation of the liver-associated natural killer activity by a streptococcal preparation (OK-432). Biomed Res 6:347–351
27. Okuno K, Jinnai H, Lee YS, et al. (1996) Interleukin-12 augments the liver-associated immunity and reduces liver metastases. Hepato-gastroenterology 43:1196–1202
28. Hashimoto W, Takeda K, Anzai R, et al. (1995) Cytotoxic $NK1.1Ag^+$ $\alpha\beta T$ cells with intermediate TCR induced in the liver of mice by IL-12. J Immunol 154:4333–4340
29. Kawamura T, Takeda K, Mendiratta SK, et al. (1998) Critical role of $NK1^+$ T cells in IL-12-induced immune responses in vivo. J Immunol 160:16–19
30. Asano Y, Kaneda K, Hiragushi J, et al. (1997) The tumor-bearing state induces augmented responses of organ-associated lymphocytes to high-dose interleukin-2 therapy in mice. Cancer Immunol Immunother 45:63–70

31. Vujanovic NL, Polimeno LP, Azzarone A, et al. (1995) Changes of liver-resident NK cells during liver regeneration in rats. J Immunol 154:6324–6338
32. Itoh H, Abo T, Sugawara A, et al. (1988) Age-related variation in the proportion and activity of murine liver natural killer cells and their cytotoxicity against regenerating hepatocytes. J Immunol 141:315–323

# Part III
# Liver Diseases and Hepatic Sinusoidal Cells

# Changes in Adhesion Molecules of Sinusoidal Endothelial Cells in Liver Injury

HIROMASA OHIRA[1], TAKATO UENO[2], KYUICHI TANIKAWA[2], and REIJI KASUKAWA[1]

*Summary.* Interactions between leukocytes and sinusoidal endothelial cells have been known to be involved in the pathogenesis of acute liver injury. In these cell-to-cell interactions, various adhesion molecules play a key role, and the expression of these adhesion molecules is mainly regulated by inflammatory cytokines such as tumor necrosis factor-$\alpha$ (TNF-$\alpha$), interleukin-1 (IL-1), and interferon-$\gamma$ (IFN-$\gamma$). Sinusoidal endothelial cells express intercellular adhesion molecule-1 (ICAM-1), ICAM-2, leukocyte function-associated-3 (LFA-3), very late antigen-5 (VLA-5), and CD44 in normal liver. However, in patients with acute or chronic liver disease, ICAM-1 and vascular cell adhesion molecule-1 (VCAM-1) expression on sinusoidal endothelial cells is markedly enhanced in the inflamed liver tissue. In one of our studies, the in vitro expression of ICAM-1 on cultured rat sinusoidal endothelial cells which had been stimulated with TNF-$\alpha$ or IL-1$\alpha$ increased in a dose- and time-dependent manner. In addition, the number of neutrophils that adhered to sinusoidal endothelial cells pretreated with TNF-$\alpha$ increased in a dose-dependent manner, and significantly decreased upon incubation with anti-ICAM-1 antibody. In vivo, following endotoxin-induced rat liver injury, the number of neutrophils infiltrating the sinusoids increased after plasma TNF and IL-8 peaked. In addition, ICAM-1 expression on sinusoidal endothelial cells strongly increased from 8 h after endotoxin exposure, and adhered to neutrophils which expressed both LFA-1 and Mac-1. These findings suggest that sinusoidal endothelial cells may mediate the direct interaction between leukocytes and sinusoidal endothelial cells by expressing adhesion molecules regulated by inflammatory cytokines.

*Key words.* ICAM-1, Inflammatory cytokines, Endotoxin, sICAM-1, sVCAM-1

[1] Internal Medicine II, Fukushima Medical University School of Medicine, 1-Hikarigaoka, Fukushima 960–1295, Japan
[2] The Second Department of Internal Medicine, Kurume University School of Medicine, 67 Asahi-machi, Kurume, Fukuoka 830-0011, Japan

# Introduction

Cellular adhesion and recognition mechanisms are among the most basic require-
ments for the evolution of multicellular organisms. Such cell-to-cell or cell-to-matrix
interactions involve an antigen-independent receptor–ligand interaction mediated by
adhesion molecules. Currently, adhesion molecules are classified into four major
families, according to common structural features, i.e., the cadherin, integrin,
immunoglobulin, and selectin familes [1, 2]. In addition, the expression of several
adhesion molecules is known to be regulated by various cytokines such as TNF-$\alpha$,
interleukin-1 (IL-1), and interferon-$\gamma$ (IFN-$\gamma$) [3, 4]. In the liver, inflammatory cells
pass through the sinusoidal endothelial cells to accumulate at the inflammatory sites.
Consequently, leukocyte–sinusoidal endothelial cell interaction may play an important role in the control of the immune response [5]. In liver injury, the expression of
adhesion molecules on sinusoidal endothelial cells is up-regulated and the production
of inflammatory cytokines increases [6, 7]. In the present study, we investigated the
relationship between changes in adhesion molecules on sinusoidal endothelial cells
and cytokine levels in vitro and in vivo. In this chapter, we focus primarily on
intercellular adhesion molecule-1 (ICAM-1), which is believed to be a very important
molecule in leukocyte–endothelial interactions.

## Expression of Adhesion Molecules on Sinusoidal Endothelial Cells

Immunohistochemical analysis using biopsy specimens from patients with liver disease and healthy controls has revealed that various adhesion molecules are expressed
on sinusoidal endothelial cells [7–9]. As shown in Table 1, ICAM-1, ICAM-2 (belonging to the immunoglobulin superfamily), leukocyte function-associated-3 (LFA-3),
very late antigen-5 (VLA-5) (integrin family), and CD44 are expressed on sinusoidal
endothelial cells in normal liver. On the other hand, in patients with acute or chronic
liver disease, the expression of these adhesion molecules is up-regulated and new
adhesion molecules such as E-selectin or P-selectin are expressed. In particular,
ICAM-1 and vascular cell adhesion molecule-1 (VCAM-1) expression on sinusoidal

TABLE 1. Expression of adhesion molecules on sinusoidal endothelial cells

| Adhesion molecules | | Healthy controls | Liver disease |
|---|---|---|---|
| Selectin family | E-selectin ⌐ P-selectin ⌐ | – | + |
| Immunoglobulin family | ICAM-1 | + | + + |
| | ICAM-2 | + | + |
| | VCAM-1 | – | + + |
| | LFA-3 | + | + |
| Integrin family | VLA-5 | + | + |
| | CD44 | + | + |

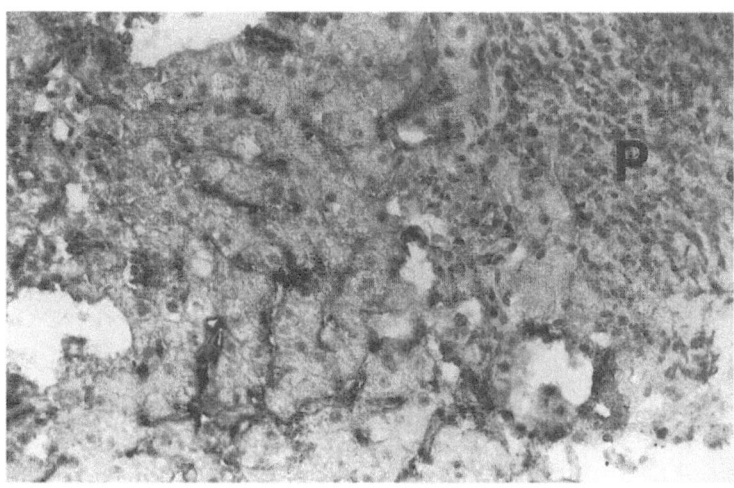

FIG. 1. Immunoperoxidase staining of intercellular adhesion molecule-1 (ICAM-1) in liver tissue biopsy from a patient with chronic hepatitis C. Remarkable localization of ICAM-1 is observed on sinusoidal lining cells in the area of priportal inflammation. *P*, portal tract. ×200

endothelial cells is markedly enhanced in inflammed liver tissue (Fig. 1). The expression of other adhesion molecules, such as cadherin or neural cell adhesion molecule (NCAM) which is known to express on vascular endothelial cells, has not been confirmed on sinusoidal endothelial cells.

The ligands of these adhesion molecules exist primarily on the surface of leukocytes [3], which strongly suggests that the interactions between sinusoidal endothelial cells and leukocytes via adhesion molecules play an important role in the pathogenesis of liver injury. The adhesion pathways between leukocytes and sinusoidal endothelial cells, such as the E-selectin ligand-1 (ESL-1)-E-selectin pathway, P-selectin glycoprotein ligand-1 (PSGL-1)-P-selectin pathway, LFA-1/Mac-1-ICAM-1 pathway, and VLA-4-VCAM-1 pathway, are involved in leukocyte infiltration and hepatocyte injury. Recently, Fas-mediated apoptosis and perforin-mediated injury have been reported to be associated with the pathogenesis of hepatocyte injury in chronic hepatitis due to hepatitis B or hepatitis C virus [10–12]. In these systems, cell-to-cell adhesion is needed, and these adhesion pathways play a crucial role for Fas-mediated apoptosis and perforin-mediated injury.

## Cytokines and Adhesion Molecules

The expression of adhesion molecules on sinusoidal endothelial cells is mediated by several substances such as thrombin, lipopolysaccharide (LPS), and histamine, and various cytokines. E-selectin, ICAM-1, and VCAM-1 are up-regulated by inflammatory cytokines such as TNF-$\alpha$, IL-1, and IFN-$\gamma$ [13]. These cytokines are induced by adjacent Kupffer cells, lymphocytes, sinusoidal endothelial cells, activated platelets

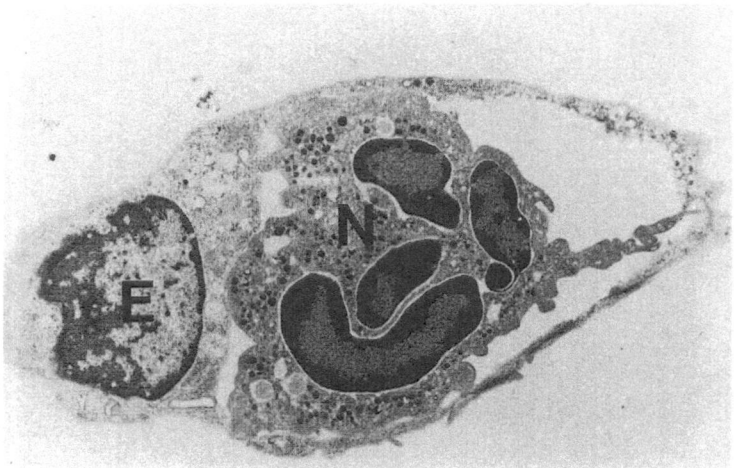

FIG. 2. Transmission electron micrograph showing a neutrophil adhering tightly to a sinusoidal endothelial cell treated with tumor necrosis factor-$\alpha$ (TNF-$\alpha$). Sinusoidal endothelial cells were isolated from male Wistar rats by collagenase perfusion and centrifugal elutriation. After incubation for 24 h on a type-1 collagen-coated dish with William's medium E containing 10% fetal calf serum, these cells were treated with 100 U/ml of TNF-$\alpha$ for 8 h. The culture was then overlaid with neutrophils purified from rat venous blood. After 20 min incubation, the culture was washed three times and fixed with 2% glutaraldehyde for electron microscopy. E, sinusoidal endothelial cell; N, neutrophil. ×8000

that have adhered to damaged sinusoidal endothelial cells, and spleen cells, which probably results in a state that promotes the adhesion of leukocytes to sinusoidal endothelial cells [6, 14–17]. P-selectin is expressed on the surface of Weibel–Palade bodies in vascular endothelial cells and is rapidly induced by histamine and thrombin [18].

In our study of the expression of ICAM-1 in cultured rat sinusoidal endothelial cells, using the immunogold technique and a cytofluorometer, ICAM-1 expression increased in a dose-dependent manner 8 h after either TNF-$\alpha$ or IL-1$\alpha$ stimulation [19]. Kinetics analysis revealed that the expression of ICAM-1 on sinusoidal endothelial cells treated with these cytokines gradually increased from the beginning of stimulation to 24 h [19].

In addition, neutrophils adhered to cultured rat hepatic sinusoidal endothelial cells treated with these cytokines in vitro (Fig. 2), with the number of neutrophils adhering to sinusoidal endothelial cells pretreated with TNF-$\alpha$ for 8 h increasing in a dose-dependent manner. Moreover, the number of neutrophils that adhered to the cells significantly decreased upon incubation with anti-ICAM-1 antibody (Fig. 3).

These findings are similar to those for other vascular endothelial cells and therefore, like vascular endothelial cells, hepatic sinusoidal endothelial cells may be closely involved in inflammation associated with liver disease via surface expression of various adhesion molecules.

FIG. 3. The number of neutrophils adhering to cultured rat sinusoidal endothelial cells treated with tumor necrosis factor-α (*TNF-α*) for 8 h. Following TNF-α treatment, neutrophils were co-cultured with sinusoidal endothelial cells for 20 min. After washing three times, adhered neutrophils were stained with chloroacetate esterase and the number of neutrophils adhering to 200 sinusoidal endothelial cells (SECs) was counted. **$P < 0.01$

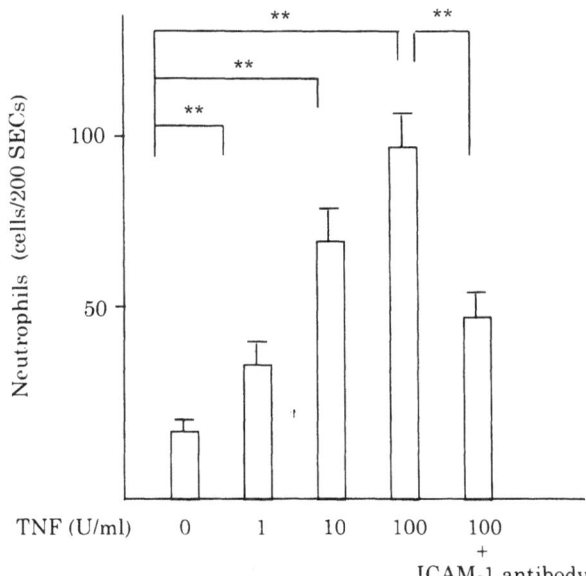

The process of molecular recognition between neutrophils and vascular endothelial cells is considered to proceed through at least three sequential steps, which are mediated by corresponding adhesion molecules and several cytokines [13, 20]. In the first step, which is called "rolling", ESL-1 and PSGL-1 on neutrophils recognize E- and P-selectin on vascular endothelial cells. In the second step, these neutrophils are activated by chemoattractants such as IL-8. In the third step, a firm adhesion is formed in which LFA-1, Mac-1, and VLA-4 on neutrophils bind to ICAM-1 or VCAM-1 on vascular endothelial cells.

In addition, we examined the relationships between the expression of adhesion molecules on sinusoidal endothelial cells and infiltrated neutrophils in the liver, and the plasma levels of TNF and IL-8 in LPS-induced acute liver injury in rats [21]. In that study, plasma TNF peaked at 1 h ($23.3 \pm 11.4$ IU/ml), and IL-8 peaked at 3 h ($343.1 \pm 110.5$ ng/ml) after LPS exposure (2 mg/kg intravenously in 0.2 ml). IL-8, which appeared to be induced in response to the increase in TNF, not only acts as a chemoattractant for neutrophils, but also induces the translocation of Mac-1 from the intercellular storage pool onto the surface of neutrophils [22]. In our previous study [21], and as shown in Fig. 4, the number of neutrophils infiltrating the sinusoids increased after plasma TNF and IL-8 peaked, indicating that these cytokines may participate in the activation of neutrophils and up-regulation of adhesion molecules. Immunohistochemical studies have revealed that the expression of ICAM-1 on sinusoidal endothelial cells and hepatocytes strongly increases from 8 h after LPS exposure, and that both LFA-1 and Mac-1 are expressed on neutrophils that have adhered to sinusoidal endothelial cells (Fig. 5). These data suggest that neutrophil–sinusoidal endothelial cell and neutrophil–hepatocyte interactions via adhesion molecules and related to inflammatory cytokines such as TNF and IL-8 play an important role in the pathogenesis of acute liver injury.

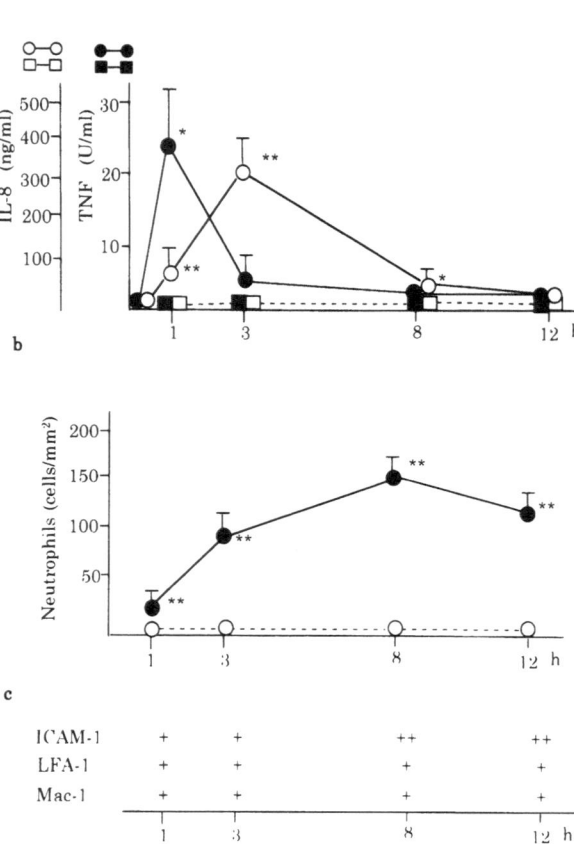

FIG. 4. The relationships among **a** plasma levels of TNF and IL-8, **b** the number of neutrophils in the liver, and **c** the expression of the adhesion molecules on sinusoidal endothelial cells (ICAM-1) and infiltrated neutrophils (LFA-1 and Mac-1) in lipopolysaccharide (LPS)-induced liver injury in rats. Male Wistar rats were administered 2 mg/Kg LPS intravenously. Liver and blood samples were obtained at 1, 3, 8, and 12 h after LPS exposure. Plasma TNF and IL-8 levels were measured using a bioassay and specific ELISA, respectively. The number of neutrophils in the liver was determined by microscopic examination and expressed as cells/mm². Frozen sections of liver fixed in periodate-lysine-paraformaldehyde were immunohistochemically analyzed using specific monoclonal antibodies to LFA-1, Mac-1, and ICAM-1. *Solid line*, LPS exposure group (*n* = 5); *dashed line*, control group (*n* = 5). **P < 0.01 and *P < 0.05 compared with controls

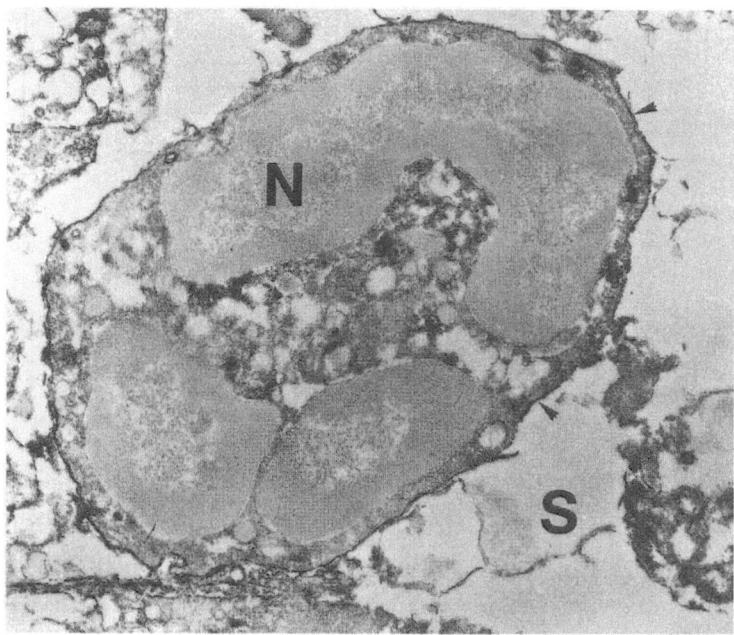

FIG. 5. Electron micrograph showing immunoreactive products for Mac-1 antibody on the surface of neutrophils (*arrowheads*) adhered to a degenerated sinusoidal endothelial cell after lipopolysaccharide treatment. *S*, sinusoid; *N*, neutrophil. ×14 000

## Soluble Form of Adhesion Molecules

Circulating soluble forms of adhesion molecules have been detected in several conditions, including inflammatory diseases and malignant diseases [23, 24]. In patients with chronic liver diseases, the serum levels of the soluble forms of ICAM-1 (sICAM-1), sVCAM-1, and sLFA-3 are elevated, with the sICAM-1 level correlating with serum asparate aminotransferase levels, which suggests that the serum sICAM-1 level is indicative of hepatocellular damage [25]. However, immunohistochemical studies have demonstrated the surface expression of ICAM-1, VCAM-1, and LFA-3 on sinusoidal lining cells as well as on hepatocytes in chronic hepatitis [26], and thus the source of these soluble forms of adhesion molecules in the sera of chronic liver disease may be nonparenchymal cells, including sinusoidal endothelial cells.

In one of our previous studies, the mean serum levels of sICAM-1 and sVCAM-1 were significantly higher in patients with chronic viral hepatitis (1213.9 ± 168.7 ng/ml and 1006.3 ± 103.9 ng/ml, respectively) than in the healthy controls (315.9 ± 93.5 ng/ml and 418.0 ± 70.2 ng/ml, respectively). In patients with acute viral hepatitis, the mean serum levels of these molecules generally increased (4824.6 ± 572.2 ng/ml

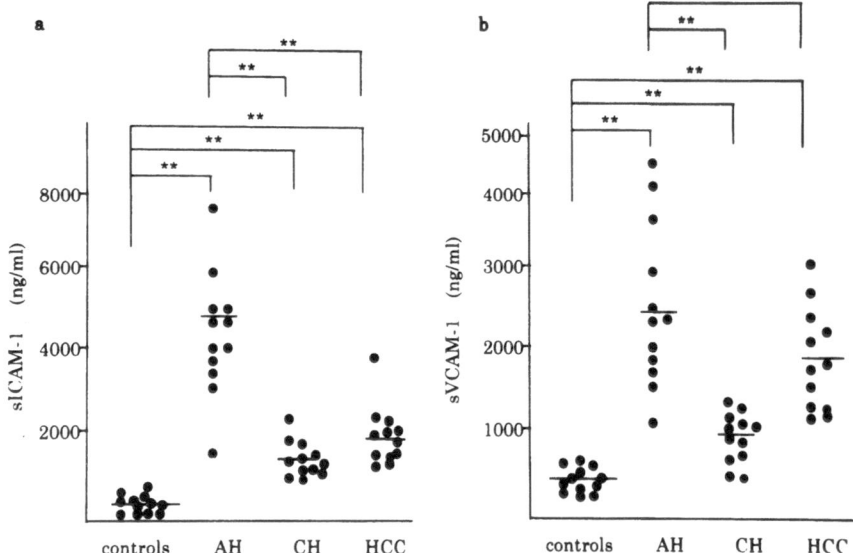

FIG. 6. Serum concentration of **a** sICAM-1 and **b** sVCAM-1 in normal subjects ($n = 12$), and in patients with acute hepatitis (*AH*, $n = 12$), chronic hepatitis (*CH*, $n = 12$), and hepatocellular carcinoma (*HCC*, $n = 12$). \*\**P* < 0.01

and 2374.6 ± 328.6 ng/ml, respectively), as shown in Fig. 6a and 6b, respectively. In addition, the serum concentration of these molecules was elevated in patients with hepatocellular carcinoma, which was similar to results in another report [27]. However, circulating sICAM-1 in HCC patients is thought to be shaded from HCC cells but not from sinusoidal endothelial cells. Naturally, there is the possibility that the levels of the soluble forms of adhesion molecules such as sE-, sP-selectin, and sCD31 are elevated in sera of various liver diseases, but this has yet to be determined.

The role of the soluble forms of adhesion molecules in liver disease remains unclear. However, these soluble forms of adhesion molecules are believed to suppress cell-to-cell adhesion and inhibit the surplus host's immune reaction by binding with their ligands [28]. Indeed, sP-selectin and sE-selectin chimeras have been found to be benefical effects in experimental models [29, 30].

In conclusion, adhesion molecules play a key role in many liver diseases, and sinusoidal endothelial cells may be highly involved in liver injury via expression of various adhesion molecules regulated by inflammatory cytokines.

## References

1. Frenett PS, Wagner DD (1996) Adhesion molecules. New Engl J Med 334:1526–1529
2. Ruoslahti E, Obrink B (1996) Common principles in cell adhesion. Exp Cell Res 227:1–11
3. Springer TA (1990) Adhesion receptor of the immune system. Nature 346:425–434

4. Pober JS, Gimbrone MA Jr, Lagierre LA, et al. (1986) Overlapping patterns of activation of human endothelial cells by interleukin-1, tumor necrosis factor and immune interferon. J Immunol 137:1893–1896
5. Rieder H, Meyer zum Buschenfelde K-H, Ramadori G (1992) Functional spectrum of sinusoidal endothelial liver cells—filtration, endosytosis, synthetic capacities and intercellular communication. J Hepatol 15:237–250
6. Stephen WC, Pauline DT, Daniel GR, et al. (1991) In vivo biologic and immunohistochemical analysis of interleukin 1 alpha, beta and tumor necrosis factor during experimental endotoxemia-kinetics, Kupffer cell expression, and gulcocorticoid effects. Am J Pathol 138:395–402
7. Volpes R, van den Oord JJ, Desmet VJ (1992) Vascular adhesion molecules in acute and chronic liver inflammation. Hepatology 15:269–275
8. Volpes R, van den Oord JJ, Desmet VJ (1991) Distribution of the VLA family of integrins in normal and pathological human liver tissues. Gastroenterology 101:200–206
9. Steinhoff G, Behrend M, Schrader B, et al. (1993) Expression patterns of leukocyte adhesion ligand molecules on human liver endothelia—lack of ELAM-1 and CD62 inducibility on sinusoidal endothelia and distinct distribution of VCAM-1, ICAM-1, ICAM-2 and LFA-3. Am J Pathol 142:481–488
10. Ando K, Hiroishi K, Kaneko T, et al. (1997) Perforin, Fas/Fas ligand, and TNF-pathway as specific and bystander killing mechanisms of hepatitis C virus-specific human CTL. J Immunol 158:5283–5291
11. Hiramatsu N, Hayashi N, Katayama K, et al. (1994) Immunohistochemical detection of Fas antigen in liver tissue of patients with chronic hepatitis C. Hepatology 19:1354–1359
12. Mochizuki K, Hayashi N, Hiramatsu N, et al. (1996) Fas antigen expression in liver tissues of patients with chronic hepatitis B. J Hepatol 24:1–7
13. Bucher EC (1991) Leukocyte–endothelial cell recognition—three (or more) steps to specificity and diversity. Cell 67:1033–1036
14. Khoruts A, Stahnke L, McClain CJ, et al. (1991) Circulating tumor necrosis factor, interleukin-1 and interleukin-6 concentrations in chronic alcoholic patients. Hepatology 13:267–276
15. Mizoguchi Y, Ichikawa Y, Kamada N, et al. (1990) Effects of arachidonic acid metabolites and platelet-activating factor (PAF) on interleukin-1 synthesis from mouse hepatic sinusoidal endothelium. Acta Hepatol Jpn 31:139–145
16. Chojkier M, Fierer J (1985) D-galactosamine hepatotoxin is associated with endotoxin sensitivity and mediated by lymphoreticular cells in mice. Gastroenterology 88:115–121
17. Hawrglowicz CM, Howells GL, Feldmann M (1991) Platelet-derived interleukin-1 induces human adhesion molecule expression and cytokine production. J Exp Med 174:785–790
18. McEver RP, Beckstead JH, Moore KL, et al. (1989) GMP-140, a platelet alpha-granule membrane protein, is also synthesized by vascular endothelial cells and is localized in Weibel–Palade bodies. J Clin Invest 84:92–99
19. Ohira H, Ueno T, Shakado S, et al. (1994) Cultured rat hepatic sinusoidal endothelial cells express intercellular adhesion molecule-1 (ICAM-1) by tumor necrosis factor-$\alpha$ or interleukin-1$\alpha$ stimulation. J Hepatol 20:729–734
20. Carlos TM, Harian JM (1994) Leukocyte–endothelial adhesion molecules. Blood 84:2068–2101
21. Ohira H, Ueno T, Torimura T, et al. (1995) Leukocyte adhesion molecules in the liver and plasma cytokine levels in endotoxin-induced rat liver injury. Scand J Gastroenterol 30:1027–1035
22. Sengelvo H, Kjeldsen L, Diamond MS, et al. (1993) Subcellular localization and dynamics of Mac-1 (alpha m beta 2) in human neutrophils. J Clin Invest 92:1467–1476

23. Furukawa S, Imai K, Matsubara T, et al. (1992) Increased levels of circulating ICAM-1 in Kawasaki disease. Arthritis Rheum 35:672–677
24. Harning R, Mainolfi E, Bystryn J-C, et al. (1991) Serum levels of circulating intercellular adhesion molecule 1 in human malignant melanoma. Cancer Res 51:5003–5005
25. Zöhrens G, Armbrust T, Pirzer U, et al. (1992) Intercellular adhesion molecule-1 concentration in sera of patients with acute and chronic liver disease: Relationship to disease activity and cirrhosis. Hepatology 18:798–802
26. Autsschbach F, Meuer SC, Moebius U, et al. (1991) Hepatocellular expression of lymphocyte function-associated antigen 3 in chronic hepatitis. Hepatology 14:223–230
27. Shimizu Y, Minemura M, Tsukishiro T, et al. (1995) Serum concentration of intercellular adhesion molecule-1 in patients with hepatocellular carcinoma is a marker of the disease progression and prognosis. Hepatology 22:525–531
28. Becker JC, Termeer C, Schmit RE, et al. (1993) Soluble intercellular adhesion molecule-1 inhibits MHC-restricted specific T cell/tumor interaction. J Immunol 151:385–392
29. Mulligan MS, Watoson SR, Fennie C, et al. (1993) Protective effects of selectin chimerasin neutrophil-mediated lung injury. J Immunol 151:6410–6417
30. Watson SR, Fennie C, Lasky LA (1991) Neutrophil influx into an inflammatory site inhibited by a soluble homing receptor ligand. Nature 349:164–167

# The Role of Hepatic Sinusoidal Cells in the Development of Massive Liver Necrosis

SATOSHI MOCHIDA and KENJI FUJIWARA

*Summary.* Massive liver necrosis develops as a result of microcirculatory disturbance due to fibrin deposition in the hepatic sinusoids through the derangement of blood coagulation equilibrium. Such mechanisms might be involved in the development of fulminant viral hepatitis as well as primary graft nonfunction following orthotopic liver transplantation. In rat models of massive liver necrosis, fibrin deposition occurred in association with endothelial cell injury in the hepatic sinusoids. Such endothelial cell injury was caused by hepatic stellate cell damage or activation of Kupffer cells and hepatic macrophages. Activated Kupffer cells and hepatic macrophages produced sinusoidal fibrin deposition in two different ways. When hepatic macrophages were activated through a cytokine network of interleukin (IL)-18, interferon (IFN)-$\gamma$, and IL-2, they expressed increased CD14, a receptor for lipopolysaccharide and its binding protein complex, and destroyed sinusoidal endothelial cells by releasing cytotoxic mediators such as tumor necrosis factor (TNF)-$\alpha$ and superoxide anions following endotoxin stimulation. In contrast, Kupffer cells activated by overloading of gut-derived substances showed marked expression of tissue factor, an initiator of the blood coagulation cascade. Although such Kupffer cells expressed less CD14 and cytotoxic mediators, they provoked sinusoidal fibrin deposition following endotoxin stimulation. The hepatic sinusoids have the unique characteristic that endothelial cells express minimal tissue factor pathway inhibitor and thrombomodulin compared with those in other organs. This may contribute to the development of sinusoidal fibrin deposition in both models. Thus, the supplementation with both factors would be a therapeutic strategy for massive liver necrosis associated with sinusoidal fibrin deposition. Also, selective bowel decontamination to inhibit bacterial translocation into the portal blood would be a promising candidate.

*Key words.* Endotoxin, Kupffer cells, Sinusoidal endothelial cells, Sinusoidal fibrin deposition, Orthotopic liver transplantation

Third Department of Internal Medicine, Saitama Medical School, 38 Morohongo, Moroyama-cho, Iruma-gun, Saitama 350-0495, Japan

# Introduction

It is accepted that liver necrosis develops in viral hepatitis during the process of viral eradication from hepatocytes by cytotoxic T lymphocytes (CTL) as a result of apoptosis through Fas and Fas–ligand systems [1]. Such mechanisms, however, seem less likely in the development of massive liver necrosis in fulminant viral hepatitis, since the CTLs infiltrating into the liver are too few to injure a large number of hepatocytes at the same time. Rake et al. [2] demonstrated that fibrin deposition exists in the hepatic sinusoids of patients with fulminant viral hepatitis. Microcirculatory disturbance due to sinusoidal fibrin deposition might contribute to the development of fulminant viral hepatitis. This postulation was strengthened by our clinical trial using antithrombin III concentrate, in which survival periods in patients with fulminant viral hepatitis were significantly improved with attenuation of blood hypercoagulopathy by the therapy [3, 4].

Primary graft nonfunction is still a critical complication following orthotopic liver transplantation using cadaveric liver as the transplant [5], the cause of which is unclear. Patients with this complication take a clinical course similar to that for fulminant viral hepatitis with massive liver necrosis [6]. Blood hypercoagulability has been suggested to occur immediately after blood reflow of the graft in patients undergoing orthotopic liver transplantation because of increased plasma concentration of thrombin–antithrombin III complex (TAT) [7, 8]. Experimentally, endothelial cell damage in the hepatic sinusoids has been observed in cold preserved liver [9]. Thus, microcirculatory disturbance due to sinusoidal fibrin deposition might develop following orthotopic liver transplantation and cause primary graft nonfunction.

In this chapter, the mechanisms of sinusoidal fibrin deposition are presented on the basis of our experimental results, especially focusing on blood coagulation equilibrium in the hepatic sinusoids. Also, novel anticoagulant therapies for the prevention of fulminant viral hepatitis as well as primary graft nonfunction following orthotopic liver transplantation are proposed.

# Blood Coagulation Equilibrium in the Hepatic Sinusoids

Blood coagulation cascade is initiated by a complex of tissue factor and activated coagulation factor VII (VIIa) through activation of coagulation factor IX or X on membrane phospholipid bilayers [10]. Activated monocytes and macrophages produce tissue factor abundantly [11–13]. In the hepatic sinusoids, activated Kuppfer cells can similarly become thrombogenic [14, 15]. On the other hand, blood coagulation is suppressed by a variety of anticoagulant factors expressed on endothelial cells [16]. Tissue factor pathway inhibitor (TFPI) and thrombomodulin are considered to be the most important anticoagulants acting on the upper and lower streams of the blood coagulation cascade. TFPI inhibits catalytic activity of the tissue factor and factor VIIa complex on factor IX or X in a two-step feedback reaction with the participation of the resultant activated factor IX or X [17, 18], while thrombomodulin not only inactivates thrombin activity, but its complex with thrombin can also increase antithrombogenic activity on endothelial cells through the activation of protein C [16].

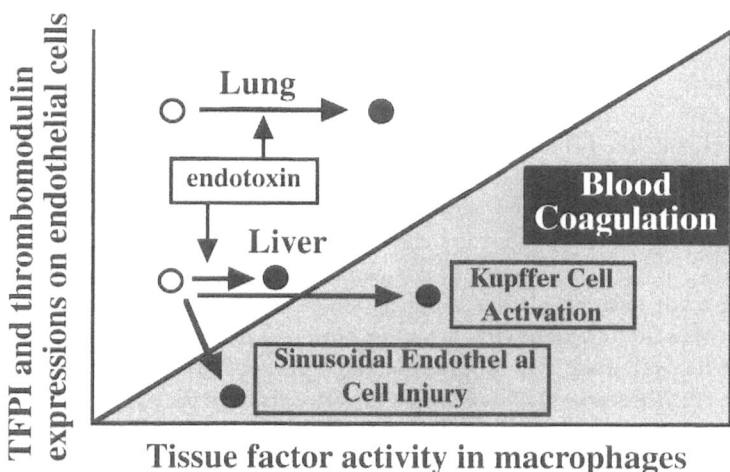

FIG. 1. Blood coagulation equilibrium in peripheral vessels TFPI, tissue factor pathway inhibitor

The hepatic sinusoid is a unique microcirculation system in blood coagulatory regulation as well as in structure. The endothelial cells express minimal TFPI and thrombomodulin compared with those in the peripheral vessels in other organs [14, 15, 18]. In normal rats, blood coagulation equilibrium may be maintained in the hepatic sinusoids despite such decreased antithrombogenic activity in endothelial cells, since the increase in tissue factor activity following endotoxin stimulation is less in Kupffer cells compared with macrophages from other organs [15]. However, blood coagulation equilibrium might easily be deranged in the hepatic sinusoids when Kupffer cells and hepatic macrophages are activated to express increased tissue factor (Fig. 1).

## Sinusoidal Fibrin Deposition as a Cause of Massive Liver Necrosis

Massive liver necrosis develops in rats given carbon tetrachloride ($CCl_4$) or dimethylnitrosamine (DMN). Although prothrombin time prolongation was similar in both groups, plasma levels of TAT and soluble fibrin monomar complex were significantly higher in DMN-treated rats than in $CCl_4$-treated rats [19]. Electron microscopic examination revealed that fibrin deposition was present in the hepatic sinusoids as well as in the necrotic areas in DMN-treated rats, but only in the necrotic areas in $CCl_4$-treated rats [19]. Sinusoidal endothelial cell injury was observed only in DMN-treated rats [19]. Moreover, intravenous infusion of antithrombin III concentrate attenuated liver injury and blood coagulation disorders in a dose-related manner in DMN-treated rats but not in $CCl_4$-treated rats, although plasma antithrombin III activity was similarly increased in both groups [19]. These results suggested that fibrin deposition in the necrotic areas occurred as a result of massive liver necrosis, whereas fibrin deposition in the hepatic sinusoids developed in association with endothelial cell injury and caused microcirculatory disturbance leading to massive liver necrosis.

On electron microscopic examination of the liver, performed serially in DMN-treated rats, the initial abnormal finding was apoptosis of hepatic stellate cells which reinforce sinusoidal endothelial cells as pericytes [20]. DMN also induced apoptosis of hepatic stellate cells in primary culture (unpublished data). Thus, in the DMN model, it is likely that apoptosis of hepatic stellate cells produced sinusoidal endothelial cell destruction leading to the onset of massive liver necrosis through microcirculatory disturbance due to sinusoidal fibrin deposition.

In patients with fulminant viral hepatitis, however, electron microscopy shows no hepatic stellate cell damage [21], while marked injuries of sinusoidal endothelial cells are observed [22]. Also, peripheral mononuclear cells have been reported to be activated in patients with fulminant viral hepatitis [23, 24]. We found that serum tumor nacrosis factor (TNF)-$\alpha$ concentration was considerably increased in some patients with fulminant viral hepatitis [25].

## Sinusoidal Fibrin Deposition in Endotoxin-Induced Liver Injury

When rats received heat-killed *Propionibacterium ances* (*P. acnes: Corynebacterium parvum*) intravenously, a marked infiltration of macrophages developed, with granuloma formation in the liver 7 days later [26, 27]. In these rats, massive liver necrosis was induced by an injection of endotoxin at a dose which is nontoxic to normal rats [26, 27]. Similar necrosis was also provoked by endotoxin administration in rats which underwent 70% hepatectomy 48 h earlies [28, 29]. In both models, electron microscopy showed endothelial cell destruction and fibrin deposition in the hepatic sinusoids preceding hepatocyte injury [27, 28]. Antithrombin III concentrate infused concomitantly with endotoxin attenuated both liver injuries [27, 28], suggesting that sinusoidal fibrin deposition contributed to massive liver necrosis through microcirculatory disturbance.

Serum TNF-$\alpha$ concentration was markedly increased following endotoxin administration in rats pretreated with heat-killed *P. acnes* [30]. Liver perfusion with nitro-blue tetrazolium (NBT) and phorbol 12-myristate 13-acetate (PMA) can determine in situ the ability of Kupffer cells and hepatic macrophages to produce superoxide anions by the extent of deposition of formazan converted from NBT [31, 32]. Formazan deposition was found extensively in hepatic macrophages throughout the liver of *P. acnes*-treated rats [32] and in Kupffer cells in 70% hepatectomized rats [28]. In both cases, pretreatment with gum arabic, which can block macrophage activation [33], reduced the extent of formazan deposition with attenuation of liver injuries [28, 34]. In contrast, eradication of circulating neutrophils by polyclonal antibody did not affect the extent of either of these liver injuries [34, 35]. It seems likely that activated Kupffer cells and hepatic macrophages, but not neutrophils, provoked fibrin deposition and endothelial cell injury in the hepatic sinusoids following endotoxin stimulation in the *P. acnes* and partial hepatectomy animals.

# Mechanisms of Sinusoidal Fibrin Deposition Induced by Activated Kupffer Cells and Hepatic Macrophages

Alanine aminotransferase (ALT) activity is exclusively present in hepatocytes, while purine nucleoside phosphorylase (PNP) activity exists in hepatocytes as well as in sinusoidal cells including endothelial cells (30). Considering the fact that the ratio of ALT activity to PNP activity is about 5:1 in isolated hepatocytes [4], the extent of sinusoidal cell injury can be evaluated by measuring both PNP and ALT activities in serum and liver perfusate [30, 36]. To clarify the cells targeted by activated Kupffer cells and hepatic macrophages, an ex vivo liver perfusion system with solutions containing no plasma would be useful, because sinusoidal fibrin deposition could not occur. The liver was perfused with Dulbecco's modified Eagle medium (DMEM) containing heat-inactivated fetal calf serum (FCS) as well as endotoxin to provoke excitation of Kupffer cells and hepatic macrophages [37]. The flow rate was maintained at 1.4 ml/min/g liver, the physiological flow rate in normal rat liver [36], in order to avoid liver cell injury due to increased perfusion pressure in the hepatic sinusoids.

When *P. acnes*-treated rats received endotoxin, the serum activities of PNP and ALT were increased following a transient peak of TNF-$\alpha$ activity [30]. Administration of antiserum against TNF-$\alpha$ as well as superoxide dismutase (SOD) significantly attenuated this liver injury [27, 38], suggesting that TNF-$\alpha$ and superoxide anions released from activated hepatic macrophages were responsible for the development of massive liver necrosis. When the liver of *P. acnes*-treated rats was perfused with endotoxin, PNP activity was similarly increased in the perfusate, but ALT activity was unchanged [30]. In these rats, electron microscopy showed sinusoidal endothelial cell injury [30]. Moreover, the increase in PNP activity in the perfusate was significantly reduced by pretreatment of the rats with gadolinium chloride, which can eradicate activated hepatic macrophages [30]. Thus, activated macrophages in the *P. acnes* model were shown to destroy endothelial cells through cytotoxic mediators and provoke fibrin deposition in the hepatic sinusoids (Figs. 1 and 2). It is concluded that hepatocyte injury developed as a result of microcirculatory disturbance due to sinusoidal fibrin deposition (Fig. 2).

In the partial hepatectomy model, serum PNP and ALT activities were similarly increased [35, 39]. However, when 70% resected rat liver was perfused with DMEM with no addition of endotoxin, both PNP and ALT activities were increased slightly in the liver perfusate. Sinusoidal endothelial cells as well as hepatocytes might be more susceptible to low flow hypoxia in 70% resected rat liver compared with *P. acnes*-treated rat liver. However, both PNP and ALT activities were unchanged in the perfusate when the liver was perfused with endotoxin [35, 39], indicating that liver cell injury was not provoked by activated Kupffer cells after endotoxin stimulation. Thus, activated Kupffer cells seemed to produce sinusoidal fibrin deposition in the partial hepatectomy model through different mechanisms. Sinusodial endothelial cells as well as hepatocyes may be injured in vivo as a result of microcirculatory disturbance due to sinusoidal fibrin deposition.

Tissue factor activity was measured in Kupffer cells isolated from 70% hepatectomized rats and cultured in the presence or absence of endotoxin. The activ-

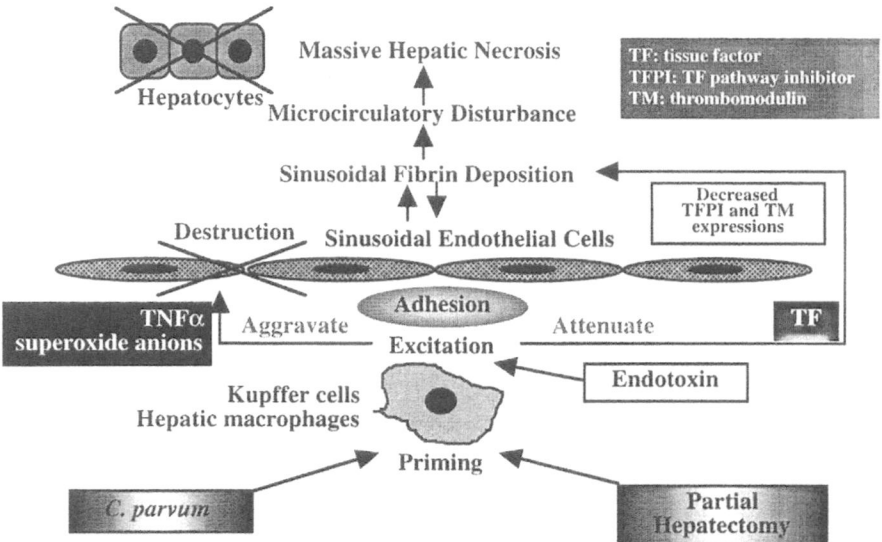

FIG. 2. Mechanisms of massive liver necrosis induced by endotoxin in heat-killed *Propionibacterium acnes*-treated and 70% hepatectomized rats

ity was much higher in 70% hepatectomized rats than in normal rats irrespective of the presence of endotoxin [15, 35, 39]. Coagulopathy in the hepatic sinusoids following endotoxin administration would easily occur in the partial hepatectomized rats. When recombinant human TFPI was given to these rats concomitantly with endotoxin, liver injury and blood coagulation disorders were significantly attenuated compared with the controls [35, 39]. Similar results were also obtained when recombinant human thrombomodulin was given [35, 39]. We conclude that blood coagulation equilibrium in the hepatic sinusoids is disturbed by increased tissue factor activity in activated Kupffer cells, and this disturbance provokes fibrin deposition (Fig. 2). The unique characteristic of the hepatic sinusoids that endothelial cells express minimal TFPI and thrombomodulin could also be a contributing factor (Fig. 1).

## Activation Mechanisms of Kupffer Cells and Hepatic Macrophages

Activated Kupffer cells in the partial hepatectomy model produced fewer cytotoxic mediators such as superoxide anions and TNF-$\alpha$ in response to endotoxin than activated hepatic macrophages in the *P. acnes* model [35], but tissue factor activity was reversed in both models [35, 39]. Both cells can release large amounts of superoxide anions after stimulation with PMA [28, 32]. Hepatic mRNA expression of CD14, a receptor for lipopolysaccharide and its binding protein complex, was markedly increased in *P. acnes*-treated rat liver compared with nomral liver, but decreased

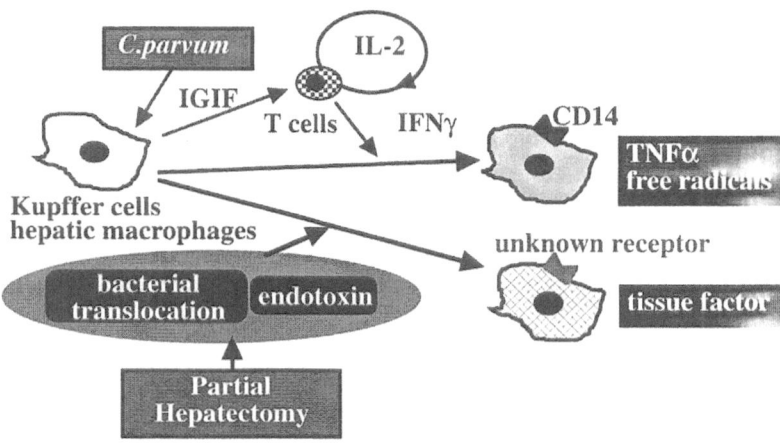

FIG. 3. Activation mechanisms of Kupffer cells and hepatic Macrophages in heat-killed *Propionibacterium acnes*-treated and 70% hepatectomized rats

in 70% resected rat liver [40]. Other endotoxin receptors than CD14 might be expressed on activated Kupffer cells in 70% hepatectomized rats in intracellular signal transduction for inducing tissue factor.

In *P. acnes*-treated rats, hepatic macrophages were activated through a cytokine network of interleukin (IL)-18 (formerly called interferon (IFN)-$\gamma$ inducing factor: IGIF), IFN-$\gamma$ and IL-2 [40, 41], while this network did not operate during the activation process of Kupffer cells in 70% hepatectomized rats [40]. The overloading of gut-derived substances seemed to be responsible for Kupffer cell activation in 70% hepatectomized rats, since oral administration of polymyxin B sulfate, an unabsorbable antibiotic which can inactivate lipopolysaccharide, reduced Kupffer cell activation and attenuated liver injury following endotoxin administration [42]. Such a difference in activation mechanisms between Kupffer cells and hepatic macrophages might cause functional differences in both cells (Fig. 3).

## Adhesion Molecules and Sinusoidal Fibrin Deposition

Because of the difference in function between activated hepatic macrophages in *P. acnes*-treated rats and Kupffer cells in partially hepatectomized rats, the interaction of macrophages with endothelial cells would be different in both models. Hepatic expressions of intercellular adhesion molecule-1 (ICAM-1) and lymphocyte function-associate antigen-1$\alpha$ (LFA-1$\alpha$) were examined immunohistochemically in *P. acnes*-treated and 70% hepatectomized rats. In both groups, light microscopy showed that the expressions of ICAM-1 and LFA-1$\alpha$ along the hepatic sinusoids were increased compared with those of normal rats [34]. When the rats received endotoxin, both expressions became more prominent preceding the development of massive liver necrosis. The cells expressing ICAM-1 and LFA-1$\alpha$ were electron microscopically identified as endothelial cells and Kupffer cells/macrophages, respectively [34].

ICAM-1 expression was not found on the surface of hepatocytes in either model [34]. Although the up-regulation of ICAM-1 expression after cytokine stimulation was reported to occur in hepatocytes and sinusoidal endothelial cells in vitro [43], similar results were not seen in hepatocytes in vivo [44, 45]. ICAM-1 expression developed on the surface of hepatocytes due to the dissociation of cell-to-cell contact in rats following liver perfusion with Hank's balanced salt solution at a threefold physiological flow rate or with collagenase or ethyleneglycoltelsaacetic acid (EGTA) [44]. Also, ICAM-1 expression was found on degenerative hepatocytes in CCl$_4$-intoxicated rats with no increase in the serum concentration of TNF-$\alpha$ [45]. ICAM-1 expression may develop on the surface of in vivo hepatocytes only as a result of cell injury [44, 45].

As mentioned above, activated Kupffer cells and hepatic macrophages may adhere to sinusoidal endothelial cells, but not to hepatocytes, through ICAM-1 and LFA-1$\alpha$ before the development of massive liver necrosis in the P. acnes and partial hepatectomy models. When monoclonal antibodies against rat-ICAM-1 [46] and LFA-1$\alpha$ [47] were administered to rats in the P. acnes model, the extent of liver injury was significantly attenuated without changes in macrophage infiltration into the liver or in the stimulatory state of macrophages [34]. The adhesion of hepatic macrophages to sinusoidal endothelial cells might increase the concentration of cytotoxic mediators on the surface and destroy sinusoidal endothelial cells (Fig. 2). Activated hepatic macrophages cannot destroy hepatocytes directly in the P. acnes model [30] because of less contact between the cells through these adhesion molecules. In contrast, a similar administration of both antibodies significantly aggravated the extent of liver injury in the partial hepatectomy model [35]. The adhesion between activated Kuppffer cells and sinusoidal endothelial cells may protect against blood coagulation imbalance in the hepatic sinusoids in the presence of minimal cytotoxic mediators (Fig 2), probably because endothelial cells are the only cells that have antithrombogenic activity in the hepatic sinusoids even though TFPI and thrombomodulin expressions are decreased.

# Mechanisms of Liver Injury Following Orthotopic Liver Transplantation

The liver from cadaveric donors is inevitably exposed to both warm and cold ischemia during orthotopic liver transplantation, suggesting that primary graft nonfunction may develop as a result of reperfusion injury of the liver following warm or cold ischemia. When rat liver was perfused with Eagle's MEM solution following warm and cold ischemia, both PNP and ALT activities were increased in the perfusate depending on the duration of ischemia [36]. The ratio of ALT activity to PNP activity in the perfusate after warm ischemia was very similar to that in isolated hepatocytes, and was significantly higher than that in the perfusate after cold ischemia [36], suggesting that hepatocytes were mainly injured in rat liver during reperfusion following warm ischemia, but cells injured after cold ischemia were sinusoidal endothelial cells. The stimulation stage of Kupffer cells evaluated in situ by formazan deposition following liver perfusion with NBT and PMA was elevated after cold ischemia for longer than 1h, but not after warm ischemia [36]. In conrast, the degree of oxidative stress in hepatocytes assessed by formazan deposition following liver perfusion with NBT alone [48] was greater after warm ischemia than after cold ischemia [36]. Blood coagulation equilibrium in the hepatic sinusoids regulated by Kupffer cells and endothelial cells may be disturbed during liver reperfusion following cold ischemia, but not following warm ischemia.

When rat livers were preserved at 1°C in University of Wisconisn (UW) solution, sinusoidal endothelial cells remained almost intact for 12 h [49]. The disruption of the cells which developed after 12 h and became prominet at 18 h [49]. Northern blot analysis revealed that mRNA expression of vascular endothelial growth factor (VEGF) had increased in the liver 12 h after cold preservation compared with that in normal liver, while mRNA expression of *KDR/flk-1*, a receptor for VEGF, had markedly decreased (unpublished data). VEGF is not only a growth factor which can induce proliferation of sinusoidal endothelial cells [50, 51], but also a factor which is essential for the maintenance of cell viability [50]. Sinusoidal endothelial cells might be injured as a result of the disappearance of intracellular signal transduction through VEGF receptors in cold-preserved liver. Also, rat liver preserved in could UW solution showed the detachment of endhothelial cells into the sinusoidal lumen at 18 h or later [49]. This detachment was accompanied by the degeneration of adjacent hepatic stellate cells, and both cell abnormalities progressed in parallel to each other in degree [49], suggesting that hepatic stellate cell damage may cause endothelial cell detachment.

Anticoagulant function was decreased in the hepatic sinusoids of cold-preserved liver compared with those of normal liver [14] due to the disruption and detachment of sinusoidal endothelial cells [49]. On the other hand, Kupffer cells we activated to express tissue factor in recipient rats when cold-preserved liver was orthotopically transplanted [14]. The increase of tissue factor in Kupffer cells was caused by the

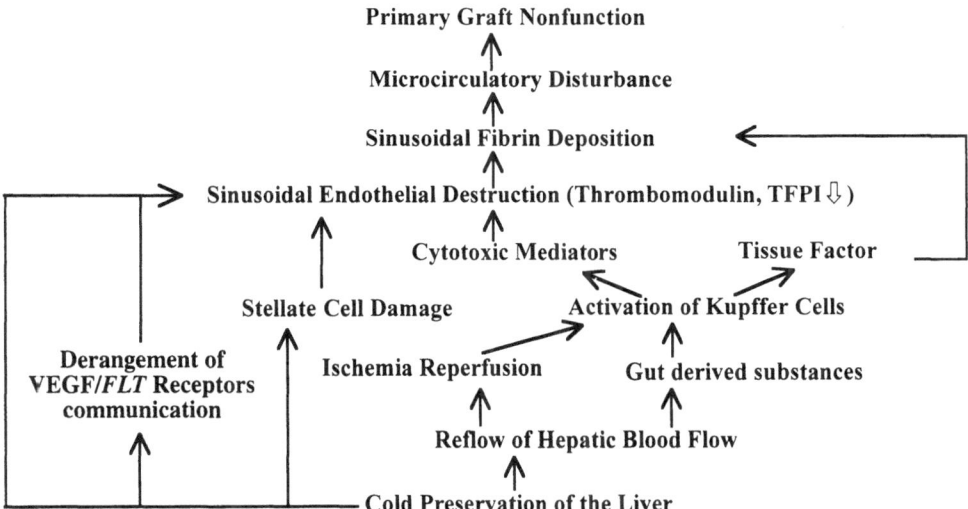

FIG. 4. Possible mechanisms of primary graft nonfunction following orthotopic liver transplantation

overloading of gut-derived substances as well as reoxygenation following hypoxia [14, 52, 53]. In these rats, electron microscopy showed sinusoidal fibrin deposition in the liver 5 h after orthotopic liver transplantation [54, 55]. Moreover, intravenous administration of antithrombin III concentrate immediately and 12 h after the operation significantly attenuated later liver injury and blood coagulation disorders [55]. It is likely that the derangement of blood coagulation equilibrium in the hepatic sinusoids regulated by Kupffer cells and sinusoidal endothelial cells produced fibrin deposition and liver necrosis in such lvier (Fig. 4).

## Treatment of Sinusoidal Fibrin Deposition

Antithrombin III concentrate is effective for liver injury associated with sinusoidal fibrin deposition [19, 27, 28]. However, its use in surgical patients, especially following liver transplantation, is not desirable, because bleeding from the operative wound would be an inevitable adverse effect. A device for increasing anticoagulant activity or decreasing thrombogenic activity exclusively in the hepatic sinusoids is required.

In patients undergoing orthotopic liver transplantation, intestinal wall congestion developing during the ahepatic phase of the operation may induce bacterial translocation from the gut to the portal blood after portal blood reflow. As already mentioned, the overloading of gut-derived substances was responsible for the increase of tissue factor activity in Kupffer cells in rats [14, 52]. When rats received oral administration of polymyxin B sulfate for 7 days, bacterial flora was significantly altered in the gut: Enterobacteriaceae diminished and anaerobes such as *Bifidobacterium* and *Lactobacillus* increased in number compared with those in the control rats [53]. Also, such treatment significantly reduced endotoxin concentration in the portal blood 30 min after blood reflow following portal vein occlusion [53]. When orthotopic liver transplantation was performed in recipient rats pretreated with polymyxin B sulfate, the increase in tissue factor activity in Kupffer cells was markedly attenuated compared with that in the controls [53]. In these recipients, the extent of liver necrosis was also attenuated at 24 h after the operation [53]. Selective bowel decontamination of recipients with polymyxin B sulfate could be a candidate for an anticoagulant therapy exclusively for the hepatic sinusoids.

Another approach is an anticoagulant therapy using recombinant human TFPI. When recombinant human TFPI was intravenously injected into rats, it disappeared rapidly from the circulation, but was detected on the surface of sinusoidal endothelial cells and microvilli of hepatocyets in the space of Disse [18]. In these rats, the TFPI reappeared in the circulation after an intravenous injection of heparin sodium with reduced immunohistochemical staining of the TFPI along the hepatic sinusoids [18]. Thus, exogenous TFPI can increase anticoagulant activity on the hepatic sinusoidal walls by binding to heparinoids on the cell surface. TFPI may act effectively even in the hepatic sinusoids, where endothelial cells are significantly destroyed following cold preservation of the liver, without inducing bleeding from the operative wound [56].

We propose two anticoagulant therapies for liver injury in patients undergoing orthotopic liver transplantation: (1) selective bowel decontamination of the recipient with polymyxin B sulfate before the operation; (2) anticoagulant therapy targeting the hepatic sinusoidal walls with recombinant human TFPI after the operation.

## References

1. Chisari FV (1995) Hepatitis B virus in transgenic mice: Insights into the virus and the disease. Hepatology 22:1316–1325
2. Rake MO, Fluite PT, Pannell G, et al. (1970) Intravascular coagulation in acute hepatic necrosis. Lancet 1970:533–537
3. Fujiwara K, Okita K, Akamatsu K, et al. (1988) Antithrombin III concentrate in the treatment of fulminant hepatic failure. Gastroenterol Jpn 23:423–427
4. Tomiya T, Fujiwara K (1989) Inhibition of thrombin generation in fulminant hepatic failure by treatment of antithrombin III. Biomed Prog 3:39–40
5. Quiroga J, Colina I, Demetris AJ, et al. (1991) Cause and timing of first allograft failure in orthotopic liver transplantation: A study of 177 consecutive patients. Hepatology 14:1054–1062
6. Maddrey WC, Van Thiel DH (1988) Liver transplantation: An overview. Hepatology 8:948–959
7. Harper PL, Luddington RJ, Jennings I, et al. (1989) Coagulation changes following hepatic revascularization during liver transplantation. Transplantation 48:603–607
8. Barker CM, Metselaar HJ, Gomes MJ, et al. (1993) Intravascular coagulation in liver transplantation: Is it present or not? A comparison between orthotopic and heteroptopic liver transplantation. Thromb Haemostas 69:25–28
9. Caldwell-Kenkel JC, Currin RT, Tanaka Y, et al. (1991) Kupffer cell activation and endothelial cell damage after storage of rat liver. Hepatology 13:83–95
10. Nemerson Y (1988) Tissue factor and hemostasis. Blood 71:1–8
11. Conkling PR, Greenberg CS, Weinberg JB (1988) Tumor necrosis factor induces tissue factor-like activity in human leukemia cell line and U937 and peripheral blood monocytes. Blood 72:128–133
12. Geczy CL, Farram E, Moon DK, et al. (1983) Macrophage procoagulant activity as a measure of cell-mediated immunity in the mouse. J Immunol 130:2743–2749
13. Car BD, Slauson DO, Sunemoto MM, et al. (1991) Expression and kinetics of induced procoagulant activity in bovine pulmonary alveolar macrophages. Exp Lung Res 17:939–957
14. Arai M, Mochida S, Ohno A, et al. (1994) Coagulability in the sinusoids of orthotopically transplanted livers in rats. Transplant Proc 26:913–915
15. Arai M, Mochida S, Ohno A, et al. (1995) Blood coagulation equilibrium in rat liver microcirculation as evaluated by endothelial cell thrombomodulin and macrophage tissue factor. Thromb Res 80:113–123
16. Esmon CT (1989) The role of protein C and thrombomodulin in the regulation of blood coagulation. J Biol Chem 264:4743–4746
17. Bromze GJ Jr (1995) Tissue factor pathway inhibitor and the current concept of blood coagulation. Blood Coagul Fibrinol 6:S7–S13
18. Yamanobe F, Mochida S, Ohno A, et al. (1997) Recombinant human tissue facto pathway inhibitor as a possible anticoagulant targeting hepatic sinusoidal walls. Thromb Res 85:493–501
19. Fujiwara K, Ogata I, Ohta Y, et al. (1988) Intravascular coagulation in acute liver failure in rats and its treatment with antithrombin III. Gut 29:1103–1108
20. Hirata K, Ogata I, Ohta Y, et al. (1989) Hepatic sinusoidal cell destruction in the development of intravascular coagulation in acute liver failure of rats. J Pathol 158:157–165

21. Bernard PH, Le Bail B, Carled J, et al. (1996) Morphology of hepatic stellate cells in patients with fulminant or subfulminant hepatitis requiring liver transplantation. J Submicrosc Cytol Pathol 28:5–12

22. Le Bail B, Bioulac Sage P, Sanuita R, et al. (1990) Fine structure of hepatic sinusoids and sinusodial cells in disease. J Electron Microsc Technol 1990:257–282

23. Muto Y, Nouria Aria KT, Meager A, et al. (1988) Enhanced tumor necrosis factor and interleukin-1 in fulminant hepatic faiure. Lancet 2:72–74

24. De la Mata M, Meager A, Rolando N, et al. (1990) Tumor necrosis factor production in fulminant hepatic failure: Relation to aetiology and superimposed microbial infection. Clin Exp Immnuol 82:479–484

25. Fujiwara K, Mochida S, Tomiya T, et al. (1994) Coagulopathy in fulminant hepatitis. In: Okita K (eds) Frontier in hepatology '93. Axel Springer Japan, Tokyo, pp 42–48

26. Ferluga J, Allison AC (1978) Role of mononuclear infiltrating cells in pathogenesis of hepatitis. Lancet 2:610–611

27. Yamada S, Ogata I, Hirata K, et al. (1989) Intravascular coagulation in the development of massive hepatic necrosis induced by *Corynebacterium parvum* and endotoxin in rats. Scand J Gastroenterol 24:293–298

28. Mochida S, Ogata I, Hirata K, et al. (1990) Provocation of massive hepatic necrosis by endotoxin after partial hepatectomy in rats. Gastroenterology 99:771–777

29. Fujiwara K, Ogata I, Mochida S, et al. (1990) Activated Kupffer cells as a factor of massive hepatic necrosis after liver resection. Hepato-Gastroenterol 37:194–197

30. Arai M, Mochida S, Ohno A, et al. (1993) Sinusoidal endothelial cell damage by activated macrophages in rat liver necrosis. Gastroenterology 104:1466–1471

31. Ogata I, Mochida S, Fujiwara K (1988) Formazan formation in hepatic macrophages after nitro blue tetrazolium perfusion into rat liver. Biomed Res 9:113–117

32. Mochida S, Ogata I, Ohta Y, et al. (1989) In situ evaluation of the stimulatory state of hepatic macrophages based on their ability to produce superoxide anions in rats. J Pathol 158:67–71

33. Fujiwara K, Mochida S, Nagoshi S, et al. (1995) Regulation of hepatic macrophage function by oral administration of Xiao-Chai-Hu-Tang in rats. J Ethnopharmacol 46:107–114

34. Mochida S, Ohno A, Arai M, et al. (1996) Role of adhesion molecules in the development of massive hepatic necrosis in rats. Hepatology 23:320–328

35. Mochida S, Ohno A, Arai M, et al. (1995) Role of adhesion between activated macrophages and endothelial cells in the development of two types of massive hepatic necrosis in rats. J Gastroenterol Hepatol 10:S38–S42

36. Mochida S, Arai M, Ohno A, et al. (1994) Oxidative stress in hepatocytes and stimulatory state of Kupffer cells after reperfusion differ between warm and cold ischemia in rats. Liver 14:234–240

37. Wright SD, Ramos RA, Tobias PS, et al. (1990) CD14, a receptor for complexes of lipopolysaccharide (LPS) and LPS binding protein. Science 249:1431–1433

38. Nagakawa J, Hishinuma I, Hirota K, et al. (1990) Involvement of tumor necrosis factor-α in the pathogenesis of activated macrophage-mediated hepatitis in mice. Gastroenterology 99:758–765

39. Mochida S, Arai M, Ohno A, et al. Deranged blood coagulation equilibrium as a factor of massive liver necrosis following endotoxin administration in partially hepatectomized rats. (submitted for publication)

40. Toshima K, Mochida S, Ishikawa K, et al. (1998) Contribution of CD14 to endotoxin-induced liver injury may depend on types of macrophage activation in rats. Biochem Biophys Res Commun 246:731–735

41. Okamura H, Tsutsui H, Komatsu T, et al. (1995) Cloning of a new cytokine that induces IFN-γ production by T cells. Nature 378:88–91

42. Mochida S, Ohta Y, Ogata I, et al. (1992) Gut-derived substances in activation of hepatic macrophages after partial hepatectomy in rats. J Hepatol 16:266–272

43. Van Oosten M, Van de Bilt E, Vries HE, et al. (1995) Vascular adhesion molecule-1 and inter cellular adhesion molecule-1 expression on rat liver cells after lipopolysaccharide administration in vivo. Hepatology 22:1538–1546
44. Ohno A, Mochida S, Arai M, et al. (1995) ICAM-1 expression in hepatocytes following dissociation of cell-to-cell contact in rats. Biochem Biophys Res Commun 214:1225–1231
45. Mochida S, Ohno A, Fujiwara K (1997) Pitfall in the implication of intercellular adhesion molecule-1 expression on isolated hepatocytes. Hepatology 25:1546
46. Tamatani T, Miyasaka M (1990) Identification of monoclonal antibodies reactive with the rat homology of ICAM-1, and evidence for a differential involvement of ICAM-1 in the adherence of resting versus activated lymphocyts to high endothelial cells. Int Immunol 2:165–171
47. Tamatani T, Kotani M, Miyasaka M (1991) Characterization of the rat leukocyte integlin, CD11/CD18, by use of LFA-1 subunit-specific monoclonal antibodies. Eur J Immunol 21:627–633
48. Mochida S, Ogata I, Ohta Y, et al. (1992) In situ detection of oxidative stress in rat hepatocytes. J Pathol 167:83–89
49. Ohno A, Mochida S, Arai M, et al. (1994) Fat-storing cell abnormalities associated with endothelial cell damage after cold ischemic storage of rat liver in UW solution. Dig Dis Sci 39:861–865
50. Yamane A, Seetharam L, Yamaguchi S, et al. (1994) A new communication system between hepatocyes and sinusoidal endothelial cells in liver through vascular endothelial growth factor and FLT tyrosine kinase receptor family (Flt-1 and KDR/Flk-1). Oncogene 9:2683–2690
51. Mochida S, Ishikawa K, Inao M, et al. (1996) Increased expression of vascular endothelial growth factor and its receptors, *flt-1* and *KDR/flk-1*, in regenerating rat liver. Biochem Biophys Res Commun 176–179
52. Mochida S, Arai M, Ohno A, et al. (1997) Bacterial translocation from gut to portal blood as a factor of hypercoagulation in the hepatic sinusoids after orthotopic liver transplantation in rats. Transplant Proc 29:874–875
53. Arai M, Mochida S, Ohno A, et al. (1998) Selective bowel decontamination of recipients for prevention against liver injury following orthotopic liver transplantation: Evaluation with rat models. Hepatology 27:123–127
54. Fujiwara K, Mochida S, Ohno A, et al. (1995) Possible cause of primary graft nonfunction after orthotopic liver transplantation: A hypothesis with rat model. J Gastroenterol Hepatol 10:S88–S91
55. Arai M, Mochida S, Ohno A, et al. (1996) Blood coagulation in the hepatic sinusoids as a factor of liver injury following orthotopic liver transplantation in rats. Transplantation 62:1398–1401
56. Mochida S, Arai S, Yamanobe F, et al. (1998) Anticoagulant targeting hepatic sinusoidal walls for prevention against hypercoagulopathy in cold preserved rat liver. Transplant Proc 30:45–48

# Sinusoidal Endothelial Cells in Liver Regeneration

Kenji Fujiwara and Satoshi Mochida

*Summary.* Vascular endothelial growth factor (VEGF) has been shown to induce proliferation of sinusoidal endothelial cells in primary culture. Northern blot analysis revealed that VEGF mRNA was expressed in hepatocytes immediately after isolation from normal rats. In contrast, nonparenchymal cells, including sinusoidal endothelial cells, expressed mRNAs of VEGF receptors *flt-1* and *KDR/flk-1*, suggesting that a communication system associated with VEGF may contribute to sinusodial endothelial cell regeneration following partial liver resection and liver injury. When rat hepatocytes were cultured on plastic dishes, VEGF mRNA expression diminished following a transient slight increase in its expression. In these cells, the expression increased again following a peak of DNA synthesis when cultured with epidermal growth factor (EGF) or hepatocyte growth factor (HGF). In 70% resected livers, mitosis was maximal at 36h after the operation in hepatocytes and at 96h in sinusoidal endothelial cells. In these livers, VEGF mRNA expression increased in hepatocytes at the G1 phase of the cell cycle and became prominent in the cells which experienced mitosis. Also, mRNA expression of VEGF receptors was up-regulated in the liver following 70% resection. When liver injury was provoked in rats by $CCl_4$ administration, mRNA expressions of both VEGF and its receptors were significantly increased in the liver compared with those in normal rat liver. VEGF expression was minimal in Kupffer cells isolated from normal rats, but was marked in activated Kupffer cells and hepatic macrophages from $CCl_4$-intoxicated rats. VEGF mRNA expression was also increased in activated stellate cells from $CCl_4$-intoxicated rats and in stellate cells from normal rats activated by primary culture. Thus, VEGF expressed in regenerating hepatocytes may induce proliferation of sinusoidal endothelial cells in partially resected liver, probably through VEGF receptors up-regulated on the cells. In injured liver, this proliferation may also be produced by VEGF derived from activated Kupffer cells, hepatic macrophages, and stellate cells.

*Key words.* Liver regeneration, Sinusoidal endothelial cells, VEGF, *flt-1*, *KDR/flk-1*

Third Department of Internal Medicine, Saitama Medical School, 38 Morohongo, Moroyama-cho, Iruma-gun, Saitama 350-0495, Japan

# Introduction

Much attention has been paid to the role of hepatic sinusoidal cells as a regulatory factor in liver regeneration. Recently, Taub et al. reported that mice with interleukin (IL)-6 gene disruption had impaired regeneration of hepatocytes following partial hepatectomy [1]. In these mice, the activation of signal transducer and activator of transcription protein 3 (STAT3) was absent in hepatocytes, and administration of recombinant IL-6 induced STAT3 activation leading to attenuation of this impaired hepatocyte proliferation [1]. Faust et al. also demonstrated that similar retardation of hepatocyte proliferation was observed in mice deficient in type I tumor necrosis factor (TNF) receptor [2]. In such knockout mice, activation of NF$\kappa$B as well as STAT3 failed to occur in the liver following partial hepatectomy, and administration of IL-6 attenuated impaired hepatocyte proliferation through the activation of STAT3 without affecting NF$\kappa$B activity [2]. Thus, IL-6 and TNF-$\alpha$ released from Kupffer cells seem to initiate hepatocyte proliferation in partially resected liver as well as in injured liver (Fig. 1). Moreover, hepatocyte growth factor (HGF) produced by Kupffer cells, sinusoidal endothelial cells, and hepatic stellate cells can act as a mitogen for hepatocytes in a paracrine manner [3]. Similar hepatotrophic action was found in heparin-binding epidermal growth factor (EGF)-like growth factor (HB-EGF) produced by Kupffer cells and sinusoidal endothelial cells [4]. In contrast, hepatic

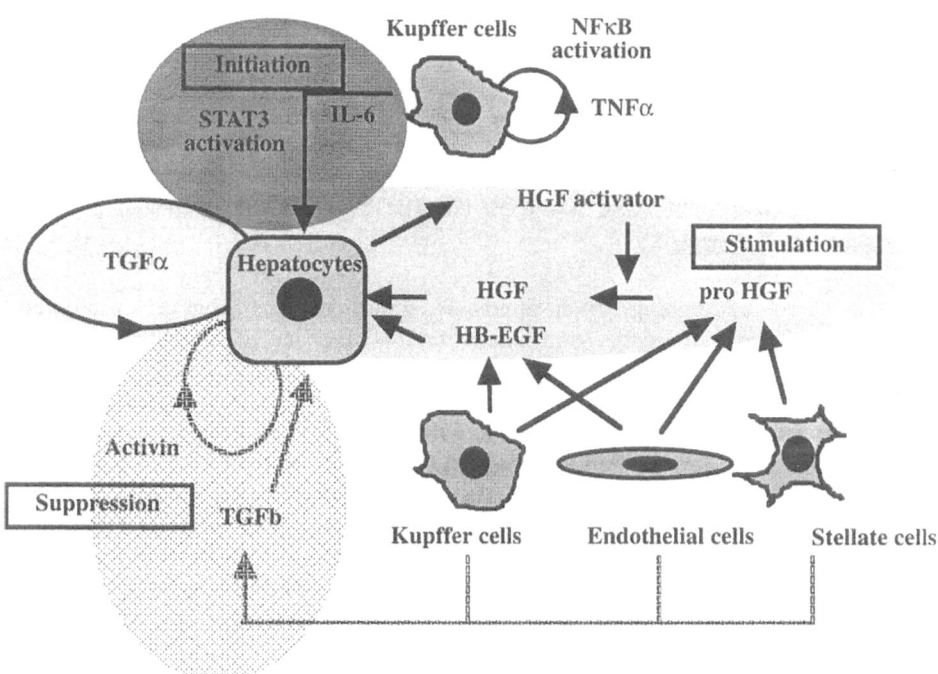

FIG. 1. The role of sinusoidal cells in hepatocyte proliferation during liver regeneration

stellate cells as well as Kupffer cells can produce transforming growth factor (TGF)-$\beta$ abundantly after activation and suppress hepatocyte proliferation [5]. Thus, it seems likely that hepatocyte proliferation is regulated by a variety of cytokines and growth factors released from sinusoidal cells during liver regeneration (Fig. 1).

Hepatic sinusoidal cells not only regulate hepatocyte proliferation, but also increase in number during liver regeneration following partial resection and injury. Among sinusoidal cells, endothelial cells are assumed to be the most important for liver regeneration, as the cells play a role in the maintenance of blood flow in the hepatic sinusoids by regulating coagulation equilibrium and by supplying blood to hepatocytes [6, 7]. However, the regulatory mechanisms of sinusoidal endothelial cell proliferation are yet to be elucidated. Although platelet-derived growth factor (PDGF) and fibroblast growth factor (FGF) are powerful angiogenic factors for vascular endothelial cells, both factors are ineffective for maintenance as well as proliferation of sinusoidal endothelial cells in primary culture [8]. Recently, vascular endothelial growth factor (VEGF), originally isolated as vascular permeability factor (VPF) by Senger et al. [9], has been shown to increase the number of endothelial cells in primary culture of any type, including sinusoidal endothelial cells [8, 10], but not the number of epithelial and mesenchymal cells [11]. VEGF are expressed in epithelial cells, including hepatocytes as well as hepatocellular carcinoma cells [8, 11, 12], and their receptors in sinusoidal endothelial cells [8, 10]. Exudative macrophages in the peritoneal cavity have also been reported to express VEGF [13], suggesting that hepatic sinusoidal cells such as Kupffer cells might express VEGF after activation. These observations led us to postulate that a communication system associated with VEGF in liver cells might contribute to sinusoidal endothelial cell proliferation during liver regeneration after injury as well as after partial resection.

## Sinusoidal Endothelial Cell Regeneration in Partially Resected Liver

In adult rats undergoing 70% hepatectomy, sinusoidal endothelial cells proliferate following hepatocyte regeneration; a peak of mitosis is observed in hepatocytes at 36 h and in sinusoidal endothelial cells at 96 h after the operation [14]. If VEGF expression is increased in regenerating hepatocytes, such hepatocytes might induce proliferation of sinusoidal endothelial cells through VEGF in a paracrine manner. Thus, we studied the expressions of VEGF and two molecules belonging to the Flt tyrosine receptor family, *flt-1* and *KDR/flk-1*, which are responsible for VEGF signal transduction in the proliferation of endothelial cells [8, 15], using rat hepatocytes in primary culture and partially resected liver.

Hepatocytes isolated from adult male F344 rats by Seglen's method [16] were immediately subjected to Northern blot analysis, and also suspended in Williams' medium E containing 10% heat-inactivated fetal calf serum (FCS), $10^{-6}$ M insulin and $10^{-5}$ M dexamethasone. They were seeded in plastic dishes at a density of $5 \times 10^4$ cells/ cm$^2$, and incubated at 37°C under an atmosphere of 5% $CO_2$ and 95% air for 2 h. Following removal of nonadherent cells by washing with Hank's balanced salt solu-

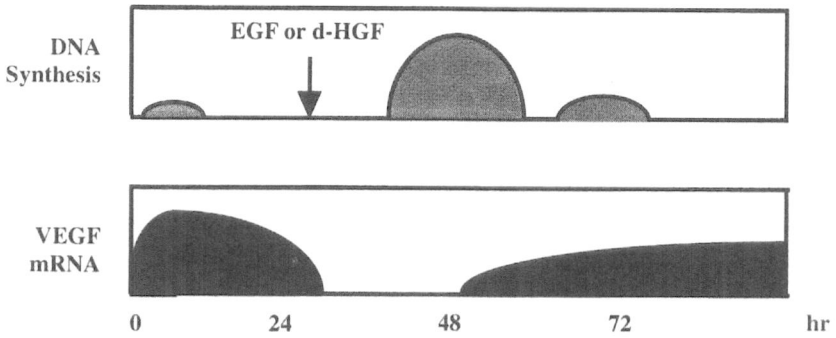

FIG. 2. Cell cycle and VEGF mRNA expression in rat hepatocytes in primary culture

tion without $Ca^{2+}$ and $Mg^{2+}$, adherent hepatocytes were further cultured in Williams' medium E containing 10% heat-inactivated FCS. Adherent hepatocytes were subjected to Northern blot analysis at 2, 12, 24, 48, 72, and 96h of culture. Northern blotting was performed using cDNA fragments of rat VEGF [17], *flt-1* [15], and *KDR/flk-1* [2].

Immediately after isolation, hepatocytes expressed VEGF mRNA. In these cells, *flt-1* and *KDR/flk-1* mRNA expressions were not seen. When isolated hepatocytes were cultured on plastic dishes, VEGF mRNA expression increased, with a peak between 2 and 12h of culture, but decreased after 24h and almost disappeared at 72h. When 50 ng/mL EGF or 10 ng/mL deletion variant of HGF (d-HGF) was added to the culture medium at 24h of culture, VEGF mRNA expression at 48h became detectable, and was markedly increased between 72 and 96h compared with that of the controls with no added growth factors (Fig. 2). Considering the facts that a small peak of DNA synthesis was found between 8 and 16h and at 45h after isolation in hepatocytes cultured without growth factors, and that active DNA synthesis occurred later than 12h after EGF or d-HGF addition [18], VEGF mRNA expression seemed to increase in cultured hepatocytes in association with DNA synthesis [19]. Hepatocytes, especially when moving into the S phase of the cell cycle, may actively express VEGF mRNA (Fig. 2).

It is well known that rat hepatocyes in primary culture seldom move into the M phase of the cell cycle, even when EGF or d-HGF is added to the culture medium. Partial resected liver could provide a key to clarifying the relationship of VEGF expression to the cell cycle. F344 rats underwent 70% liver resection according to the method of Higgins and Anderson [20]. They were killed either immediately or at 12, 24, 48, 72, or 168h after the operation, and the livers were excised for Northern blot analysis of VEGF and its receptors.

Normal rat liver expressed *flt-1* and *KDR/flk-1* mRNAs, as well as VEGF mRNA [19]. Since hepatocytes isolated from normal rats did not express both *flt-1* and *KDR/flk-1* mRNAs, mRNA expressions of VEGF receptors seemed to originate from sinusoidal cells, including endothelial cells [19]. In 70% resected liver, where hepatocyte mitosis peaks at 36h after the operation [14], VEGF mRNA expression had increased significantly at 72h compared with that of normal rat liver (Fig. 3). When

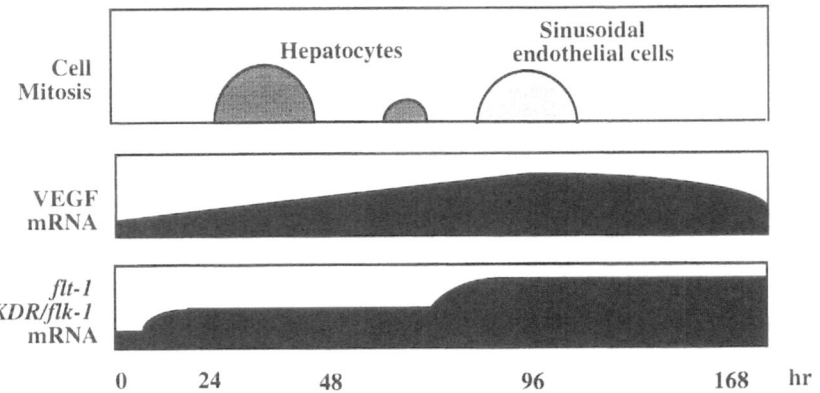

FIG. 3. Cell mitosis and mRNA expressions of VEGF and its receptors in rat liver following partial resection

hepatocytes were isolated from partially resected liver, VEGF mRNA expression had increased in hepatocytes later than 12h after the operation, and became more prominent in the cells between 72 and 168h (unpublished data). These observations are comparable with the results using hepatocytes in primary culture (Fig. 2). VEGF mRNA expression is likely to increase gradually in hepatocytes entering into the G1 phase of the cell cycle and become prominent in the cells after the S or M phase. Such an increase in VEGF expression in regenerating hepatocytes was also supported by

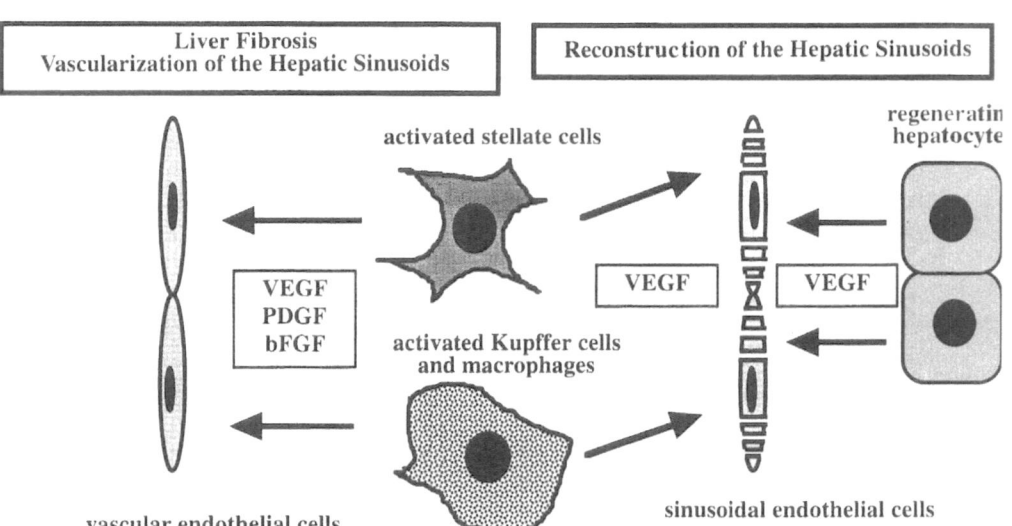

FIG. 4. Possible mechanisms of sinusoidal endothelial cell regeneration in partial resected and injured rat liver

imunohistochemical findings that VEGF protein expression was marked in the cytoplasma of hepatocytes in rats 72 h after 70% hepatectomy compared with that in normal rats (unpublished data). On the other hand, *flt-1* mRNA expression had increased significantly later than 12 h after the operation, and *KDR/flk-1* mRNA expression had increased between 72 and 168 h in partially resected liver compared with normal liver (Fig. 3). During this period, sinusoidal endothelial cells have been shown to increase mitosis, with a peak at 96 h [14]. It would be reasonable to conclude that VEGF expressed in regenerating hepatocytes may contribute to the proliferation of sinusoidal endothelial cells in rat liver after partial resection, probably through *flt-1* and *KDR/flk-1* receptors up-regulated on sinusoidal endothelial cells (Fig. 4).

## Expressions of VEGF and Its Receptors in Hepatic Sinusoidal Cells

Activated Kupffer cells and hepatic macrophages as well as hepatic stellate cells can induce proliferation of vascular endothelial cells through production of angiogenic factors such as PDGF and basic FGF [21]. However, the contribution of these sinusoidal cells to sinusoidal endothelial cell proliferation is yet to be elucidated. Hepatic sinusoidal cells were isolated from male F344 rats by gradient centrifugation in 18% metrizamide solution following digestion of the liver with collagenase and pronase E [22]. Kupffer cells and hepatic stellate cells were further purified from sinusoidal cells by adhesion to plastic dishes [22] and by gradient centrifugation in 13% metrizamide solution [23], respectively. Isolated cells were subjected to Northern blot analysis immediately after isolation and culture in Dulbecco's modified Eagle medium (DMEM) with 10% heat-inactivated FCS.

Isolated sinusodial cells expressed both *flt-1* and *KDR/flk-1* mRNAs abundantly [19]. These expressions might mainly result from the expressions in sinusoidal endothelial cells as reported by Yamane et al. [2]. Interestingly, in our experiment both hepatic stellate cells and Kupffer cells immediately after isolation also expressed mRNAs of VEGF receptors (unpublished data). The significance of such expressions in liver regeneration should be further investigated.

Yamane et al. [2] reported that VEGF mRNA was not expressed in sinusoidal endothelial cells immediately after isolation. In our experiment, however, sinusoidal cells expressed VEGF mRNA faintly immediately after isolation [19]. This prompted us to examine VEGF mRNA expression in Kupffer cells and hepatic stellate cells. Kupffer cells expressed minimal VEGF mRNA immediately after isolation, but the expression became apparent when the cells were cultured on plastic dishes for 24 h (unpublished data). Macrophages have been shown to increase phagocytic activity during culture [24], suggesting that Kupffer cells may express VEGF mRNA after activation. In hepatic stellate cells, VEGF mRNA expression was detected immediately after isolation and also at 3 days after culture (unpublished data). It is widely accepted that hepatic stellate cells cultured for 3 days are quiescent and similar in function to in vivo cells [23], suggesting that the slight VEGF mRNA expression in sinusoidal cells immediately after isolation is derived from hepatic stellate cells. When hepatic stellate cells were cultured on plastic dishes for 10 days, VEGF mRNA expression became more prominent compared with that of cells cultured for 3 days (unpublished data). Such stellate cells are considered to be activated, since they show increased smooth muscle $\alpha$ actin expression and active synthesis of DNA and collagen [23, 25]. Thus, VEGF mRNA expression may increase in hepatic stellate cells depending on the extent of activation in vitro.

## Sinuosidal Endothelial Cell Regeneration in Injured Liver

Kupffer cells and hepatic stellate cells isolated from normal rats showed increased VEGF mRNA expression following activation by culture on plastic dishes, as mentioned above. This may indicate that activated Kupffer cells, hepatic macrophages, and stellate cells in necrotic areas of injured liver can induce proliferation of sinusoidal endothelial cells.

F344 rats were orally given 10 ml/kg body weight of carbon tetrachloride ($CCl_4$) as a 20% solution in olive oil. They were killed immediately or at 1, 3, or 7 days after intoxication, and the liver was excised for Northern blot analysis of VEGF and its receptors. In these rats, hepatic VEGF mRNA expression was increased 1 day after intoxication and became more prominent 7 days later (Unpublished data). Also, mRNA expressions of *flt-1* and *KDR/flk-1* were increased in the liver between 1 and 3 days after intoxication (unpublished data).

Massive liver necrosis developed in centrilobular areas of hepatic lobules between 1 and 3 days after $CCl_4$-intoxication in rats (Fig. 5). Kupffer cells and hepatic macrophages in the necrotic areas are activated to produce a large amount of superoxide anions in phagosomes [22]. Also, hepatic stellate cells in such areas produce extracellular matrix abundantly [26]. Activated Kupffer cells, hepatic

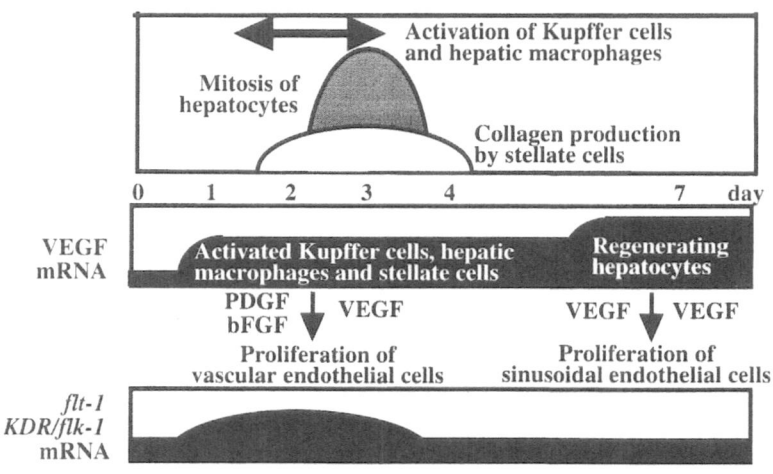

Fig. 5. Pathophysiology and mRNA expressions of VEGF and its receptors in the livers of carbon tetrachloride-intoxicated rats

macrophages, and stellate cells in necrotic areas might contribute to the increase of hepatic VEGF expression between 1 and 3 days after $CCl_4$-intoxication. Moreover, the up-regulation of VEGF receptors may develop in proliferating endothelial cells in necrotic areas. In the liver of $CCl_4$-intoxicated rats, hepatocytes increased in number with a peak at 3 days (unpublished data), and the liver became histologically normal at 7 days. It seemed that after the M phase of the cell cycle, regenerating hepatocytes increased VEGF mRNA expression.

When Kupffer cells and hepatic macrophages were isolated from rat liver after $CCl_4$-intoxication, both types of cell showed increased VEGF mRNA expression compared with that of Kupffer cells from normal rats (unpublished data). Also, activated stellate cells increased VEGF mRNA expression compared with that of stellate cells from normal rats (unpublished data). VEGF mRNA expression was higher in hepatocytes isolated from rat liver 7 days after $CCl_4$-intoxication than in hepatocytes from normal rats (unpublished data). These data strongly suggest that VEGF expressed in activated Kupffer cells, hepatic macrophages, and stellate cells, as well as regenerating hepatocytes, may contribute to sinusoidal endothelial cell proliferation in injured rat liver (Fig. 4).

Regenerating hepatocytes express VEGF exclusively among various angiogenic factors, while activated Kupffer cells, hepatic macrophages, and stellate cells have the ability to produce PDGF and basic FGF as well as VEGF [21]. In contrast to sinusoidal endotheial cells, vascular endothelial cells increase in numer in response to angiogenic factors other than VEGF. SE-1 is an antibody specific for sinusoidal endothelial cells in rats [27]. Vascular endothelial cells can be identified by the staining of thrombomodulin, an anticoagulant which inactivates thrombin [28], since thrombomodulin expression is considerably decreased in sinusoidal endotheial cells compared with that of endothelial cells in microvessels of other organs [6]. In rat liver 3 days after $CCl_4$ intoxication, the staining for SE-1 was absent in the centrilobular necrotic areas, while such staining was positive along the hepatic sinusoids of nonnecrotic areas in the periportal and midzonal areas (unpublished data). In these rats, positive staining for thrombomodulin was found in the centrizonal necrotic areas, while SE-1 was stained along the hepatic sinusoids in the centrilobular areas as well as in the periportal and midzonal areas in rats 7 days after intoxication. These data may suggest that vascular endothelial cells proliferate in necrotic areas in injured liver, while sinusoidal endothelial cell proliferation develops following absorption of such necrotic areas. Activated Kupffer cells, hepatic macrophages, and stellate cells may induce proliferation of vascular endothelial cells through production of PDGF and basic FGF as well as VEGF in injured liver (Figs. 4 and 5). Under these conditions, it is also possible that VEGF derived from regenerating hepatocytes stimulate proliferation of sinusoidal endothelial cells (Figs. 4 and 5). PDGF and basic FGF are known to stimulate proliferation of hepatic stellate cells as well as vascular endothelial cells [21]. Also, activated sinusoidal cells can promote extracellular matrix production in hepatic stellate cells by releasing TGF-$\beta$ in an autocrine or paracrine manner [21]. It seems likely that hepatic fibrosis associated with the vascularization of the hepatic sinusoids can progress when angiogenic factors are more actively produced by sinusoidal cells in injured liver. Reconstruction of the hepatic sinusoids might depend on the balance between VEGF derived from regenerating hepatocytes and PDGF and basic FGF from sinusoidal cells.

# Conclusion

VEGF expressed in regenerating hepatocytes may contribute to proliferation of sinusoidal endothelial cells in partially resected liver, probably through VEGF receptors, *flt-1* and *KDR/flk-1*, up-regulated on the cells. In injured liver, increased expression of VEGF may derive from activated Kupffer cells, hepatic macrophages, and stellate cells as well as regenerating hepatocytes. These activated sinusoidal cells might also induce proliferation of vascular endothelial cells through production of PDGF and basic FGF as well as VEGF. It seems that VEGF derived from regenerating hepatocytes is essential for sinusoidal endothelial cell proliferation leading to reconstruction of the hepatic sinusoids.

## References

1. Cressman DE, Greenbaum LE, DeAngelis RA, et al. (1996) Liver failure and defective hepatocyte regeneration in interleukin-6-deficient mice. Science 274:1379–1383
2. Yamada Y, Kirillova I, Peschon JJ, et al. (1997) Initiation of liver growth by tumor necrosis factor: Deficient liver regeneration in mice lacking type I tumor necrosis factor receptor. Proc Natl Acad Sci USA 94:1441–1446
3. Matsumoto K, Nakamura T (1991) Hepatocyte growth factor: Molecular structure and implications for a central role in liver regeneration. J Gastroenterol Hepatol 6:509–519
4. Kiso S, Kawata S, Tamura S, et al. (1995) Role of heparin binding epidermal growth factor-like growth factor as a hepatotrophic factor in rat liver regeneration after partial hepatectomy. Hepatology 22:1584–1590
5. Braun L, Mead JE, Panzica M, et al. (1988) Transforming growth factor mRNA increases during liver regeneration: A possible paracrine mechanism of growth regulation. Proc Natl Acad Sci USA 85:1539–1543
6. Arai M, Mochida S, Ohno A, et al. (1995) Blood coagulation equilibrium in rat liver microcirculation as evaluated by endothelial cell thrombomodulin and macrophage tissue factor. Thromb Res 80:113–123
7. Yamanobe F, Mochida S, Ohno A, et al. (1997) Recombinant human tissue factor pathway inhibitor as a possible anticoagulant targeting hepatic sinusoidal walls. Thromb Res 85:493–501
8. Yamane A, Seetharam L, Yamaguchi S, et al. (1994) A new communication system between hepatocytes and sinusoidal endothelial cells in liver through vascular endothelial growth factor and FLT tyrosine kinase receptor family (Flt-1 and KDR/Flk-1). Oncogene 9:2683–2690
9. Senger DR, Galli SJ, Dvorak AM, et al. (1983) Tumor cells secrete a vascular permeability factor that promotes accumulation of ascitic fluid. Science 219:983–985
10. Shibuya M (1995) Role of VEGF-FLT receptor system in normal and tumor angiogenesis. Adv Cancer Res 67:281–316
11. Ferrara N, Henzel WJ (1989) Pituitary follicular cells secrete a novel heparin-binding growth factor specific for vascular endothelial cells. Biochem Biocphys Res Commun 161:851–858
12. Mise M, Arii S, Higashitsuji H, et al. (1996) Clinical significance of vascular endothelial growth factor and basic fibroblast growth factor gene expression in liver tumor. Hepatology 23:455–464
13. Ferrara N, Leung DW, Cachianes G, et al. (1991) Purification and cloning of vascular endothelial growth factor secreted by pituitary folliculosellate cells. Methods Enzymol 198:391–405

14. Widmann J, Fahimi HD (1975) Proliferation of mononuclear phagocytes (Kupffer cells) and endothelial cells in regenerating rat liver. Am J Pathol 80:349–366
15. Shibuya M, Yamaguchi S, Yamane A, et al. (1990) Nucleotide sequence and expression of a novel human receptor-type tyrosine kinase gene (*flt-1*) closely related to the *fms* family. Oncogene 5:519–524
16. Seglen PO (1976) Preparation of isolated rat liver cells. Methods Cell Biol 13:29–83
17. Keck JP, Hauser SC, Krivi G, et al. (1989) Vascular permeability factor, an endothelial cell mitogen related to PDGF. Science 246:1309–1312
18. Yamada S, Fujiwara K, Oka Y, et al. (1987) Role of cell-surface modulator of DNA synthesis in liver regeneration. J Biochem 101:1385–1389
19. Mochida S, Ishidawa K, Inao M, et al. (1996) Increased expression of vascular endothelial growth factor and its receptors, *flt-1* and *KDR/flk-1*, in regenerating rat liver. Biochem Biophys Res Commun 226:176–179
20. Higgins GM, Anderson RM (1931) Experimental pathology of the liver. I. Restortion of the liver of the white rat following partial surgical removal. Arch Pathol 12:186–202
21. Gressner AM (1995) Cytokines and cellular crosstalk involvd in the activation of fat-storing cells. J Hepatol 22:28–36
22. Mochida S, Ogata I, Ohta Y, et al. (1989) In situ evaluation of stimulatory state of hepatic macrophages based on their ability to produce superoxide anions in rats. J Pathol 158:67–71
23. Ikeda H, Fujiwara K (1995) Cyclosporin A and FK-506 in inhibition of rat Ito cell activation in vitro. Hepatology 21:1161–1166
24. Adams DO, Levis JG, Johnson WJ (1983) Multiple modes of cellular injury by macrophages: Requirement for differential forms of effector activation. In: Yamamura Y, Tada T (eds) Progress in immunology V. Academic Press, Tokyo, pp 1009–1018
25. Inao M, Mochida S, Ikeda H, et al. (1997) Effect of neurotropic pyrimidine heterocyclic compound, MS-430, on cultured hepatic parenchymal and stellate cells. Life Sci 61:273–282
26. Ogata I, Mochida S, Tomiya T, et al. (1991) Minor contribution of hepatocytes to collagen production in normal and early fibrotic rat liver. Hepatology 14:220–224
27. Ohmura T, Enomoto K, Satoh H, et al. (1993) Establishment of a novel monoclonal antibody, SE-1, which specifically reacts with rat hepatic sinusoidal endothelial cells. J Histochem Cytochem 41:1253–1257
28. Esmon CT (1989) The role of protein C and thrombomodulin in the regulation of blood coagulation. J Biol Chem 264:4743–4746

# Angiogenesis of Cultured Rat Sinusoidal Endothelial Cells

Satoshi Shakado[1], Shotaro Sakisaka[2], Kazunori Noguchi[2], Michio Sata[2], and Kyuichi Tanikawa[2]

*Summary.* We have previously shown that rat sinusoidal endothelial cells cultured on Matrigel presented a great number of tube-like structures, forming a network, on the surface of the gel. In the present study, using this model, mimicking angiogenic processes that occur in vivo, we examined the effects of growth factors on these tube-like structures, and also the effects of extracellular matrices. Isolated sinusoidal endothelial cells were plated on culture dishes coated with type-1 collagen or Matrigel. Cultured sinusoidal endothelial cells were incubated in a medium containing various growth factors (a-FGF, b-FGF, HGF, and VEGF). Ultrastructurally, tube-like structures were formed by two or three sinusoidal endothelial cells which retained many endothelial pores on the cell surface. In morphometric analysis, acidic fibroblast growth factors (a-FGF), basic fibroblast growth factors (b-FGF), and especially hepatocyte growth factors (HGF) accelerated the formation of the tube-like structures. Vascular endothelial cell growth factor (VEGF) did not stimulated the formation of the tubes. These results suggest that growth factors which promote tube-like structures in cultured sinusoidal endothelial cells may induce regeneration of sinusoids in vivo.

*Key words.* Sinusoidal endothelial cell, Culture, Angiogenesis, Growth factor, Rat

## Introduction

The formation of new blood capillaries (angiogenesis) is a common biological process in response to physiological or pathological stimuli [1, 2]. Whereas angiogenesis of sinusoidal endothelial cells occurs in hepatic regeneration and the growth of hepatocellular carcinoma, the mechanism of angiogenesis by sinusoidal endothelial cells has not been clearly understood. Recently, extracellular matrix proteins have

---

[1] Social Insurance Tagawa Hospital, Kamihon-machi 10-18, Tagawa 826-8585, Japan
[2] The Second Department of Internal Medicine, Kurume University School of Medicine, 67 Asahi-machi, Kurume, Fukuoka 830-0011, Japan

been shown to stimulate tube formation in vitro by cultured endothelial cells from the human umbilical vein and bovine aorta [3, 4]. We have studied the tube-like structures of cultured rat sinusoidal endothelial cells in order to understand the angiogenesis of sinusoidal endothelial cells, and we have previously reported that rat sinusoidal endothelial cells cultured on Matrigel (which contains high concentrations of laminin, type-4 collagen, and various growth factors) presented a great number of tube-like structures which formed a network on the surface of the gel [5, 6]. Vascular endathelial cell growth factor (VEGF) is an endothelial cell-specific mitogen and angiogenic inducer released by a variety of tumor cells. In an experimental metastatic liver tumor, VEGF was found in all tumor cells, and their receptors for VEGF were also demonstrated in tumor endothelial cells [7]. Messenger-RNA of VEGF was demonstrated in hepatocytes but not in nonparenchymal cells [8]. In liver regeneration, VEGF from hepatocytes may be a proliferative stimulus for sinusoidal endothelial cells. In the present study, the effects of VEGF in the tube-like structure formation of cultured rat sinusoidal endothelial cells were studied and compared with those of acidic fibroblast growth factors (a-FGF), basis fibroblast growth factors (b-FGF), and hepatocyte growth factors (HGF).

## Materials and Methods

Nonparenchymal liver cells were isolated from normal male Wistar rats by the collagenase perfusion method. Sinusoidal endothelial cells were separated with a centrifugal elutriation rotor from the nonparenchymal cells [6]. Purified endothelial cells ($1 \times 10^7$ cells per culture dish) were plated onto 35-mm culture dishes coated with type-1 collagen, type-1 collagen gel, laminin gel, or Matrigel with William's medium E containing 20% fetal calf serum. Cultured cells were incubated in the medium with the addition of various growth factors (a-FGF, b-FGF, HGF, or VEGF) for 48 h, and then the cells were viewed by light and electron microscopy. The lengths of the tube-like structures formed by the cultured sinusoidal endothelial cells were morphometrically analyzed using light micrographs.

## Results

Cultured rat sinusoidal endothelial cells were attached on type-1 collagen-coated dishes and formed a cobblestone-like pattern (Fig. 1). The cells did not form tube-like structures on this culture matrix. However, cultured cells did form tube-like structures on the surface of type-1 collagen gel. On laminin gel, the cells invaded the gel and formed tube-like structure in the gel. The diameter of the tubes was about 5–10 mm. Ultrastructurally, tube-like structures were formed by two or three sinusoidal endothelial cells which retained many endothelial pores on the cell surface. Sinusoidal endothelial cells cultured on Matrigel formed a great number of tube-like structures in a network on the surface of the gel (Fig. 2), and this tube-like structure formation of cultured cells was accelerated by a-FGF, b-FGF, and (markedly) HGF, but not by VEGF (Table 1).

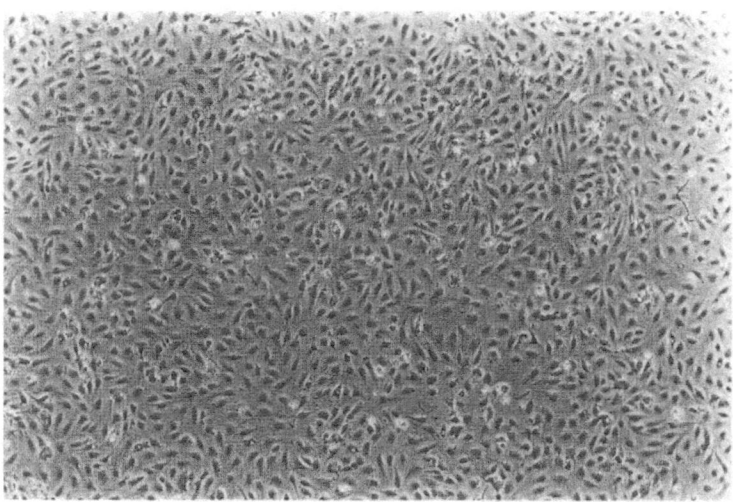

FIG. 1. Phase-contrast micrograph showed the cobblestone-like pattern formed by cultured sinusoidal endothelial cells on a type-1 collagen-coated dish

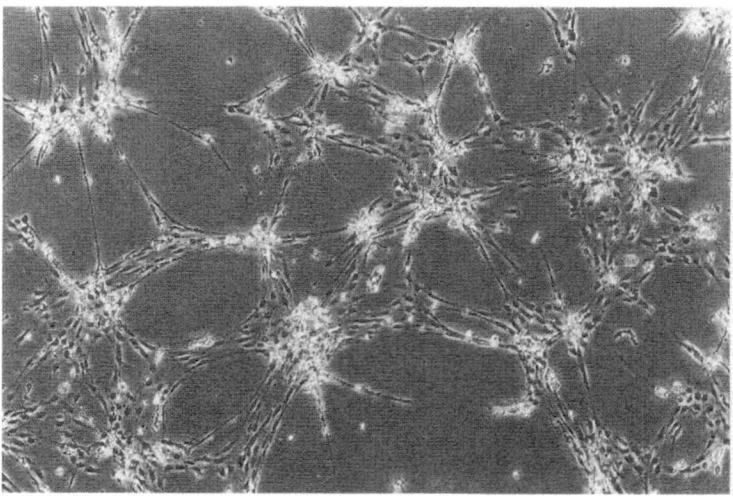

FIG. 2. Phase-contrast micrograph showing that cultured sinusoidal endothelial cells form tube-like structures with an anastomosing network on the surface of Matrigel

## Discussion and Conclusions

We have previously shown that cultured rat sinusoidal endothelial cells formed tube-like structures on the surface of Matrigel [9]. Tube-like structure formation by cultured sinusoidal endothelial cells is a phenomenon mimicking angiogenesis in vivo, as

TABLE 1. Tube-like structure formation in cultured sinusoidal endothelial cells was accelerated by a-FGF, b-FGF, and (markedly) HGF, but not by VEGF

| | |
|---|---|
| Control | 100 ± 9.3 (%) |
| a-FGF 25 ng/ml | 157.5 ± 14.4* |
| bFGF 25 ng/ml | 148.7 ± 23.6* |
| HGF 10 ng/ml | 179.3 ± 14.9* |
| VEGF 20 ng/ml | 68.6 ± 26.3* |

*$P < 0.01$.

described in other vascular endothelial cells. Thus, the factors promoting tube-like structure formation in cultured sinusoidal endothelial cells may be involved in regeneration of the sinusoid in vivo. An inducer of such tube formation in cultured sinusoidal endothelial cells may be effective as a new therapeutic drug for treating fulminant hepatitis, since fulminant hepatitis requires the active regeneration of endothelial cells as hepatocytes. Since HGF, a-FGF, and b-FGF showed stimulatory activity of tube-like structures in cultured sinusoidal endothelial cells, VEGF may be involved in the reconstruction of the sinusoid in liver regeneration, in cooperation with other growth factors.

# References

1. Montesano R, Orci L (1987) Phorbol esters induce angiogenesis in vitro from large-vessel endothelial cells. J Cell Physiol 130:284–291
2. Kubota Y, Kleinman HK, Martin GR, et al. (1988) Role of laminin and basement membrane in the morphological differentiation of human endothelial cells into capillary-like structure. J Cell Biol 107:1589–1598
3. Grant DS, Tashiro K, Segui-Real B, et al. (1989) Two different laminin domains mediate the differentiation of human endothelial cells into capillary-like structures in vitro. Cell 58:933–943
4 Iruela-Arispe KL, Hasselaar P, Sage H (1991) Differential expression of extracellular proteins is correlated with angiogenesis in vitro. Lab Invest 64:174–186
5 Shakado S, Sakisaka S, Yoshitake M, et al. (1993) The effect of extracellular matrix on an ultrastructure of cultured rat sinusoidal endothelial cells. In: D.L. Knook (eds) Cells of the hepatic sinusoid vol 4. The Netherlands Rijswijk, pp 195–197
6 Shakado S, Sakisaka S, Noguchi K, et al. (1995) Effects of extracellular matrices on tube formation of cultured rat hepatic sinusoidal endothelial cells. Hepatology 22:969–973
7 Warren RS, Yuan H, Matli MR, et al. (1995) Regulation by vascular endothelial growth factor of human colon cancer tumorigenesis. A mouse model of experimental liver metastasis. J Clin Invest 95:1789–1797
8 Yamane A, Seetharam L, Yamaguchi S (1994) A new communication system between hepatocytes and sinusoidal endothelial cells in liver through vascular endothelial growth factor and Flt tyrosine kinase receptor family (Flt-1 and KDR/Flk-1). Oncogene 9:2683–2690
9 Shakado S, Sakisaka S, Noguchi K (1995) Effect of various growth factors on tube-like structure of rat sinusoidal endothelial cells cultured on Matrigel. In: E. Wisse (ed) Cells of the hepatic sinusoid, vol 5. The Netherlands Rijswijk, pp 283–284

# The Multiple Roles of Macrophages in Hepatic Granuloma Formation in Mice

Kiyoshi Takahashi[1], Motohiro Takeya[1], Kazuhisa Miyakawa[1], Sho-Ichiro Hagiwara[1], Aye Aye Wynn[1], Makoto Naito[2], and Masahiko Yamada[3]

*Summary.* In this chapter, the multiple types of involvement of macrophages at different stages of Zymosan (glucan)-induced hepatic granuloma formation are reviewed based on our studies with different mouse models. Mice depleted of Kupffer cells show a delay in Zymosan-induced hepatic granuloma formation, indicating the importance of Kupffer cells in the initial stage. Mice depleted of blood monocytes show a delay in glucan-induced hepatic granuloma formation due to a defect in the supply of blood monocytes into the liver, and the granulomas are formed by the proliferation of Kupffer cells and their change into epithelioid and multinuclear giant cells. In op/op mice, hepatic granuloma formation is delayed due to a defect in the supply of blood monocytes and their impaired differentiation into macrophages in loco. The granulomas are mainly induced by the accumulation of immature Kupffer cells and their transformation into epithelioid and multinuclear giant cells. Daily macrophage colony-stimulating factor (M-CSF) administration induces a sufficient supply of blood monocytes, their differentiation into macrophages, and a proliferation of Kupffer cells in the hepatic granuloma formation of op/op mice. In our previous studies of nude mice, scid mice, and xid mice, T lymphocytes were shown to be involved in the activation of macrophages during hepatic granuloma formation. Granulocyte/macrophage (GM)-CSF-deficient mice show a delay in hepatic granuloma formation and a rapid disappearance of the granulomas due to GM-CSF deficiency. In interleukin-5 (IL-5) -transgenic mice, Zymosan-induced hepatic granuloma formation is enhanced. Type I and type II class A macrophage scavenger receptor (MSR-A)-deficient mice show a delay in glucan-induced hepatic granuloma formation due to a reduced uptake of glucan particles by Kupffer cells and monocyte-derived macrophages.

*Key words.* Kupffer cells, Macrophages, Monocytes, Granuloma, Mouse

[1] Second Department of Pathology, Kumamoto University School of Medicine, 2-2-1 Honjo, Kumamoto 860-0811, Japan
[2] Second Department of Pathology, Niigata University School of Medicine, 757 Asahimachidori-Ichibancho, Niigata 951-8122, Japan
[3] Department of Neurosurgery, 20-17 Kajiyacho, Kagoshima City Hospital, Kagoshima 892-0846, Japan

# Introduction

In humans and animals, the liver is the most important organ for defense mechanisms against pathogenic microorganisms invading through the portal vein and hepatic arteries. Kupffer cells are involved in the removal of a variety of macromolecular substances including such microorganisms. In cases where the invading substances are largely undigested by Kupffer cells and thus not eliminated from the liver, granulomas are formed by the accumulation of macrophages, including Kupffer cells, in the hepatic sinusoids, followed by their change into epithelioid cells and multinuclear giant cells. However, the role of macrophages, including Kupffer cells, in hepatic granuloma formation is not yet fully understood. To clarify their role in relation to hepatic granulomas, the processes of granuloma formation in a variety of mice, including those with severe monocytopenia induced by the administration of strontium-89 ($^{89}$Sr), osteopetrosis (op/op) mice defective in the production of functional M-CSF protein, GM-CSF-deficient mice, IL-5 transgenic mice, type I and type II MSR-A-deficient mice, and immunodeficient mice such as nude mice, scid mice, and xid mice, are reviewed on the basis of the results obtained in our previous and ongoing preliminary studies. Before the review, we would like to present our view on the development and differentiation of macrophages in the liver on the basis of the results of our previous in vivo and in vitro studies.

# The Development and Differentiation of Macrophages

Figure 1 shows schematic diagrams of macrophage development and differentiation during ontogeny and in adult life. During early murine ontogeny, macrophages first develop in the yolk sac hematopoiesis, and directly differentiate from hematopoietic stem cells without passing through the stage of monocytic cells [1, 2]. In the earliest embryonic stage, fetal macrophages predominate in the yolk sac hematopoiesis and are matured from immature macrophages called primitive macrophages[1–3]. In this stage, monocytic cells are absent from the blood islands of the yolk sac. After the connection of vitelline veins with the embryonic cardiovascular system, hematopoietic cells, including primitive and fetal macrophages, migrate from the yolk sac into various fetal tissues, particularly into the fetal liver [4]. There, the primitive and fetal macrophages proliferate actively and differentiate into Kupffer cells [4–7]. In the murine fetal liver, monocytic cells are few in the early stage, and have developed and expanded from the middle stage of ontogeny [8]. In the early stage of ontogeny [3], primitive and fetal macrophages circulate in the peripheral blood and show a marked proliferative capacity in fetal tissues [9]. From the early stage of yolk sac and hepatic hematopoiesis, primitive and fetal macrophages circulate in blood, migrate, and colonize in peripheral tissues [9]. However, the number of circulating macrophages reduces with gestational day in the late stage of ontogeny, and they disappear at birth [9]. At 17 or 18 fetal days, monocytes are released from the liver into peripheral blood, migrate into peripheral tissues, and differentiate into macrophages [9]. However, monocyte-derived macrophages have no proliferative capacity in fetal tissues as they do in normal unstimulated adult tissues.

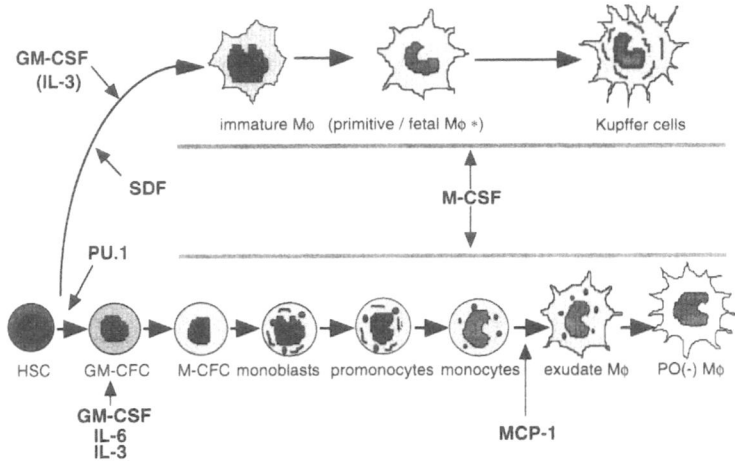

FIG. 1. A schematic representation of macrophage development, differentiation, and maturation during ontogeny and in adult life. *HSC*, hematopoietic stem cells; *GM-CFC*, granulocyte/macrophage colony-forming cells; *M-CFC*, macrophage colony-forming cells; *Mφ*, macrophages; *SDF*, stromal-derived factor; *MCP-1*, monocyte chemoattractant protein-1. *in fetal period

In adult life, the bone marrow has a peculiar mechanism for releasing macrophage precursors. After hematopoietic stem cells enter the stage of lineage-specific differentiation, they are not released from the bone marrow unless they are completely differentiated into monocytes via colony-forming unit-macrophages (CFU-M), monoblasts, and promonocytes [9, 10]. In response to chemotactic factors such as monocyte chemoattractant protein-1 (MCP-1), monocytes migrate into the liver and differentiate into exudate (monocyte-derived) macrophages [9]. In a normal steady-state condition, monocyte-derived macrophages are short-lived, have no proliferative capacity, and die by apoptosis in loco [11]. In op/op mice, monocytic cells and monocyte-derived macrophages are absent [9, 10]. In contrast, hematopoietic stem cells or immature myeloid macrophage precursor cells at the stage prior to entering monocytic cell differentiation are released from the bone marrow into peripheral blood, circulate via the blood stream, and migrate into peripheral tissues [9, 12]. Certain chemotactic factors such as stromal-derived factor-1 (SDF-1) may be involved in the migration of the hematopoietic stem cells into the tissues, and these cells differentiate into tissue macrophages in loco by the action of various growth factors such as stem cell factor (SCF), interleukin (IL)-6, IL-3, GM-CSF, and M-CSF produced in loco. As PU.1 (Spi-1, Sfpi-1) is a hematopoietic transcription factor essential for the differentiation of myeloid and B lymphoid cells, all macrophages, including tissue macrophages and osteoclasts, are completely absent in mice homozygous for the PU.1 gene mutation [13, 14]. However, a few macrophages appear in the liver of long-surviving PU.1-null mutant mice, suggesting that macrophages can develop from hematopoietic stem cells before PU.1 involvement [14]. Kupffer cells show a long life-span, have proliferative capacity, and can survive by self-renewal in the liver without a supply of blood monocytes. This differentiation pathway of tissue macrophages, including Kupffer cells, in the liver was clearly demonstrated from data obtained in previous studies of [89]Sr-induced monocytopenic mice [15] and op/op mice [9, 10]. Therefore, there exist at least two distinct macrophage populations in the liver: Kupffer cells and monocyte-derived macrophages (Fig. 1).

## The Role of Kupffer Cells in the Initial Stage of Hepatic Granuloma Formation: Studies with Mice Depleting Kupffer Cells

Since liposome-encapsulated dichloromethylene diphosphonate (lipo-MDP) is highly toxic to macrophages, Naito and co-workers [16, 17] examined the processes of Zymosan-induced hepatic granuloma formation in mice which had depleted Kupffer cells after the administration of lipo-MDP and compared them with those of lipo-MDP-untreated control mice to elucidate the role of Kupffer cells in the initial stage of granulomatous inflammation in the liver. In the control mice, cell clusters and granulomas started to form by accumulation, aggregation, and collection of macrophages in the hepatic sinusoids from 2 days after a single intravenous injection of 0.1 ml Zymosan [17]. The number and size of granulomas increased with days after injection, peaked at 10 days, and declined thereafter [17]. In these processes, macrophages collect, aggregate, and fuse with each other to develop into multinuclear giant cells of foreign-body type or Langhans type. In the lipo-MDP-injected mice, the number of Kupffer cells decreased to approximately 12% of that of normal mice at 3 days after injection [16]. Two days after Zymosan injection, no granulomas had formed, but a few small cellular clusters were detected in the liver at 3 days after injection. At 5 days, a small number of granulomas had formed, and they increased in number and size with days after Zymosan injection [16]. However, compared with the lipo-MDP-untreated control mice, the number and size of hepatic granulomas in the lipo-MDP-treated mice reduced from 3 to 28 days after Zymosan injection, and the expression of M-CSF, IL-1, MCP-1, tumor necrosis factor (TNF)-$\alpha$, and interferon (INF)-$\gamma$ messenger RNA (mRNA) was suppressed in the stage of granuloma formation [16]. These data imply that Kupffer cells are indispensable for granuloma formation, play a part as an initiator, and produce various cytokines including MCP-1 and M-CSF.

## The Role of Kupffer Cells in Hepatic Granuloma Formation in the Liver: Studies with Mice Devoid of Blood Monocytes

Administration of a bone-seeking radioisotope [89]Sr to C3H/HeN mice severely impairs the development and differentiation of hematopoietic cells, particularly monocytic cells, in bone marrow due to its exchange with calcium in the developing bones [18]. In these mice, splenectomy had been performed 1 month before [89]Sr administration to exclude the possibility of developing extramedullary hematopoiesis in the spleen [15]. In the splenectomized mice, [89]Sr administration induces severe monocytopenia without any damage to Kupffer cells in the liver and tissue macrophages in tissues other than bone and bone marrow [15, 18, 19]. From 2 weeks after administration, monocytes virtually disappear in peripheral blood in these mice, and the monocyte pool is reduced to less than 0.5% of that of the splenectomized control mice [15, 18, 19]. However, the number of Kupffer cells is not reduced in the liver of $^{89}$Sr-induced, severely monocytopenic mice, and they show a proliferative potential and a [$^3$H]thymidine labeling index of less than 10% [15, 19]. These data suggest that Kupffer cells are sustained by self-renewal without a supply of blood monocytes [15]. In the severely monocytopenic mice, hepatic granuloma formation occurred from 5 days after glucan injection onward, and the number and size of hepatic granulomas increased thereafter [15, 19]. At 5 days after glucan injection, Kupffer cells markedly proliferate, aggregate, and collect to form hepatic granulomas, together with the formation of multinuclear giant cells by the fusion of proliferating Kupffer cells [15, 19]. These findings indicate that Kupffer cells proliferate in response to inflammatory stimuli, aggregate, and collect to form hepatic granulomas without a supply of blood monocytes [15, 19].

# The Role of Immature Kupffer Cells in Hepatic Granuloma Formation in op/op Mice Defective in the Production of Functional M-CSF Protein

Breeders of (C57BL/6J × C3He/FeJ) csfm$^{op}$/csfm$^{op}$-op/op mice were supplied by Dr. Leonard D. Shultz, Jackson Laboratory (Bar Harbor, ME, USA), and op/op mice were obtained by mating of +/op heterozygotes. Op/op mice show a complete, or nearly complete, deficiency of monocytes in peripheral blood, impaired production of monocytic cells and their precursors in the bone marrow, a complete deficiency of monocyte-derived macrophages, defective differentiation of monocytes into macrophages in tissues, and a reduced number of tissue macrophages, including Kupffer cells, in the liver [9]. The Kupffer cells are small and round and show immature ultrastructure [9]. All these abnormalities result from a total lack of functional M-CSF activity due to a defect in the coding region of the Csfm gene [20]. A similar delay in hepatic granuloma formation to that of $^{89}$Sr-induced, monocytopenic mice was found in the op/op mice [21]. After Zymosan injection, granulomas started to form from 5 days on, and their number and size increased with days, although the proliferative capacity of Kupffer cells in the op/op mice was lower than in monocytopenic mice [21]. These findings indicate that immature Kupffer cells increase, aggregate, and collect to form hepatic granulomas in op/op mice without a supply of blood monocytes [21].

# The Role of Kupffer Cells and Monocyte-Derived Macrophages in Hepatic Granuloma Formation in M-CSF-Treated op/op Mice

Daily M-CSF administration into the op/op mice induces an increase in the number of Kupffer cells and monocyte-derived macrophages due to the proliferation and maturation of the Kupffer cells, an influx of macrophage precursor cells, including monocytes, and the differentiation of monocytes into macrophages [22]. In M-CSF-treated op/op mice, processes of hepatic granuloma formation similar to those of normal littermates were demonstrated by a single intravenous injection of Zymosan [21]. Zymosan injection induced an influx of monocytes into the liver and their differentiation into macrophages in loco in the early stage of hepatic granuloma formation, followed by the proliferation of Kupffer cells in its late stage [21]. These data indicate that monocytes are mobilized from bone marrow and migrate into the liver, where they differentiate into macrophages in loco, and that Kupffer cells proliferate in response to inflammatory stimuli [21].

# The Role of Macrophages in Hepatic Granuloma Formation in Mice Homozygous for the GM-CSF Mutation

Breeders of GM-CSF-deficient mice were given by Dr. Glenn Dranoff (Dana Farber Cancer Institute, Boston, MA, USA) and homozygous, heterozygous, and wild types of the mouse were distinguished by polymerase chain reaction (PCR) using GM-CSF genomic DNA. Compared with the wild type, hepatic granuloma formation in the GM-CSF-deficient mice was delayed until 5 days after Zymosan injection. The number and size of granulomas peaked at 8 days, when they reached the levels of the wild type. From 8 days after injection, hepatic granulomas declined more rapidly in the GM-CSF-deficient mice than in the wild type, and disappeared at 14 days. Compared with the wild type, the number of monocytes in the hepatic granulomas of GM-CSF-deficient mice was reduced by 5 days after injection. Investigation by reverse transcriptase (RT)-PCR revealed no significant difference in the expression of MCP-1, IL-1, TNF-$\alpha$, or INF-$\gamma$ between the homozygous and wild types. The reduced influx of monocytes/macrophages into the hepatic granulomas and the rapid disappearance of the granulomas in GM-CSF-deficient mice seem to result from a total lack of functional GM-CSF activity.

# The Effect of IL-5 on Hepatic Granuloma Formation in Transgenic Mice Overexpressing IL-5 and in IL-5-Treated Mice

To clarify the role of IL-5 in hepatic granuloma formation in vivo, glucan (0.1 mg/g body weight) was injected into the tail vein of IL-5 transgenic mice, IL-5-treated C3H/HeN mice, and C3H/HeN control mice, and the animals were killed 2, 5, 8, 10, or 14 days after injection [23]. IL-5 (1 $\mu$g/day) was injected intraperitoneally into C3H/HeN mice daily from 3 days before to 14 days after glucan injection. In the liver of IL-5 transgenic mice and IL-5-treated mice, granulomas started developing from 2 days after glucan injection, and their number and size became larger with days after injection. However, unlike the control mice, the hepatic granulomas in the transgenic and IL-5-treated mice showed marked infiltration of eosinophils, abscess formation, and necrosis, and their number and size were greater than in the control mice [23]. In both the transgenic and IL-5-treated mice, marked eosinophilia appeared in peripheral blood. In our previous studies on IL-5 inhibition with an anti-mouse monoclonal antibody against IL-5, NC17, infiltration of eosinophils, abscess formation, and necrosis were completely inhibited in the IL-5-treated mice, accompanied by reduction in the volume and number of hepatic granulomas [23]. The reduced number and volume of the hepatic granulomas are due mainly to the inhibition of eosinophil infiltration and/or the disappearance of necrosis in the granulomas [23]. In the IL-5 transgenic mice, however, NC17-pretreatment did not inhibit hepatic granuloma formation [23]. Based on these results, IL-5 seems to induce eosinophilia in peripheral blood, the migration and infiltration of eosinophils into the hepatic granulomas, and the enhancement of hepatic granuloma formation.

# The Role of T Lymphocytes in Hepatic Granuloma Formation in Immunodeficient Mice

In order to elucidate the role of T lymphocytes in hepatic granuloma formation, we used three different immunodeficient mice: nude (Hfhllnu/Hfhllnu) mice, C3H/HeN and CB-17/lcr-scid mice, and CBA/N(xid/xid) mice. Nude mice are congenitally athymic, have a profound deficiency of T cells, and lack T cell-dependent immune responses in the early stage of adult life. A single intravenous injection of Zymosan into the nude mice and control BALB/c mice induced granuloma formation in the liver, but the number and size of hepatic granulomas and the influx of monocytes into the granulomas were slightly smaller in the nude mice. Also, differentiation, maturation, and activation of macrophages in the granulomas were delayed in the nude mice compared with the controls [24]. In the nude mice, Thy 1.2-positive T cells infiltrated in the Zymosan-induced hepatic granulomas, but their percentages in the granulomas and peripheral blood were lower than in the control mice [24].

Severe combined immunodeficiency (scid) mice are a murine model of T and B cell dysfunction. In the scid mice, the development and formation of hepatic granulomas were delayed for more than a week after Zymosan injection, the influx of monocytes into the granulomas in the early stage of granuloma formation was reduced compared with the controls, and the percentages of Thy 1.2-positive T cells in the granulomas and peripheral blood were also lower than in the controls [25]. However, [$^3$H]thymidine labeling rates of macrophages in the granulomas in the nude and scid mice were not different from those of the control mice, and B220- and IgM-positive B cells were a minor cell population in the hepatic granulomas [25]. In both immunodeficient mice, T cell deficiency seems to result in a delay in hepatic granuloma formation due to a failure in the differentiation, maturation, and activation of macrophages in loco.

Xid mice are a murine model of X-linked immunodeficiency (xid) with impaired proliferation and differentiation of B cells [26]. In xid mice, however, the number of T cells is normal in peripheral blood. After Zymosan injection, the number of hepatic granulomas slightly increased in the early stage, peaked at 5 days, and rapidly declined from 8 days on [25]. The influx of monocytic cells and earlier macrophage precursors into the granulomas, the proliferative capacity of granuloma macrophages, and the phagocytosis and digestive capacity of granuloma macrophages for glucan particles were increased in the xid mice compared with the controls [25]. In the xid mice, the percentage of T cells in the granulomas was higher than in the control mice [25]. Such an increased percentage of T cells seems to result in activation of macrophages and their function in hepatic granulomas, leading to a rapid disappearance of granulomas by enhanced phagocytosis and digestion of glucan particles by macrophages in the hepatic granulomas.

The above-mentioned data shown in three different types of immunodeficient mouse indicate that T lymphocytes are involved in the activation of macrophages in hepatic granuloma formation in vivo.

## The Role of Type I and Type II Class A Macrophage Scavenger Receptors (MSR-A) in Hepatic Granuloma Formation

Among the numerous cell surface receptors of macrophages, scavenger receptors are essential for endocytosis by macrophages, together with Fc receptor and complement (C3) receptor. There are several different types of macrophage scavenger receptors (MSR), divided into classes A, B, and C. The class A macrophage scavenger receptors (MSR-A) include type I, type II, and MARCO receptors, all of which are important for the uptake of a variety of negatively charged macromolecules and bacterial antigens [27, 28]. To investigate the role of MSR-A, mice deficient in type I and type II MSR-A were generated by disrupting exon 4 of the MSR-A gene, which is essential for the formation of functional trimeric receptors [27, 29]. Mice homozygous for the MSR-A mutation were normal in both appearance and growth and were fertile like the wild type. Immunostaining of liver sections from the mice, using anti-MSR-A monoclonal antibody 2F8, demonstrated the presence of MSR-A protein in Kupffer cells and sinusoidal endothelial cells of the wild type; however, MSR-A protein was absent in the mice homozygous for the MSR-A mutation [27, 29]. To produce hepatic granulomas, 2 mg of Zymocel ($\beta$-glucan) was injected intravenously into the MSR-A-deficient mice and wild-type mice, and the animals were killed at 3, 5, 7, 10, 14, or 21 days after injection. In Zymocel-injected MSR-A-deficient mice, the hepatic granulomas were larger and more irregular than those of the wild type mice, suggesting the failure of cell adhesion in the granulomas [29]. However, the formation of compact and densely cellular hepatic granulomas was delayed in the early stage in the MSR-A-deficient mice compared with the wild type, and the influx of monocytes into the hepatic granulomas was reduced. Therefore, type I and type II MSR-A are important for hepatic granuloma formation in the early stage. In the MSR-A-deficient mice, the expression of MARCO receptor in granuloma macrophages and MARCO mRNA in the liver was demonstrated by immunostaining using a monoclonal antibody against MARCO receptor, and by RT-PCR with MARCO cDNA from the early stage of the granuloma formation. This finding indicates that the MARCO receptor is expressed on macrophages independently from type I and type II MSR-A.

## Discussion

$\beta$-glucan, a component of Zymosan, used in our studies is an intense stimulant for macrophages [30, 31] and induces increased numbers of granulocyte/macrophage colony-forming cells (GM-CFC), macrophage colony-forming cells (M-CFC), monocytic cells in bone marrow [30, 31], and extramedullary hematopoiesis [32]. It also induces increased numbers of macrophages and their proliferation in the liver by enhanced expression and production of growth factors such as M-CSF and GM-CSF in loco [17, 31]. In addition to these, other growth factors or pro-inflammatory cytokines such as MCP-1, IL-1, IL-3, TNF-$\alpha$, and INF-$\gamma$ are produced in the liver by glucan injection [18]. In this review article, we mentioned that Kupffer cells and monocyte-derived macrophages are different cell populations, are derived from macrophage precursor cells at different stages of differentiation, and show marked differences in their lifespan, proliferative capacity, and ontogenetic or post-natal differentiation.

In the liver, Kupffer cells are the first cells to protect against exogenously invading pathogenic microorganisms. If Kupffer cells are deleted from the liver by administration of lipo-MDP, granulomas are not formed in the initial stage of hepatic granuloma formation and the granuloma formation is markedly delayed. Since Kupffer cells produce M-CSF, GM-CSF, IL-3, MCP-1, and other pro-inflammatory cytokines in response to injected glucan, the production of these growth factors and cytokines are markedly reduced in mice deleted of Kupffer cells, resulting in a delay of monocyte mobilization and migration into the liver, impairment of their differentiation into macrophages, and disturbance of macrophage maturation and activation [17]. $^{89}$Sr-induced, severely monocytopenic mice cannot supply sufficient monocytes to the liver after glucan injection, which induces a marked delay in hepatic granuloma formation. In monocytopenic mice, it takes several days to induce proliferation of Kupffer cells and their granuloma formation against injected glucan particles. Since monocyte-derived macrophages produce a variety of cytokines including MCP-1, M-CSF, and GM-CSF, monocytes are considered important for hepatic granuloma formation in its early stage [17, 19].

In op/op mice defective in the production of functional M-CSF protein, similar processes are considered, although the Kupffer cells are immature and show a low proliferative capacity compared with those of normal littermates. In mice homozygous for the op mutation, hepatic granuloma formation is delayed due to a complete or nearly complete deficiency of blood monocytes, a defective monocyte supply to the liver, and impairment of their differentiation into macrophages. In mutant mice, the hepatic granulomas seem to be formed by the accumulation of immature Kupffer cells and their functional activation by GM-CSF and growth factors other than M-CSF [22]. Because M-CSF is essential for the development of monocytic cells in bone marrow, the differentiation of monocytes into macrophages, the proliferation of immature Kupffer cells, and Kupffer cell maturation, M-CSF administration induces increased levels of monocyte influx into the liver, monocyte/macrophage differentiation and maturation, and the proliferation and maturation of Kupffer cells in op/op mice which correspond to those of normal littermates [22]. Our preliminary study revealed a delay in Zymosan-induced hepatic granuloma formation in its early stage and a rapid disappearance of the granulomas in GM-CSF-deficient mice. These seem to be caused by GM-CSF deficiency, since GM-CSF is involved in the migration, proliferation, and survival of macrophages, as shown in GM-CSF transgenic mice [33] and in GM-CSF-treated op/op mice [34]. In our previous studies on hepatic granuloma formation in IL-5 transgenic and IL-5-treated mice, the infiltration of eosinophils, abscess formation, and necrosis in the granulomas were prominent features, and the number and size of the granulomas were greater than in the controls [22]. In the process of hepatic granuloma formation, no direct effects of IL-5 on granuloma macrophages were evident in vivo, although GM-CSF, IL-3, and IL-5 are known to have overlapping functions [35, 36].

It is known that in vitro, T lymphocytes produce many cytokines in response to stimuli and are involved in the activation and maturation of macrophages. In our previous and ongoing in vivo studies using nude mice and scid mice, a marked delay in Zymosan-induced hepatic granuloma formation has been demonstrated in both types of immunodeficient mouse; this seems to result from the reduction of monocyte influx into the granulomas and the low proliferative capacity of the macrophages, as well as a delay in their differentiation and activation [24, 25]. In the immunodeficient mice, the number of T cells was proved to be reduced in the hepatic granulomas, a reduction which seems to retard hepatic granuloma formation [24, 25]. In contrast with these immunodeficient mice, xid mice show X-linked immunodeficiency due to a point mutation in the Bruton's tyrosine kinase gene. The animals have a smaller peripheral B cell pool than normal animals, lack CD5-positive B (B-1) cells, and show low responses to anti-immunoglobulins and thymus-independent type 2 antigens [26]. In xid mice, the number and size of hepatic granulomas had increased by 5 days after Zymosan injection and reduced from 8 days on, compared with the control mice. These changes were parallel to the influx of monocytes and macrophage precursors into the granulomas of xid mice [25]. In addition, the proliferative capacity of macrophages and the uptake and digestion of glucan particles by macrophages were increased in the hepatic granulomas of xid mice, suggesting that granuloma macrophages are activated [25]. Compared with the control mice, the number of T cells in the hepatic granulomas of xid mice increased, which seems to induce the activation of granuloma macrophages.

Our studies revealed that glucan-induced hepatic granuloma formation in MSR-A-deficient mice was delayed in its early stage compared with that of wild-type mice [29]. These granulomas showed a loose, irregular shape in MSR-A-deficient mice [29]. These properties were caused by MSR-A deficiency, as MSR-A is known to mediate cation-independent macrophage adhesion [37]. Since type I and type II MSR-A and MARCO receptors participate in the uptake of bacterial antigens by macrophages, MSR-A deficiency seems to result in reduced uptake of glucan particles by macrophages in MSR-A-deficient mice, leading to a delay in macrophage activation. Since MARCO receptor is expressed at the protein and messenger levels on macrophages in both MSR-A-deficient and wild-type mice, it may play a major role in the uptake of glucan particles by macrophages and in granuloma formation in mutant mice. To clarify the role of MARCO and other receptors in hepatic granuloma formation, it is necessary to investigate granuloma formation in mice homozygous for a gene mutation of the MARCO receptor and other receptors involved in the endocytosis of bacteria.

In this article, we have reviewed abnormal hepatic granuloma formation in mice defective at the cellular, cytokine, and receptor levels to explain the multiple roles of macrophage involvement in the different steps of defense mechanisms against bacterial antigens exogenously invading the liver (Fig. 2).

138    K. Takahashi et al.

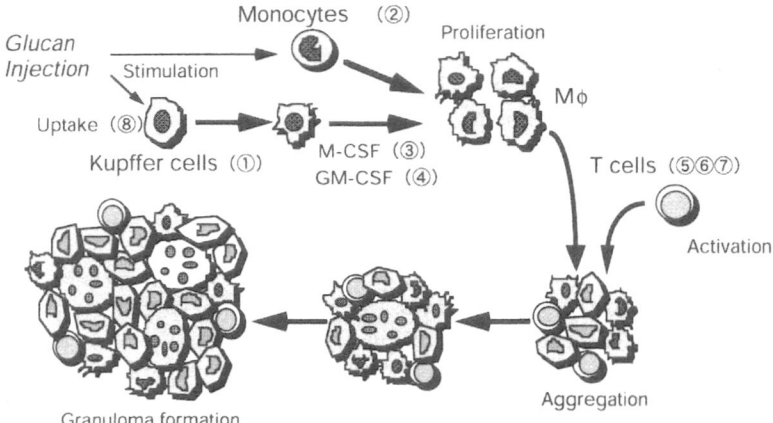

FIG. 2. A schematic representation of macrophage involvement in hepatic granuloma formation in mice. ① mice devoid of Kupffer cells after lipo-MDP; ② mice devoid of blood monocytes after $^{89}$Sr; ③ op/op mice (M-CSF deficiency); ④ GM-CSF-deficient mice (GM-CSF deficiency; ⑤ nude mice (T-cell defect); ⑥ scid mice (T and B cell defect); ⑦ xid mice (B cell abnormality); ⑧ MSR-A-deficient mice (MSR-A deficiency)

*Acknowledgments.* We thank Dr. Leonard D. Shultz, the Jackson Laboratory, Bar Harbor, Maine, USA, for supplying breeders of op/op mice, and Dr. Glenn Dranoff, Dana Farber Cancer Institute, Boston, USA, for sending breeders of GM-CSF-deficient mice.

## References

1. Takahashi K, Yamamura F, Naito M (1989) Differentiation, maturation, and proliferation of macrophages in the yolk sac: A light-microscopic, enzyme-cytochemical, immunohistochemical, and ultrastructural study. J Leukoc Biol 45:87–96
2. Takahashi K, Naito M (1993) Development, differentiation, and proliferation of macrophages in the rat yolk sac. Tissue Cell 25:351–362
3. Naito M, Yamamura F, Nishikawa S-I, et al. (1989) Development, differentiation, and maturation of fetal mouse yolk sac macrophages in cultures. J Leukoc Biol 46:1–10
4. Naito M, Takahashi K, Nishikawa S-I (1990) Development, differentiation, and maturation of macrophages in the fetal mouse liver. J Leukoc Biol 48:27–37
5. Naito M, Takahashi K, Takahashi H, et al. (1982) Ontogenetic development of Kupffer cells. In: Knook DL, Wisse E (eds) Sinusoidal liver cells. Elsevier Biochemical, Amsterdam, pp 155–164
6. Naito M, Yamamura F, Takeya M, et al. (1986) Ultrastructural analysis of Kupffer cell progenitors. In: Kirn A, Knook DL, Wisse E (eds) Cells of the hepatic sinusoid, vol 1. Kupffer Cell Foundation, Rijwijk, pp 13–20
7. Naito M, Takahashi K, Nishikawa S-I (1989) Yolk sac macrophages: A possible Kupffer cell precursor in the fetal mouse liver. In: Wisse E, Knook DL, Decker K (eds) Cells of the hepatic sinusoid, vol 2. Kupffer Cell Foundation, Rijwijk, pp 419–420
8. Morioka Y, Naito M, Sato T, et al. (1994) Immunophenotypic and ultrastructural heterogeneity of macrophage differentiation in bone marrow and fetal hematopoiesis of mouse in vivo and in vitro. J Leukoc Biol 84:27–35

9. Takahashi K, Naito M, Takeya M (1996) Development and heterogeneity of macrophages and their related cells through their differentiation pathways. Pathol Int 46:473–485
10. Naito M, Hayashi S-I, Yoshida H, et al. (1991) Abnormal differentiation of tissue macrophage populations in "osteopetrosis" (op) mice defective in the production of macrophage colony-stimulating factor. Am J Pathol 139:657–667
11. van Furth R (1989) Origin and turnover of monocytes and macrophages. In: Iverson OH (ed) Cell kinetics of inflammatory reaction. Springer Verlag, Berlin-Heidelberg, pp 125–150 .
12. Travassoli M, Yoffey JM (1983) Bone marrow: Structure and function. Alan R Liss, New York, pp 235–256
13. Tondravi MM, McKercher SR, Anderson K, et al. (1997) Osteopetrosis in mice lacking hematopoietic transcription factor PU.1. Nature 386:81–84
14. McKercher SR, Torbet BC, Anderson L, et al. (1996) Targeted disruption of the PU.1 gene results in multiple hematopoietic abnormalities. EMBO J 15:5647–5658
15. Yamada M, Naito M, Takahashi K (1990) Kupffer cell proliferation and glucan-induced granuloma formation in mice deleted of blood monocytes by strontium-89. J Leukoc Biol 47:195–205
16. Yamamoto T, Naito M, Moriyama H, et al. (1996) Repopulation of murine Kupffer cells after intravenous administration of liposome-encapsulated dichloromethylene diphosphonate. Am J Pathol 149:1271–1286
17. Moriyama H, Yamamoto T, Takatsuka H, et al. (1997) Expression of macrophage colony-stimulating factor and its receptor in hepatic granulomas of Kupffer-cell-depleted mice. Am J Pathol 150:2047–2060
18. Volkman A, Chang NC, Strausbauch PH, et al. (1983) Differential effects of chronic monocyte depletion on macrophage populations. 49:291–298
19. Naito M, Takahashi K (1991) The role of Kupffer cells in glucan-induced granuloma formation in the liver of mice depleted of blood monocytes by administration of strontium-89. Lab Invest 64:664–674
20. Yoshida H, Hayashi S-I, Kunisada T, et al. (1990) The murine mutation "osteopetrosis" (op) is a mutation in the coding region of the macrophage colony-stimulating factor (Csfm) gene. Nature 345:442–443
21. Takahashi K, Naito M, Umeda S, et al. (1994) The role of macrophage colony-stimulating factor in hepatic glucan-induced granuloma formation in the osteopetrosis mutant mouse defective in the production of macrophage colony-stimulating factor. Am J Pathol 144:1381–1392
22. Umeda S, Takahashi K, Shultz LD, et al. (1996) Effects of macrophage colony-stimulating factor on macrophages and their related cell populations in the osteopetrosis mouse defective in production of functional macrophage colony-stimulating factor protein. Am J Pathol 149:559–574
23. Takahashi K, Honda Y, Tominaga A, et al. (1995) Effects of anti-mouse IL-5 monoclonal antibody NC17 on glucan-induced hepatic granuloma formation in IL-5 transgenic mice and IL-5-treated mice. In: Wisse E, Knook DL, Wake K (eds) Cells of the hepatic sinusoid, vol 5. Kupffer Cell Foundation, Leiden, pp 300–303
24. Naito H, Honda Y, Umeda S, et al. (1993) Glucan-induced granuloma formation in the liver of osteopetrosis (op) and nude (nu) mutant mice. In: Knook DL, Wisse E (eds) Cells of the hepatic sinusoid, vol 4. Kupffer Cell Foundation, Leiden, pp 95–100
25. Takahashi K, Miyakawa K, Myint YY, et al. (1997) Zymocel-induced granuloma formation in the liver of immunodeficient mice. In: Wisse E, Knook DL, Balaband C (eds) Cells of the hepatic sinusoid, vol 6. Kupffer Cell Foundation, Leiden, pp 290–292
26. Woodland RT, Schmidt MR, Korsmeyer SJ, et al. (1996) Regulation of B cell survival in xid mice by the proto-oncogene bcl-2. J Immunol 156:2143–2154

27. Suzuki H, Kurihara Y, Takeya M, et al. (1997) A role for macrophage scavenger receptors in atherosclerosis and susceptibility to infection. Nature 386:292–296
28. Elomaa O, Kangas M, Sahlberg C, et al. (1995) Cloning of a novel bacteria-binding receptor structurally related to scavenger receptors and expressed in a subset of macrophages. Cell 80:603–609
29. Suzuki H, Kurihara Y, Takeya M, et al. (1997) The multiple roles of macrophage scavenger receptors (MSR) in vivo: Resistance to atherosclerosis and susceptibility to infection in MSR-knockout mice. J Atherosc Thromb 4:1–11
30. Deiman W, Fahimi H (1980) Induction of focal hematopoiesis in adult rat liver by glucan, a macrophage stimulator. Lab Invest 42:217–224
31. Williams DL, Pretus HA, Jones RB, et al. (1989) Glucan stimulates in vitro proliferation of murine Kupffer cells. In: Wisse E, Knook DL, Decker K (eds), Cells of hepatic sinusoid, vol 2. Kupffer Cell Foundation, Rijwijk, pp 390–393
32. Patchen Ml, D'Alesandro MM, Brook I, et al. (1987) Glucan: Mechanisms involved in its "radio-protective" effect. J Leukoc Biol 42:95–105
33. Metcalf C (1994) Granulocyte-macrophage colony-stimulating factor transgenic mice. In: Jacob CO (ed), Over-expression and knockout of cytokines in transgenic mice. Academic Press, London, pp 161–186
34. Wiktor-Jedrejczak W, Urbanowska E, Szperl M (1994) Granulocyte-macrophage colony-stimulating factor corrects macrophage deficiency, not osteopetrosis in the macrophage-stimulating factor-1-deficient op/op mouse. Endocrinology 134:1932–1935
35. Emarson SG, Yang YE, Clark SC, et al. (1988) Human recombinant granulocyte-macrophage-stimulating factor and interleukin-3 have overlapping but distinct hematopoietic activities. J Clin Invest 82:1282–1287
36. Takatsu K, Tominaga A (1991) Interleukin-5 and its receptor. Prog Growth Factor Res 3:89–102
37. Fraser I, Highes D, Gordon S (1993) Divalent cation-independent macrophage adhesion inhibited by murine scavenger receptor. Nature 364:343–346

# Roles of Sinusoidal Endothelial Cells in the Local Regulation of Hepatic Sinusoidal Blood Flow—Involvement of Endothelins and Nitric Oxide

Masaya Oda[1], Hiroaki Yokomori[2], and Yoshitaka Kamegaya[1]

*Summary.* This chapter reviews current understanding of the regulation of hepatic microcirculation, with particular reference to the authors' own work on the roles of sinusoidal endothelial cells and the mechanism of dynamic changes in the sinusoidal endothelial fenestrae (SEF) induced by the potent vasoconstrictor endothelin (ET)-1. From the viewpoint of myogenic control in microcirculation, it is considered essential for the local control of hepatic sinusoidal blood flow that the dynamic contracting and relaxing changes of the SEF correspond with those of Ito cells (hepatic stallate cells, HSCs), both of which are mediated by the sinusoidal endothelium-derived vasoconstrictor endothelins (ETs) and the vasodilator nitric oxide (NO). The contractility of the SEF and HSCs entirely depends on the intracellular $Ca^{2+}$–calmodulin–actomyosin system, in which plasma membrane $Ca^{2+}$-pump ATPase controlling the intracytoplasmic free calcium concentration $[Ca^{2+}]_i$ is one of the key modulators.

ET-1 produced and released from the sinusoidal endothelial cells acts on the HSCs via the $ET_A$ receptors as a paracrine effect, inducing a contraction of the HSCs. ET-1 also acts on the sinusoidal endothelial cells themselves via the $ET_B$ receptors as an autocrine effect, inducing a contraction of the SEF with a prompt elevation of $[Ca^{2+}]_i$ enhanced by a decrease in fenestral plasma membrane $Ca^{2+}$-pump ATPase. This elevation of $[Ca^{2+}]_i$ is markedly suppressed by pretreatment with an $ET_B$ receptor antagonist. In parallel with this process, NO produced by NO synthase (NOS) within the sinusoidal endothelial cells gets into the HSCs, inducing a relaxation of the HSCs.

*Key words.* Hepatic sinusoidal endothelium, Sinusoidal endothelial fenestrae, Endothelin-1, Endothelin receptor subtypes ($ET_A$, $ET_B$ receptor), Intracytoplasmic free calcium ions

---

[1]Department of Internal Medicine, School of Medicine, Keio University, 35 Shinanomachi, Shinjuku-ku, Tokyo 160-0016, Japan
[2]Division of Internal Medicine, Kitasato Institute Medical Center Hospital, 6-100 Arai, Kitamoto, Saitama 364-0026, Japan

The hepatic microcirculatory system consists of three microvascular components: the terminal portal venule (TPV) and the terminal hepatic arteriole (THA) as two afferent vessels, the sinusoids corresponding to the capillary bed, and the terminal hepatic venule (THV) as an efferent vessel [1]. From an ultrastructural point of view, the hepatic sinusoids located between the liver cell cords are characterized by the presence of a large number of sieve plate-like pores in the sinusoidal endothelium, i.e., the sinusoidal endothelial fenestrae (SEF) [2], and by the absence of the basement membrane beneath the sinusoidal endothelium, allowing free exchange between the sinusoidal blood and the hepatocytes via the SEF. It is noteworthy that these anastomosing sinusoids occupy the largest areas of the hepatic microvasculature, possibly contributing to the regulatory mechanism of hepatic microcirculation by changing the circulatory blood volumes in the sinusoids and microvascular tones.

In recent years, the authors have postulated that the contraction and dilatation of the SEF as well as of the sinusoids would be involved in the local regulation of hepatic sinusoidal blood flow [3, 4]. There has been increasing evidence that microvascular tones are regulated by vasoconstrictor endothelins (ETs) [5] and vasodilator nitric oxide (NO) [6] corresponding to the endothelium-derived relaxing factor (EDRF), both of which are derived from vascular endothelial cells.

The main purpose of this chapter is to review current understanding of the regulation of hepatic sinusoidal microcirculation, particularly focusing on the authors' recent work on the roles of sinusoidal endothelial cells and the mechanism of dynamic changes of the SEF induced by a potent and long-acting vasoconstrictor endothelin-1 [7].

# Morphological and Physiological Features of Hepatic Microcirculation

The hepatic microvascular system is characterized by the structure that the sinusoids, corresponding to the capillary bed in the microcirculatory system, receive the blood from two types of afferent vessels, the portal vein and the hepatic artery, both of which have different blood pressure and circulating blood volume [1] (Fig. 1). The blood circulating in the anastomosing sinusoids then empties into the efferent vessels, the terminal hepatic venules, at an angle which almost forms a right angle with the vessel walls, as has been observed by intravital and scanning electron microscopy [3].

This specialized microvascular system of the liver is peculiar in that a ratio of the precapillary (presinusoidal) to the postcapillary (postsinusoidal) resistance is much greater than in other microvascular systems [8]. Blood pressure in the hepatic sinusoids is very low [9] in comparison with that of the portal venules and of the hepatic arterioles, and the pressure gradient from the sinusoids to the hepatic venules is small [1, 8]. Based on the concept of microcirculatory autoregulation, there seems to be no distinct autoregulatory mechanism in the local control of portal venous and hepatic arterial blood flow [10].

There is no doubt, however, that the contraction and relaxation of the smooth muscle layers of the hepatic arterioles and portal venules are effectively involved in the dynamic control of the hepatic microvascular blood flow [1]. In relation to this

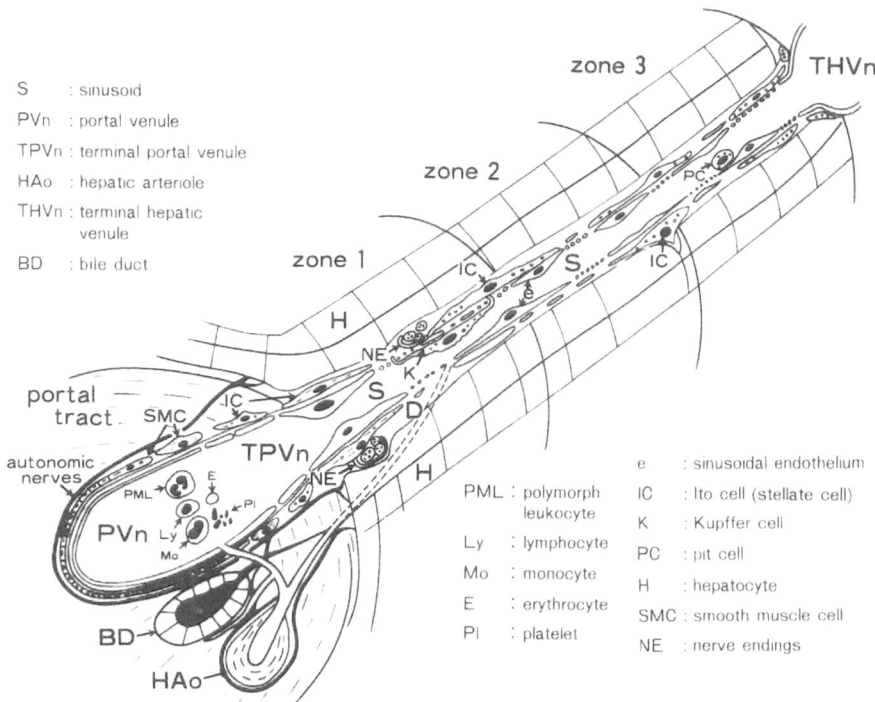

S     : sinusoid
PVn   : portal venule
TPVn  : terminal portal venule
HAo   : hepatic arteriole
THVn  : terminal hepatic
        venule
BD    : bile duct

zone 3                THVn
zone 2
zone 1

portal
tract
autonomic
nerves

PML : polymorph
      leukocyte
Ly  : lymphocyte
Mo  : monocyte
E   : erythrocyte
Pl  : platelet

e    : sinusoidal endothelium
IC   : Ito cell (stellate cell)
K    : Kupffer cell
PC   : pit cell
H    : hepatocyte
SMC  : smooth muscle cell
NE   : nerve endings

FIG. 1.  Hepatic microvasculature and sinusoidal cells

regulatory mechanism, it has been proposed that the inlet and outlet sphincters are important in the regulation of the blood flow through the sinusoids [1, 11].

In spite of a large number of ultrastructural studies, no distinct sphincter structures (such as the precapillary sphincter of the terminal arteriole identified by electron microscopy in the muscle microvasculature [12]) have been identified at the pre- or postsinusoidal junctional sites where the blood enters the sinusoids from the terminal portal venule (TPV) or drains into the terminal hepatic venule (THV).

## Relation Between Hepatic Sinusoidal Cells and Hepatic Microvasculature

It is well known that the hepatic sinusoid is composed of four different cell types, i.e., endothelial cells, Ito cells (hepatic stellate cells, HSCs) [13], Kupffer cells and pit cells (Fig. 1). It has been confirmed by scanning electron microscopy that the TPV directly connect with the sinusoids, and the endothelial cells of the TPV are continuously transformed into sinusoidal endothelial cells possessing a large number of sieve plate-like pores [3] (Fig. 1). By scanning electron microscopic analysis, HSCs have been shown to encircle the abluminal surfaces of the sinusoidal endothelial cells with their extended and interconnected cytoplasmic processes [13]. Kupffer cells stick to the luminal surfaces of the sinusoidal endothelial cells, extending their processes into the perisinusoidal space (the space of Disse) through the sinusoidal endothelial pores and attaching to the processes stretching out from the HSCs, and sometimes migrating onto the endothelial luminal surface in an ameboid movement [14, 15].

# Regulatory Factors of Hepatic Sinusoidal Blood Flow

In general, the regulatory factors of organ microcirculation are divided into three groups, i.e., myogenic, neurogenic, and humoral control (Fig. 2). This article deals with myogenic control and the surrounding hepatic microcirculation, mainly focussing on recent understanding of the regulatory mechanism of hepatic sinusoidal microcirculation.

## The Inlet Sphincter-Like Structures at the Junction Between the TPV and the Sinusoid

By scanning electron microscopy, the junctional area between the TPV and the sinusoid is occasionally found to be extremely narrow and almost occluded [3], implying the presence of an inlet sphincter-like structure which would locally control the sinusoidal blood flow. By transmission electron microscopy, the presence of a long continuous and unfenestrated endothelium surrounded by a basement membrane, with no smooth muscle layer, has been confirmed at the junction between the TPV and the sinusoid [3], as had been proposed earlier [11]. Although there are no structures specializing as a sphincter, such as an endothelial-smooth muscular junction [12], actin filaments are evident in the junctional endothelium [3].

### REGULATORY FACTORS IN ORGAN MICROCIRCULATION

1. **Myogenic Control**
2. **Nervous Control**
3. **Humoral Control**

**Diversity of the above controling systems in each organ**

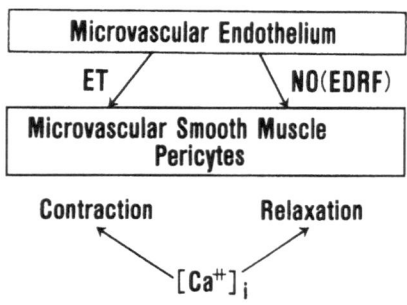

FIG. 2. Involvement of microvascular endothelium-derived vasoconstrictor endothelins (*ETs*) and vasodilator nitric oxide (*NO*) in myogenic control of organ microcirculation. Intracytoplasmic free calcium ion concentration $[Ca^{2+}]_i$ is a key modulator of the contraction and relaxation of microvascular endothelial cells and pericytes

Furthermore, there is recent evidence that HSC-like pericytes exist in close contact with the junctional endothelium between the TPV and the sinusoid [16, 17]. Based on a previous report on endothelial contractility [18], these findings suggest that this junctional portion would make a local circular contraction by the coordinative contractility of the transitional endothelium and the Ito cell-like pericyte [16, 17], possibly occluding the erythrocytes flowing into the sinusoids and locally regulating the sinusoidal blood flow [3].

## The Role of Terminal Hepatic Arterioles (THAs) in Hepatic Sinusoidal Microcirculation

Not only the intrahepatic distribution of the hepatic artery but also the blood supply ratio of the hepatic artery to the portal vein vary from one species to another. The THAs have branches in four different locations. Some of the THAs form microvascular plexuses around bile ducts in the portal tract, and some have branches which connect with the sinusoids [19]. Other branches from the THAs make anastomoses directly with the TPV, providing the vasa vasorum for branches of the portal vein.

The direct connections of hepatic arteriolar capillaries with the sinusoids in the periportal (zone 1) and middle (zone 2) zones, originally observed by intravital microscopy [1, 11, 19], have been confirmed both by scanning electron microscopy using corrosion cast preparations [20] and by an enzymohistochemical technique [21]. There seem to be no smooth muscle sphincters at the junction of the arteriolar capillaries with the sinusoids or TPV [19]. Even after ligation of the hepatic artery in the rat, hepatic blood flow measured by hydrogen gas clearance or the laser Doppler method is reduced by only 20%, whereas it is completely stopped after ligation of the portal trunk, indicating that hepatic sinusoidal blood flow mainly depends on the portal blood flow.

## Contraction and Relaxation of Hepatic Sinusoidal Endothelial Fenestrae (SEF) and Sinusoids

Based on in vivo studies [3, 4], it has been postulated that the hepatic sinusoids and SEF contract or dilate in response to a decrease or an increase in hepatic sinusoidal blood flow induced by neuroamines and neuropeptides, contributing to the homeostatic control of hepatic microcirculation. There is no doubt that the plasma flowing inside the sinusoidal vascular lumens variably transits the sinusoidal endothelial lining cells via the SEF in response to a variety of sinusoidal blood flow states. Thus the diameters and numbers of the SEF are considered not to be static but to be dynamic, regulating the transition of sinusoidal circulating plasma into the perisinusoidal space.

A question has been raised as to whether these dynamic changes in diameter in the SEF and sinusoids are active or passive phenomena. In an attempt to resolve this question, sinusoidal endothelial cells isolated from rat liver by the collagenase-perfusion method were subjected to primary monolayer culture, and then studied in vitro [4, 22–24]. The results showed that the SEF contract in in vitro culture conditions without blood flow after the addition of an $\alpha$-adrenoceptor agonist such as norepinephrine [4], neuropeptide Y (NPY) to the culture medium [4], or serotonin

[24], whereas they dilate after the addition of a $\beta$-adrenoreceptor agonist such as isoproterenol [4], or a muscarinic acetylcholine receptor ($M_2$) agonist such as acetylcholine [4], a vasoactive intestinal polypeptide (VIP) [4], or prostaglandin $E_1$ [23].

All these changes in fenestral diameters in vitro are considered to be mediated by receptors on the endothelial cell surface. Therefore, the contraction and dilatation of the SEF may not always be a secondary effect of the changes in sinusoidal blood flow volumes and resistances, but may also be actively induced by the actions of vasoactive substances.

## The $Ca^{2+}$-Calmodulin–Actomyosin System in the Hepatic Sinusoidal Endothelium

By immunofluorescence, immunoperoxidase, and electron microscopy, actin filaments are evident in the hepatic sinusoidal endothelial cells not only in primary culture but also in liver tissue [22, 25]. These microfilaments are specifically coated with heavy meromyosin [4], and are bound with fluorescein isothiocyanate (FITC)-labeled phalloidin. By electron microscopy, this coating has been shown to be particularly enriched around the labyrinth-like structures of the SEF [22, 24, 26], forming a cytoskeleton ring composed of actin and myosin [24], and providing a mechanical contractile basis for the SEF. Furthermore, by immunoelectron microscopy, a $Ca^{2+}$-binding protein calmodulin has also been found in the sinusoidal endothelium.

It has been shown that the addition of calcium ionophore to the culture medium causes an increase in intracytoplasmic free calcium ion concentration $[Ca^{2+}]_i$, determined by microfluorometric digital image analysis using fura-2 AM [27, 28], concomitant with a contraction of the SEF in the primary monolayer-cultured sinusoidal endothelium [22, 24]. On the other hand, an actin-depolymerizing agent, cytochalasin B, as well as a $Ca^{2+}$-binding protein calmodulin antagonist, W-7, cause dilation of the SEF in primary monolayer culture [4, 22]. However, it remains to be explained why the numbers of SEF are increased by prolonged treatment with cytochalasin B [29]. In addition, a $Ca^{2+}$-chelating agent EGTA and $Ca^{2+}$-channel blockers prevent a serotonin-induced contraction of the SEF [24].

Based on all the data described above, the $Ca^{2+}$-calmodulin–actomyosin system within the sinusoidal endothelium clearly plays a major role in the regulation of the contraction and dilatation of SEF. In this contractile process, myosin light chain kinase (MLCK) is a $Ca^{2+}$-calmodulin-dependent key enzyme for inducing the association of actin and myosin and the activation of myosin $Mg^{2+}$-ATPase [30]. The calmodulin antagonist (W-7)-induced dilatation of SEF is considered to be mainly due to the inhibition of $Ca^{2+}$-calmodulin-dependent phosphorylation of MLCK [31].

## Contractility of Ito Cells (Hepatic Stellate Cells) as Pericytes

As has been shown in other microvascular pericytes [32], it is essential for Ito cells (hepatic stellate cells, HSCs) to possess contractility as pericytes in providing tone to the hepatic sinusoids and maintaining a constant sinusoidal blood flow. Microfluorometric digital image analysis has revealed that a $Ca^{2+}$-agonist-induced elevation of intracytoplasmic free calcium ion concentration $[Ca^{2+}]_i$ results in a contraction of the HSCs isolated from human liver in primary monolayer culture [33].

This type of contraction in the HSCs isolated from rat liver has been shown to be enhanced by the addition of endothelin-1 to the culture medium according to the reduction rate of the areas of cells [34], the formation of wrinkles in the agar matrix [35], and time-lapse cinematography [36].

## Vascular Endothelium-Derived Vasoconstrictor Endothelins and Vasodilator Nitric Oxide

In recent years there has been accumulating evidence that hepatic microcirculation is controlled at least in part by the vasoconstricting and relaxing effects of endothelins (ETs) [5] and nitric oxide (NO) [6] (Fig. 2). The ETs can be divided into three isopeptides, ET-1, ET-2, and ET-3 [7]. Continuous infusion of ET-1 via the portal vein in the rat causes a decrease in hepatic sinusoidal blood flow measured by a laser Doppler flow metry [37], and this is concomitant with a reduction of the SEF both in diameter and in number shown by scanning electron microscopy [23] (Fig. 3a,b).

At the same time, as fluorescence microscopy had suggested in the isolated perfused rat liver [38], scanning electron microscopy revealed that hepatic sinusoids are locally constricted along the HSCs situated beneath the sinusoidal endothelial cells [23] (Fig. 3c,d). Furthermore, as had previously been shown in vivo by infusion of norepinephrine and NPY [4], hepatic sinusoids were also shown by intravital microscopy to be reduced in diameter following ET-1 infusion [39]. However, there is still a possibility that the terminal portal venules (TPVs) directly connecting with the sinusoids contract most intensely in response to ET-1 in the hepatic microvessels, thus reducing the sinusoidal blood flow, and as a result the sinusoids collapse rather than actively contract. Therefore, it seems unlikely that hepatic sinusoids themselves contract sufficiently to diminish red blood cell velocity.

On the other hand, nitric oxide (NO) produced and released from vascular endothelial cells would act on the HSCs, making them relaxed and leading to a reduction of vascular tone in the hepatic sinusoids [40]. It has recently been reported that carbon monoxide (CO) produced by the action of heme oxygenase in the degradation process of heme may be involved in a contraction of the HSCs [41]. The relation between NO and CO needs to be further elucidated.

## Local Regulatory Mechanisms of Hepatic Sinusoidal Microcirculation

From the viewpoint of myogenic control in the microcirculation, it is considered to be essential for the local regulation of hepatic sinusoidal blood flow that the dynamic contracting and relaxing of the sinusoidal endothelial cells and SEF should correspond with those of the HSCs, both of which are mediated by the sinusoidal endothelium-derived ETs and NO. According to a radioimmunoassay study [42], ET is released from primary cultured sinusoidal endothelial cells. In addition, it has recently been shown that NO is produced by the sinusoidal endothelial cells through the enzyme action of endothelial cell NO synthase (ecNOS) [43]. Contractility of the SEF and HSCs entirely depends on the intracellular $Ca^{2+}$–calmodulin–actomyosin system.

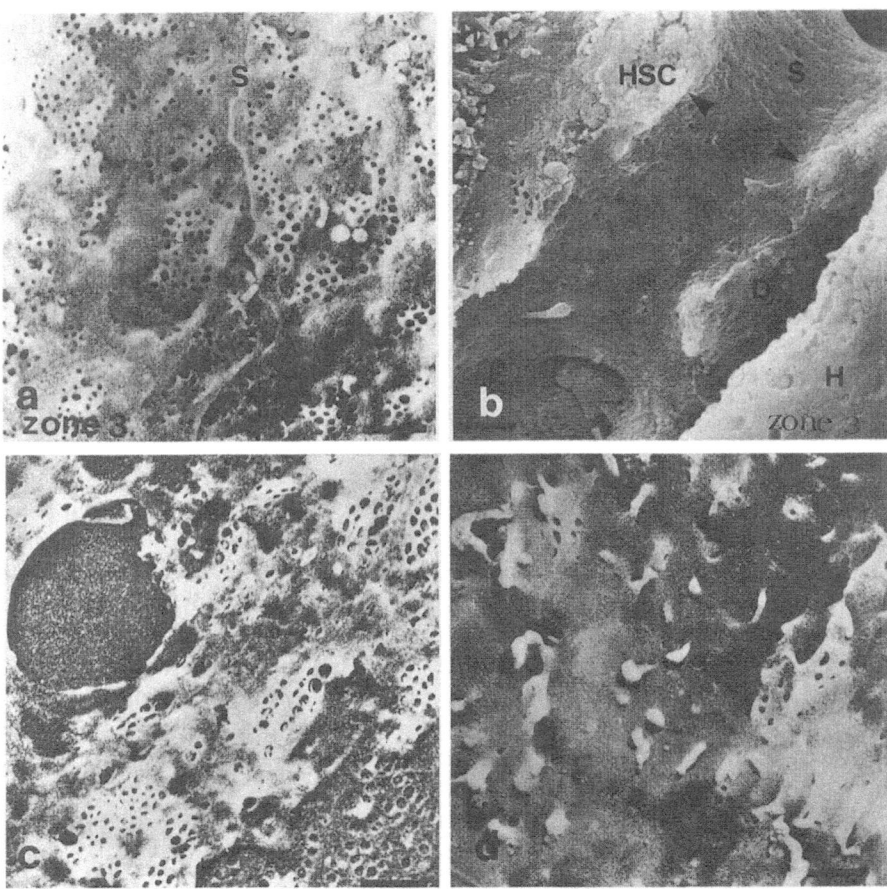

FIG. 3a–d. Scanning electron micrographs showing the effects of endothelin (ET)-1 on hepatic sinusoidal endothelial fenestrae (SEF) in vivo and in vitro. Each bar denotes 1 μm. **a** An internal view of the sinusoid in a control rat liver. There are a large number of SEF, approximately 90 nm in diameter, in zone 3. **b** An ET-1-infused rat liver. Note that the SEF are markedly decreased in diameter and in number in zone 3. The sinusoid (*S*) appears focally narrowed (*arrowheads*) along the hepatic stellate cell (*HSC*) beneath the sinusoidal endothelium. Compare with **a**. *D*, the space of Disse; *H*, hepatocyte. **c** A non-treated primary monolayer-cultured sinusoidal endothelium isolated from rat liver. There are a large number of SEF, as shown in **a**. **d** An ET-1-treated sinusoidal endothelium in primary monolayer culture. Note that the SEF are reduced in diameter and in number, as shown in vivo in **b**. Compare with **c**

# Intracytoplasmic Free Calcium Ions and $Ca^{2+}$-Pump ATPase

In the primary monolayer-cultured sinusoidal endothelium, the concentration of intracytoplasmic free $Ca^{2+}$ $[Ca^{2+}]_i$, determined by microfluorometric digital image analysis using fura-2 AM (Fig. 4), is immediately elevated by the addition of ET-1 to the culture medium [23] (Fig. 5a).

In general, it has been well documented that the plasma membrane $Ca^{2+}$-ATPase plays a major role in maintaining a very low concentration of intracellular free $Ca^{2+}$ by extruding $Ca^{2+}$ from the cytoplasm against a high concentration of extracellular free $Ca^{2+}$, thus contributing to the homeostatic control of intracellular free calcium ion concentration ($[Ca^{2+}]_i$) [44]. According to a recent report [45], this $Ca^{2+}$-pump ATPase is located in the caveolae of vascular endothelium. It is intriguing to note that the $Ca^{2+}$-pump ATPase is localized on the fenestral plasma membrane in the hepatic sinusoidal endothelium, which corresponds to the deeply and tortuously invaginated labyrinth structure of the sinusoidal endothelial plasma membrane [23]. Moreover, it is noteworthy that electron cytochemistry shows that plasma membrane $Ca^{2+}$-ATPase activities are also evident on the fenestral plasma membrane [23] (Fig. 6a). Although these $Ca^{2+}$-ATPase activities on the fenestral membrane may represent an ectoenzyme, as shown on the bile canalicular membrane [46], there is a possibility that these cytochemical $Ca^{2+}$-ATPase activities may parallel the $Ca^{2+}$-pump ATPase activities for active extrusion of $Ca^{2+}$ from the cytoplasm, since the structure of $Ca^{2+}$-pump ATPase is of the membrane-penetrating type [47]. Accordingly, the attenuation of fenestral plasma membrane $Ca^{2+}$-ATPase activities by ET-1 [23] (Fig. 6b) would cause an elevation of $[Ca^{2+}]_i$, possibly due to an inhibition of extrusion of intracytoplasmic $Ca^{2+}$, resulting in a contraction of the SEF.

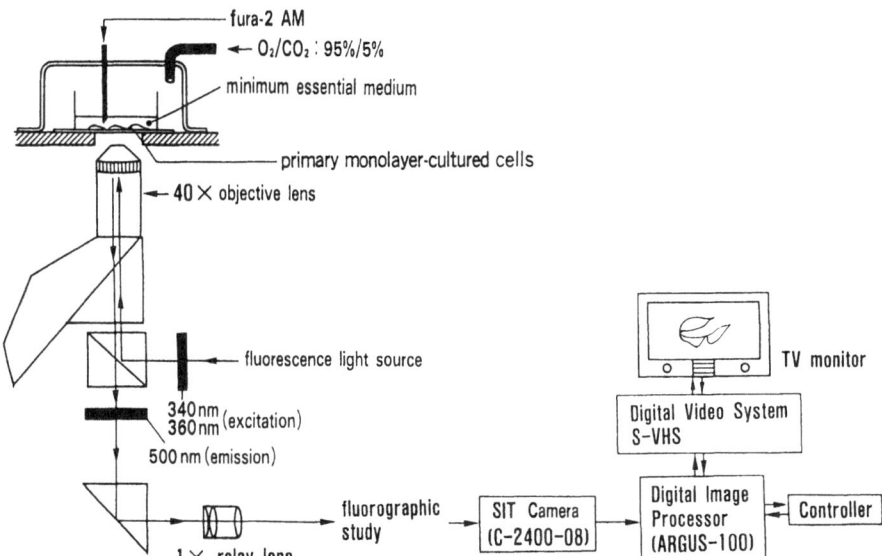

FIG. 4. Experimental design for microfluorometric digital image analysis of intracytoplasmic free calcium ion concentration $[Ca^{2+}]_i$ in primary monolayer-cultured sinusoidal endothelium

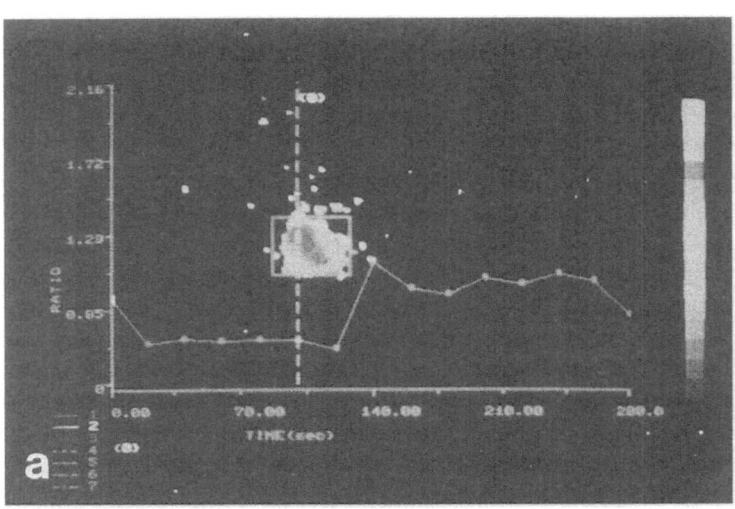

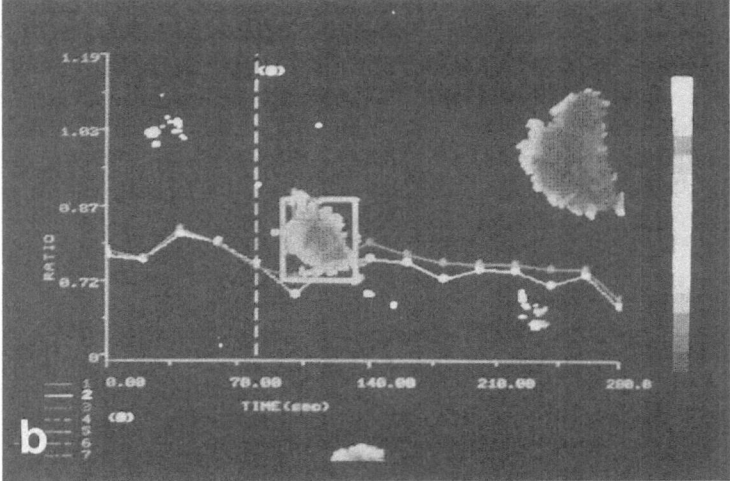

FIG. 5a,b. The time course changes of $[Ca^{2+}]_i$ in the primary monolayer-cultured sinusoidal endothelium by microfluorometric digital image analysis. **a** $[Ca^{2+}]_i$ is immediately elevated by the addition of ET-1 to the culture medium. **b** An ET-1-induced elevation of $[Ca^{2+}]_i$ is suppressed by pretreatment with $ET_B$ receptor antagonist (BQ788)

## Endothelin Receptor Subtypes: $ET_A$ and $ET_B$ Receptors

The pharmacological effects of ETs are transducted into a cell via receptors on the outer surface of the cell plasma membrane. $ET_A$ and $ET_B$ receptors are well documented as ET receptor subtypes [48]. $ET_A$ receptors show much stronger affinity to ET-1 and ET-2 than to ET-3, while $ET_B$ receptors possess almost equal affinity to

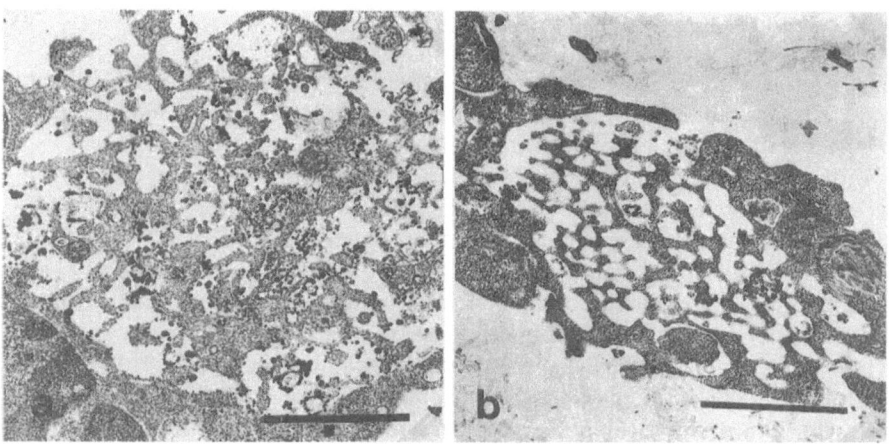

FIG. 6a,b. Transmission electron microscopic alterations of the $Ca^{2+}$-ATPase activities and the diameter of SEF by ET-1 treatment in the primary monolayer-cultured sinusoidal endothelium [23]. Each bar denotes 1 μm. **a** The electron-dense reaction products showing the presence of $Ca^{2+}$-ATPase activities are localized on the fenestral plasma membrane in the nontreated sinusoidal endothelium. **b** $Ca^{2+}$-ATPase activities are markedly decreased in the fenestral plasma membrane of the contracted SEF by treatment with ET-1

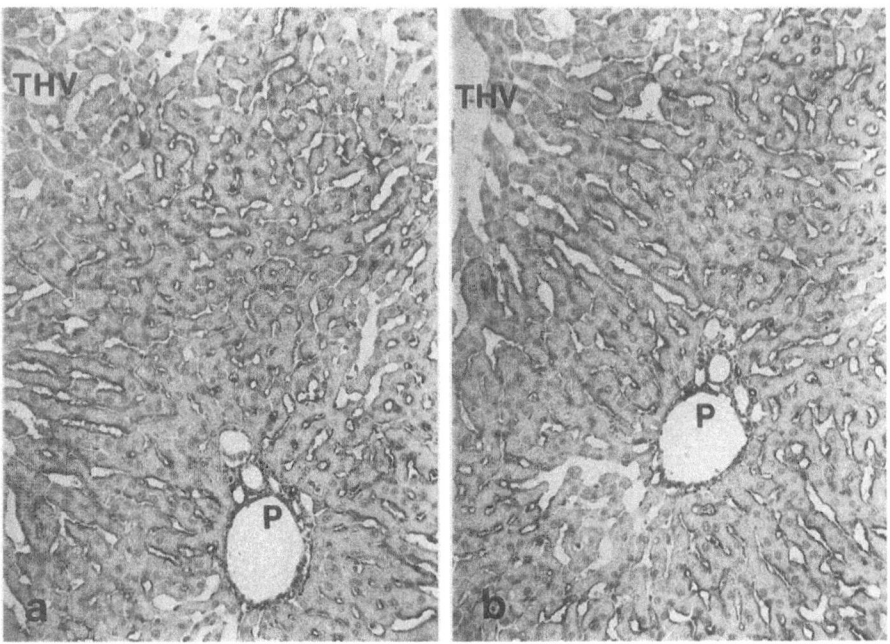

FIG. 7a,b. Immunohistochemical localizations of $ET_A$ and $ET_B$ receptors in rat liver. **a** At low magnification, the immunopositive substances showing the presence of $ET_A$ receptors can be seen localized on the sinusoidal lining cells. At high magnification, they are chiefly on the hepatic stellate cells (HSCs) and partly on the sinusoidal endothelial cells. *P*, portal tract; *THV*, terminal hepatic venule. **b** $ET_B$ receptors are evident mainly on the sinusoidal endothelial cells

ET-1, ET-2, and ET-3. These two types of receptor are distributed in tissue in different ways. $ET_A$ receptors are known to be localized mainly on vascular smooth muscle cells, while $ET_B$ receptors are present on many other types of cell.

In the microvasculature of rat liver, immunohistochemistry has shown that $ET_A$ receptors are evident most intensely on the sinusoidal lining cells (Fig. 7a). Under high magnification, they are found to be mainly located on the HSCs, and also to some extent on the sinusoidal endothelial cells. These localizations of $ET_A$ receptors have been shown ultrastructurally by immunoelectron microscopy. On the other hand, immunohistochemical and immunoelectron microscopy have shown that $ET_B$ receptors are expressed chiefly on the sinusoidal endothelial cells (Fig. 7b).

An ET-1-induced increase in intracytoplasmic free calcium ion concentration $[Ca^{2+}]_i$ in primary cultured sinusoidal endothelium isolated from rat liver is markedly suppressed by pretreatment with an $ET_B$ receptor antagonist (BQ788) (Fig. 5b), whereas this increase in $[Ca^{2+}]_i$ is partly attenuated by pretreatment with an $ET_A$ receptor antagonist (BQ645). Therefore, ET-1 mainly acts on the sinusoidal endothelium via $ET_B$ receptors on the cell surface.

## Interactions Between Hepatic Sinusoidal Endothelial Cells and Stellate Cells

As described, hepatic sinusoidal endothelial cells are closely associated with hepatic stellate cells (HSCs) both morphologically and functionally, since they are involved in the local control of sinusoidal blood flow. As shown schematically in Fig. 8, ETs produced and released from the sinusoidal endothelial cells would act on the HSCs via the $ET_A$ receptors as a paracrine effect [49], inducing an increase in $[Ca^{2+}]_i$ through the activation of inositol triphosphate ($IP_3$) transduced by GTP (guanine triphosphate)-binding protein (G protein), and then resulting in a contraction of the HSCs following

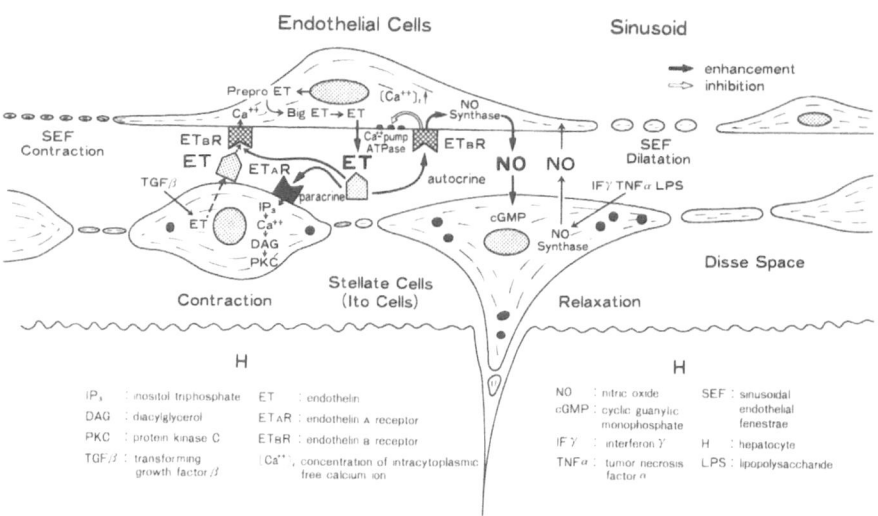

FIG. 8. Local regulatory mechanisms of hepatic sinusoidal microcirculation

the activation of the $Ca^{2+}$-calmodulin–actomyosin system and providing contractile tone to the sinusoids. At the same time, ETs would act on the sinusoidal endothelial cells via the $ET_B$ receptors as an autocrine effect, inducing a contraction of the SEF and possibly of the sinusoidal endothelial cells themselves, as has been indicated in capillary endothelial contraction [18, 50], and resulting in an increase in sinusoidal resistance (Fig. 8). An autoradio-graphic study has revealed that $^{125}I$-ET binds the sinusoidal endothelial cells as well as the HSCs [51].

In addition, in this autocrine effect, NO is produced by the action of NO synthase within the sinusoidal endothelium and released into the space of Disse, going through the plasma membrane of the HSC, followed by the production of cyclic GMP through the activation of guanylate cyclase [52].

This cyclic GMP is considered indirectly to activate $Ca^{2+}$-pump ATPase activity, with a subsequent reduction of $[Ca^{2+}]_i$ and a suppression of myosin phosphorylation, inducing a relaxation of the HSC (Fig. 8).

In liver cirrhosis, not only a contraction of the HSCs but also a reduction in the diameter and number of SEF would be induced by ETs excessively released from the sinusoidal endothelial cells, thus increasing sinusoidal vascular resistance and contributing to the pathogenesis of portal hypertension [52, 53].

## References

1. Rappaport AM (1973) The microcirculatory hepatic unit. Microvasc Res 6:212–228
2. Wisse E (1970) An electron microscopic study of fenestrated endothelium lining of rat liver sinusoids. J Ultrastruct Res 31:125–150
3. Oda M, Nakamura M, Watanabe N, et al. (1983) Some dynamic aspects of the hepatic microcirculation: Demonstration of sinusoidal endothelial fenestrae as a possible regulatory factor. In: Tsuchiya M, Wayland H, Oda M, et al. (eds) Intravital observation of organ microcirculation. Excerpta Medica, Amsterdam, pp 105–138
4. Oda M, Azuma T, Watanabe N, et al. (1990) Regulatory mechanisms of the hepatic microcirculation. Involvement of the contraction and dilatation of sinusoids and sinusoidal endothelial fenestrae. Prog Appl Microcirc 17:103–128
5. Yanagisawa M, Kurihara H, Kimura S, et al. (1988) A novel potent vasoconstrictor peptide produced by vascular endothelial cells. Nature 332:411–415
6. Palmer RMJ, Ferrige AG, Moncada S (1987) Nitric oxide release accounts for the biological activity of endothelium-derived relaxing factor. Nature 327:524–526
7. Yanagisawa M (1994) The endothelin system. A new target for therapeutic intervention. Circulation 89:1320–1322
8. Lautt WW, Greenway CV (1987) Conceptual review of the hepatic vascular bed. Hepatology 7:952–963
9. Nakata K, Leong GF, Brauer RW (1961) Direct measurement of blood pressures in minute vessels of the liver. Am J Physiol 199:1181–1188
10. Hanson KM, Johnson PC (1966) Local control of hepatic arterial and portal venous flow in the dog. Am J Physiol 211:712–720
11. McCuskey RS (1966) A dynamic and static study of hepatic arterioles and hepatic sphincters. Am J Anat 119:455–478
12. Rhodin JAG (1967) The ultrastructure of mammalian arterioles and precapillary sphincters. J Ultrastruct Res 18:181–223
13. Ito T (1987) Participation of Ito cells in sinusoidal blood flow. In: Tsuchiya M, Asano M, Mishima Y, et al. (eds) Microcirculation—an update. vol 2. Excerpta Medica, Amsterdam, pp 321–324

14. McCuskey RS (1986) Hepatic microvascular dysfunction during sepsis and end-otoxemia. In: Tsuchiya M, Kawai K, Kitajima M, et al. (eds) Cytoprotection and cytobiology. vol 3. Excerpta Medica, Amsterdam, pp 3–17
15. Oda M, Nishida J, Honda K, et al. (1991) Relation between sinusoidal endothelial cells and Kupffer cells in hepatic defence mechanisms. In: Tsuchiya M, Nagura H, Hibi T, et al. (eds) Frontiers of mucosal immunology. vol. 2. Excerpta Medica, Amsterdam, pp 193–196
16. Oda M, Kaneko H, Suematsu M, et al. (1993) A new aspect of the hepatic microvasculature: Electron microscopic evidence for the presence of Ito cells around portal and hepatic venules as pericytes. Prog Appl Microcirc 19:25–39
17. Suematsu M, Oda M, Suzuki H, et al. (1993) Intravital and electron microscopic observation of Ito cells in the rat hepatic microcirculation. Microvas Res 46:28–42
18. Majno G, Shea SM, Leventhal M (1969) Endothelial contraction induced by histamine-type mediators. J Cell Biol 41:657–672
19. Rappaport AM, Schneiderman JH (1976) The function of the hepatic artery. Rev Physiol Biochem Pharmacol 76:129–175
20. Kardon RH, Kessel RG (1980) Three-dimensional organization of the hepatic microcirculation in the rodent as observed by scanning electron microscopy of corrosion casts. Gastroenterology 79:72–81
21. Kazemoto S, Oda M, Kaneko H, et al. (1992) Enzymohistochemical demonstration of arterial capillaries in rat liver. Microcirc Annual 8:109–110
22. Oda M, Kazemoto S, Kaneko H, et al. (1993) Involvement of $Ca^{2+}$-calmodulin-actomyosin system in contractility of hepatic sinusoidal endothelial fenestrae. In: Knook DL, Wisse E (eds) Cells of the hepatic sinusoid. vol 4. Kupffer Cell Foundation, Leiden, pp 174–178
23. Oda M, Kamegaya Y, Yokomori H, et al. (1997) Roles of plasma membrane $Ca^{2+}$-ATPase in the relaxation and contraction of hepatic sinusoidal endothelial fenestrae-effects of prostaglandin $E_1$ and endothelin 1. In: Wisse E, Knook DL, Balabaud C (eds) Cells of the hepatic sinusoid. vol 6. Kupffer Cell Foundation, Leiden, pp 313–317
24. Gatmaitan Z, Varticovski L, Ling L, et al. (1996) Studies on fenestral contraction in rat liver endothelial cells in culture. Am J Pathol 148:2027–2041
25. Oda M, Tsukada N, Komatsu H, et al. (1986) Electron microscopic localization of actin, calmodulin and calcium in the hepatic sinusoidal endothelium in the rat. In: Kirn A, Knook DL, Wisse E (eds) Cells of the hepatic sinusoid. vol 1. Kupffer Cell Foundation, Rijswijk, pp 511–512
26. Braef F, De Zanger R, Baekeland M, et al. (1995) Structure and dynamics of the fenestrae-associated cytoskeleton of rat liver sinusoidal endothelial cells. Hepatology 7:1230–1238
27. Wier WG, Cannell MB, Berlin JR, et al. (1987) Cellular and subcellular heterogeneity of $[Ca^{2+}]_i$ in single heart cells revealed by fura 2. Science 235:325–328
28. Oda M, Watanabe N, Komatsu H, et al. (1988) Electron microscopic demonstration of free calcium in the capillary endothelium in comparison with computerized image analysis using fura 2-AM. J Clin Electron Microsc 21:558–559
29. Braef F, De Zanger R, Jans D, et al. (1996) Microfilament-disrupting agent latrunculin A induces an increased number of fenestrae in rat liver sinusoidal endothelial cells: comparison with cytochalasin B. Hepatology 24:627–635
30. Arias IM (1990) The biology of hepatic endothelial cell fenestrae. In: Popper H, Schaffner S (eds) Progress in liver diseases. vol 9. Grune and Stratton, New York, pp 11–26
31. Nishihama M, Nanaka T, Hidaka H (1980) $Ca^{2+}$-calmodulin-dependent phosphory-lation and platelet secretion. Nature 287:883–885
32. Kelley C, D'Amore P, Hechtmann HB, et al. (1987) Microvascular pericyte contractility in vitro: Comparison with other cells of the vascular wall. J Cell Biol 104:483–490

33. Pinzani M, Faun P, Reocco U, et al. (1992) Fat storing cells as liver-specific pericytes. Spatial dynamics of agonist-stimulated intracellular calcium transients. J Clin Invest 90:642–646

34. Sakamoto M, Ueno T, Kin M, et al. (1993) Ito cell contraction in response to endothelin-1 and substance P. Hepatology 18:978–983

35. Kawada N, Tran-Thi TA, Klein H, et al. (1993) The contraction of hepatic stellate (Ito) cells stimulated with vasoactive substances. Possible involvement of endothelin 1 and nitric oxide in the regulation of the sinusoidal tonus. Eur J Biochem 213:815–823

36. Kamegaya Y, Oda M, Kazemoto S, et al. (1995) Evidence for the spontaneous contractility of Ito cells. Time-lapse cinematography and couputerized image analysis. In: Wisse E, Knook DL, Wake K (eds) Cells of the hepatic sinusoid. vol 5. Kupffer Cell Foundation, Leiden, pp 306–307

37. Kamegaya Y, Oda M, Yokomori H, et al. (1997) Effect of endothelin-1 on hepatic microcirculation—relation between the changes in hepatic sinusoidal endothelial fenestrae and intracytoplasmic free calcium ion. Microcirc Annual 13:163–164

38. Zhang JX, Pegoli WJ, Clemens MG (1994) Endothelin-1 induces direct constriction of hepatic sinusoids. Am J Physiol 266:G624–G632

39. Okumura S, Takei Y, Kawano S, et al. (1994) Vasoactive effect of endothelin-1 on rat liver in vivo. Hepatology 19:155–161

40. Rockey DC, Chung JJ (1995) Inducible nitric oxide synthase in rat hepatic lipocytes and the effect of nitric oxide on lipocyte contractility. J Clin Invest 95:1197–1206

41. Suematsu M, Goda N, Sano T, et al. (1995) Carbon monoxide: An endogenous modulator of sinusoidal tone in the perfused rat liver. J Clin Invest 96:2431–2437

42. Rieder H, Ramadori G, Meyer zum Buschenfelde KH (1991) Sinusoidal endothelial liver cells in vitro release endothelin augmentation by transforming growth factor beta and Kupffer cell-conditioned media. Klin Wochenschr 69:387–391

43. Rockey DC, Chung JJ (1998) Reduced nitric oxide production by endothelial cells in cirrhotic rat liver: Endothelial dysfunction in portal hypertension. Gastroenterology 114:344–351

44. Carafoli E (1991) Calcium pump of plasma membrane. Physiol Rev 71:129–153

45. Fujimoto T (1993) Calcium pump of the plasma membrane is located in caveolae. J Cell Biol 120:1147–1157

46. Lin PH (1990) Liver plasma membrane ectoATPase. Ann NY Acad Sci 603:394–400

47. Verma AK, Filoteo AG, Stanford DK, et al. (1988) Complete primary structure of a human plasma membrane $Ca^{2+}$ pump. J Biol Chem 263:14152–14159

48. Sakurai T, Yanagisawa M, Masaki T (1992) Molecular characterization of endothelin receptors. Trends Pharmacol Sci 13:103–108

49. Housset C, Rockey DC, Bissell DM (1993) Endothelin receptors in rat liver lipocytes as a contractile target for endothelin 1. Proc Natl Acad Sci USA 90:9266–9270

50. Rangen DMS, Schmidt EE, MacDonald IC, et al. (1988) Spontaneous cyclic contractions of the capillary wall in vivo, impeding red cell flow—A quantitative analysis. Evidence for endothelial contractility. Microvasc Res 36:13–30

51. Gondo K, Ueno T, Sakamoto M, et al. (1993) The endothelin-1 binding site in rat liver tissue: Light- and electron-microscopic, autoradiographic studies. Gastroenterology 104:1745–1749

52. Rocky D (1997) The cellular pathogenesis of portal hypertension: Stellate cell contractility, endothelin, and nitric oxide. Hepatology 25:2–5

53. Oda M, Azuma T, Nishizaki Y, et al. (1989) Alterations of hepatic sinusoids in liver cirrhosis—involvement in the pathogenesis of portal hypertension. J Gastroenterol Hepatol 4 (Suppl. 1):111–113

# Hepatic Innervation and Hepatic Sinusoidal Cells

Takato Ueno,[1] Ryuichiro Sakata,[1] Takuji Torimura,[1]
Seishu Tamaki,[1] Masaharu Sakamoto,[1] Kazuhisa Gondo,[1]
Michio Sata,[1] and Kyuichi Tanikawa[2]

*Summary.* The innervation of the human liver is distributed throughout the hepatic lobules from the portal spaces to the centralobular spaces. Nerve endings in the intralobular spaces are localized mainly in the Disse spaces, and are closely related to hepatic stellate cells (HSCs). Various neurotransmitters such as substance P exist in these nerve endings. Substance P induces contraction in HSCs. In addition, HSCs possess endothelin (ET) receptors, and contract in response to ET-1 treatment. Moreover, $\alpha$-smooth muscle actin ($\alpha$-SMA) is localized in the cytoplasm of HSCs. $\alpha$-SMA is closely related to the contractility of smooth muscle cells. Nitric oxide (NO) inhibits the contraction of HSCs. HSCs thus appear to be involved in the regulation of hepatic sinusoidal microcirculation by contraction and relaxation. In the human cirrhotic liver, intralobular innervation is decreased or absent, but ET, ET receptors, and NO are overexpressed in the HSCs. These phenomena indicate that HSCs in the human cirrhotic liver may play an important role in the sinusoidal microcirculation through agents such as ET or NO rather than through intralobular innervation.

*Key words.* Hepatic innervation, Vasoactive agents, Hepatic sinusoidal microcirculation, Hepatic sinusoidal cells

## Introduction

The human liver is innervated by splanchnic nerves (sympathetic nerves) originating in the sixth to ninth level of the thoracic spine and vagal nerves originating in the medulla oblongata. Efferent and afferent pathways are formed by these splanchnic and vagal nerves. The efferent pathway has an important role in the regulation of hepatic microcirculation as well as in glycogen, protein, and lipid metabolism, and in biliary function. The afferent pathway provides sensory function through

[1] The Second Department of Internal Medicine, Research Center for Innovative Cancer Therapy, Kurume University School of Medicine, 67 Asahi-machi, Kurume, Fukuoka 830-0011, Japan
[2] International Institute for Liver Research, Kurume Research Center, 2432-3 Aikawa-machi, Kurume, Fukuoka 839-0861, Japan

osmoreceptors, baroreceptors, and glucose receptors [1]. Previous studies of hepatic innervation have produced different findings according to the spaces [2]. In this chapter, we discuss the relationship between hepatic innervation and intralobular innervation and hepatic sinusoidal cells in the human liver.

## Intralobular Innervation and Nerve Endings in the Human Liver

The human liver shows an intralobular innervation similar to that of guinea pigs, cats, and tupaias [1]. Generally, branches of vagal nerves, splanchnic nerves, and some-times phrenic nerves enter the human liver. In the human liver, a mainly adrenergic type of innervation is seen, and some cholinergic innervation is also localized [3–6]. In addition, innervation mediated by various neurotransmitters such as substance P (SP), vasoactive intestinal peptide (VIP), somatostatin, cholecystokinin, neurotensin, and neuropeptide Y has been reported to exist in the human liver [7–10].

In the portal and centrolobular spaces, a single axon or axon bundles with or without a Schwann sheath are seen close to fibroblasts or myofibroblasts localized around blood vessels and bile ducts (Fig. 1a,b). In the intralobular spaces, nerve bundles run in the Disse spaces, and nerve endings are visible close to hepatic stellate cells (HSCs) and hepatocytes. However, these endings are associated with the sinusoidal endothelial cells for a short distance (Fig. 1c). Nerve endings with vesicles containing neurotransmitters such as SP or VIP are often visible close to HSCs (Fig. 2). In certain respects, HSCs around the sinusoidal endothelial cells which form the hepatic sinusoids resemble pericytes around a capillary (Fig. 1d). It has thus been suggested that HSCs have contractility, and are involved in the regulation of hepatic sinusoidal microcirculation.

## Vasoactive Substances and Hepatic Sinusoidal Cells

Substances such as SP, angiotensin II, norepinephrine, and thrombin have been shown to have significant effects on HSC contractility.

Vasoactive substances such as endothelin (ET) [11] and nitric oxide (NO) [12] have been identified, and the characteristics of these substances have been clarified.

ET is a peptide composed of 21 amino acids that has been isolated from the supernatant obtained after the culture of porcine aortic endothelial cells [11]. ET has potent vasoconstrictive effects on smooth muscle cells. ET has three isoforms (ET-1, -2, and -3) with different sequences of amino acids [13]. Isopeptides arise through proteolytic cleavage of prepropeptides to the proendothelins (big-ET), which are converted to activate peptides by ET-converting enzyme.

ET receptors were confirmed by the identification and cloning of the $ET_A$ receptor (vasoconstricting) and the $ET_B$ receptor (vasodilatory), that both belong to the superfamily of G protein-coupled receptors [14]. In addition, a third receptor, $ET_C$, has recently been cloned [15]. The function and distribution of $ET_C$ are unknown.

The $ET_A$ receptor binds ET-1 and ET-2 with a higher affinity than ET-3, but the $ET_B$ receptor displays similar affinity for all three isopeptides. The binding of ET to both $ET_A$ and $ET_B$ receptors leads to an increase in cytosolic calcium ($Ca^{2+}$) through the release of $Ca^{2+}$ from intracellular stores consequent to the production of inositol triphosphate ($IP_3$) by activated phospholipase C [16]. In addition, the stimulation of

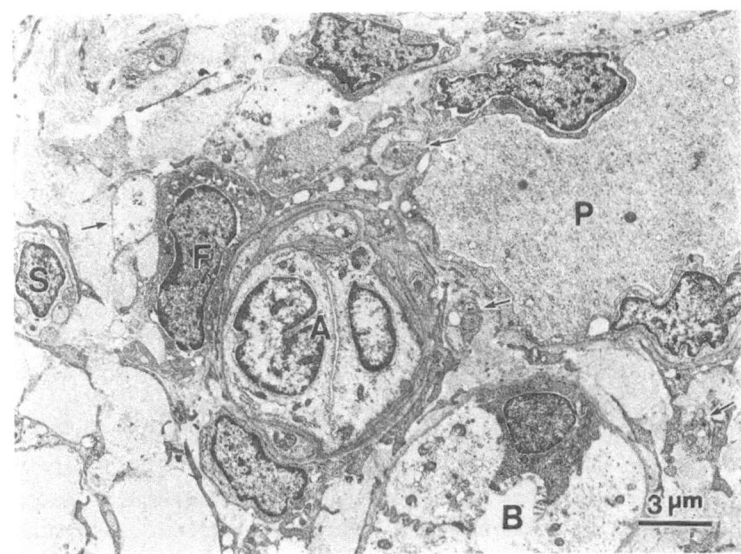

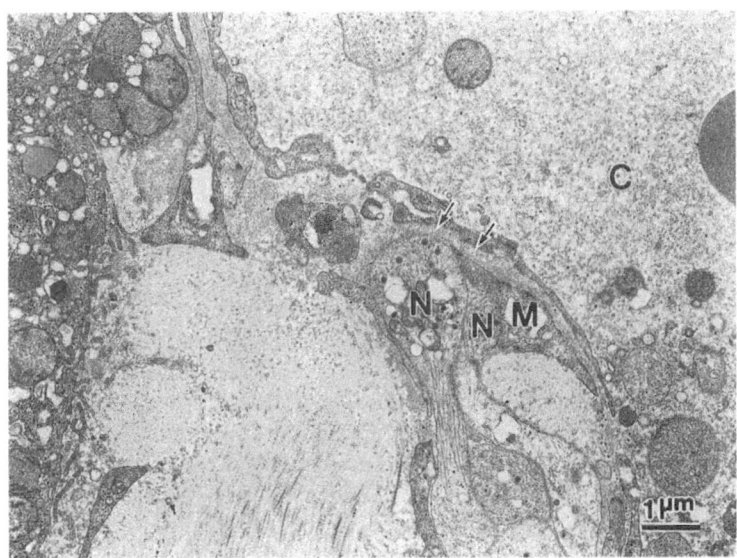

Fig. 1a–d. Electron micrographs of a human liver. **a** Nerve bundles (*arrows*) are visible close to fibroblasts (*F*) around the portal vein (*P*), hepatic artery (*A*), and bile duct (*B*). *S*, Schwann cell. (From [2], with permission). **b** Nerve endings (*N*) are visible close to the surface of myofibroblasts (*M*). The distal end of the nerve ending is closely associated with the basal lamina (*arrows*) of an endothelial cell of the central vein (*C*). (From [2], with permission). **c** Nerve endings (*arrows*) are observed close to a hepatic stellate cell (HSC) (*S*) and hepatocyte (*H*). The nerve endings are associated with a sinusoidal endothelial cell (*E*) for a short distance. *Si*, sinusoid. (From [2], with permission). **d** Sinusoidal endothelial cells with fenestrae (*arrows*) in the cytoplasm are enfolded by the cytoplasmic processes of HSCs (*S*). A nerve bundle (*N*) closely apposes the process of an HSC. *Si*, sinusoid. (From [2], with permission)

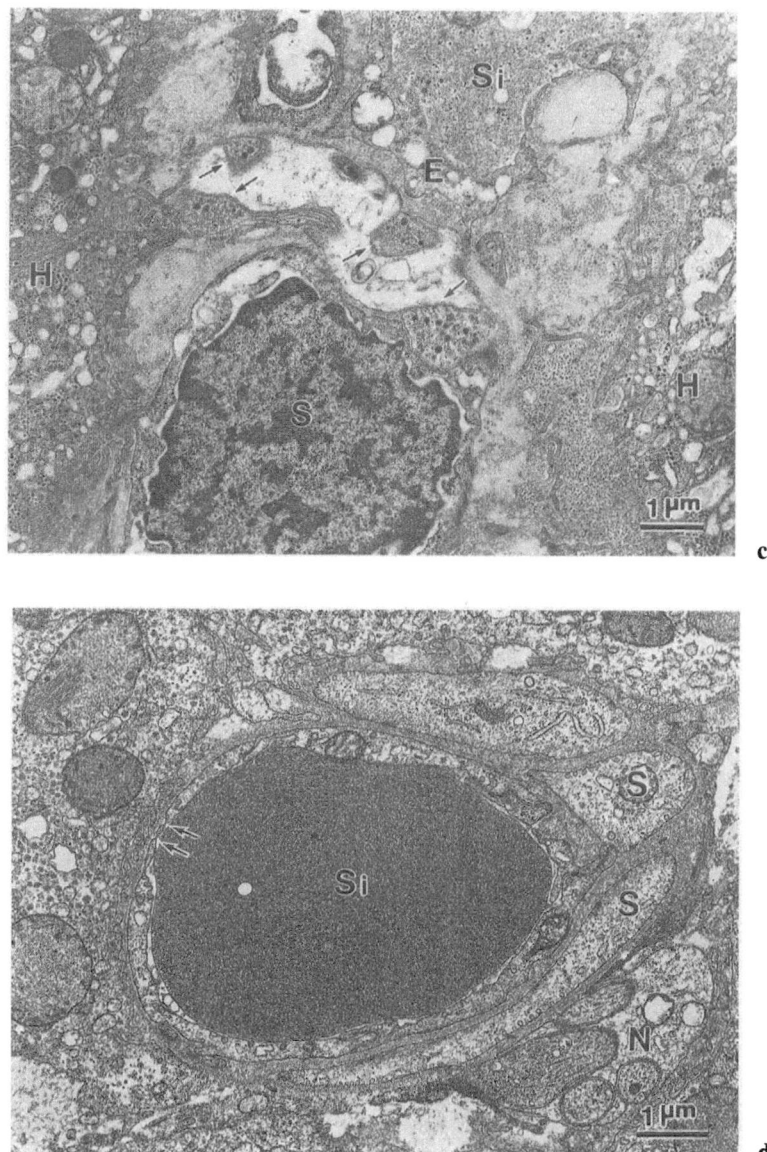

FIG. 1. *Continued*

$ET_A$ receptors increases the cyclic adenosine 3',5'-monophosphate (cAMP) level in the cells, while the $ET_B$ receptor is associated with an inhibition of the adenyl cyclase system [17]. $ET_B$ receptor also activates a $Ca^{2+}$-dependent stimulation of constitutive NO synthase [18]. In addition, in the heterogeneity of $ET_B$ receptor, the existence of two $ET_B$ receptor subtypes, i.e., $ET_{B1}$ and $ET_{B2}$, has recently been postulated [19]. Douglas et al. reported that $ET_A$ and $ET_{B1}$ receptors may induce the contraction of

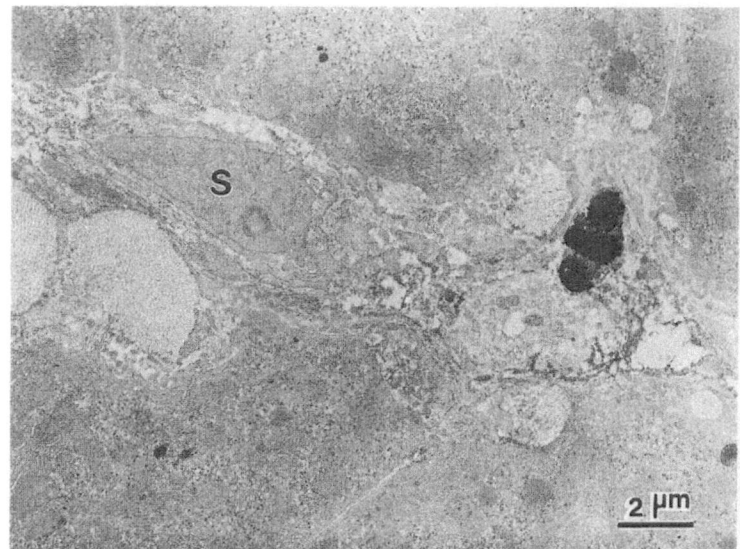

FIG. 2a,b. Electron micrographs showing the immunolocalization of substance P (SP) and vasoactive intestinal peptide (VIP) in the human liver. **a** Nerve endings containing SP-immunoreactive vesicles are observed close to an HSC (*S*). (From [8], with permission). **b** Nerve endings containing VIP-immunoreactive vesicles are observed in the Disse space. *Si*, sinusoid; *S*, hepatic stellate cell; *E*, sinusoidal endothelial cell. (From [8], with permission)

vascular smooth muscle cells, while $ET_{B2}$ receptors of endothelial cells promote vasodilation through the production of diffusible NO [19].

ET-1 binding sites in the rat liver are located mainly in the sinusoidal lining cells of hepatic lobules, and are weakly expressed in the luminal space of the portal and central veins [20]. In the intralobular spaces, the binding sites are greatest in the

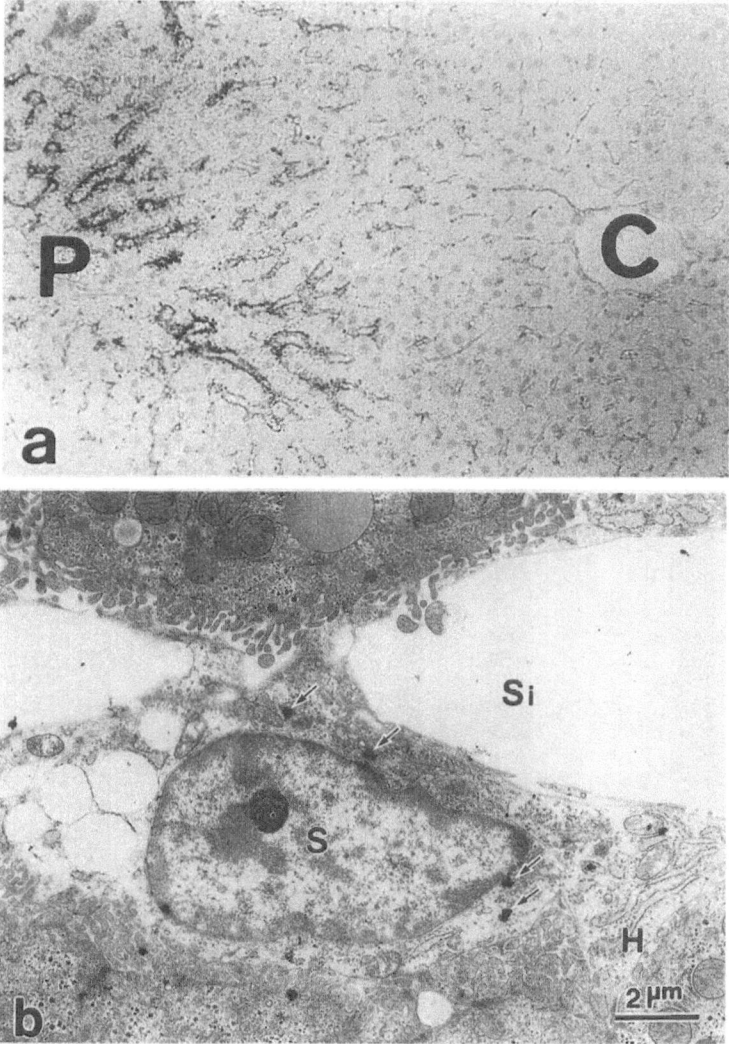

FIG. 3a,b. Light and electron microscopic autoradiographs showing [125]I-ET-1 binding sites in the rat liver. **a** Many more [125]I-ET-1 grains are observed in sinusoidal lining cells of the periportal space compared with the midzonal and pericentral spaces. *C*, central vein; *P*, portal vein. ×100. (From [20] with permisson). **b** [125]I-ET-1 grains (*arrows*) are observed on a hepatic stellate cell (*S*). *Si*, sinusoid; *H*, hepatocyte. (From [20], with permission)

periportal region (Fig. 3a). An ultrastructural analysis showed that about 35% of ET-1 binding sites are located on the HSCs (Fig. 3b), and that some of the binding sites are located on endothelial cells or Kupffer cells [21]. The heterogeneity of ET-1 binding sites in hepatic lobules appears to parallel the blood flow pattern in hepatic sinusoids. Stable regulation of blood flow is required in the periportal spaces compared with that in the midzonal and centrolobular spaces. A few recent studies of HSCs and ET in the human liver are informative; Pinzani et al. [22] reported that ET-1 immunolocalization was visible in nonparenchymal cells along hepatic sinusoids, hepatocytes, cells of the portal tract stroma, bile ducts, and vessels. Mallat et al. [23] reported that $ET_A$ (20%) and $ET_B$ (80%) receptors were identified in human HSCs.

NO is synthesized from L-arginine via the catalytic action of a group of enzymes, i.e., the NO synthases (NOSs). Three isoforms of NOS have been identified by the use of biochemical, immunohistochemical, and molecular biological techniques [24]. Constitutive calcium–calmodulin-dependent isoforms were initially localized to neuron (nNOS or NOSI) and vascular endothelial cells (eNOS or NOS III). A cytokine-inducible calcium-independent isoform (iNOS or NOS II) is present in macrophages. The principal target of NO is soluble guanylate cyclase, the cells of which result in an increased level of intracellular guanosine 3′,5′-cyclic monophosphate (cGMP). We observed that cultured rat HSCs overexpressed iNOS and cGMP and relaxed under the condition of interleukin (IL)-1$\beta$ treatment [25].

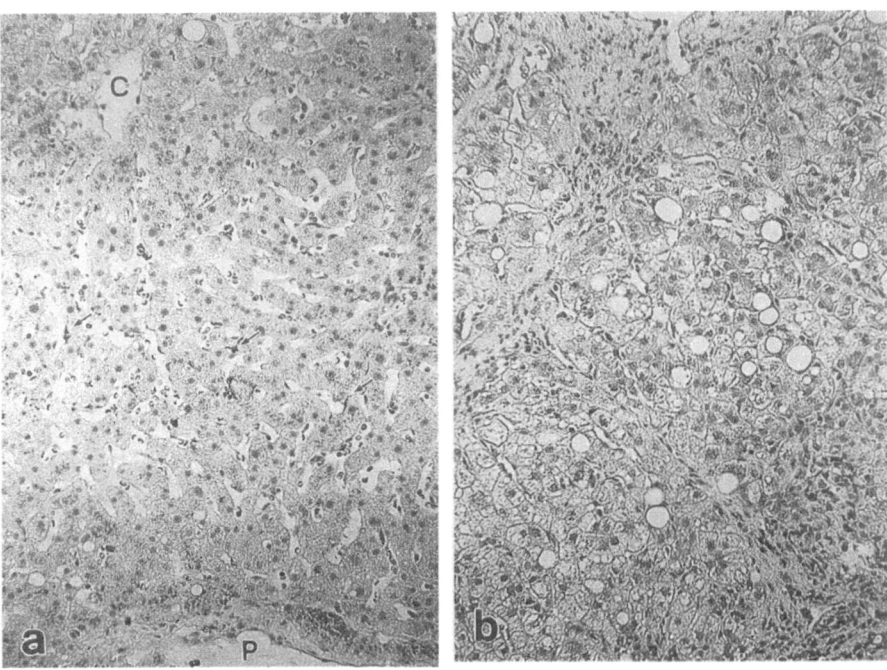

FIG. 4a,b. Immunolocalization of anti-S-100 protein in normal and cirrhotic livers. S-100 protein is a marker of peripheral nerve fibers. Immunoreactive products of anti-S-100 protein (*arrows*) in intralobular spaces are abundant in the normal liver (**a**) compared with the cirrhotic liver (**b**). *P*, portal vein; *C*, central vein. ×300. (From [26], with permission)

## Changes in Hepatic Innervation and Hepatic Stellate Cells in Human Liver Cirrhosis

In human liver cirrhosis, intralobular innervation is decreased [7, 9, 26] (Fig. 4), whereas the expression of $\alpha$-smooth muscle actin ($\alpha$-SMA), which is related to cell contraction, is increased on the HSCs [26, 27] (Figs. 5 and 6). ET-1 is overexpressed and exerts multiple effects on HSCs [22] in liver cirrhosis. In human liver cirrhosis, $\alpha$-SMA-positive HSCs seem to be deeply involved in the hepatic sinusoidal microcirculation through various vasoactive agents such as ET-1 and NO, rather than through intralobular innervation. In addition, the expression of ET receptors is clearly enhanced along the sinusoidal walls, especially on HSCs in human cirrhotic liver compared with normal liver [22, 26] (Figs. 7 and 8). Moreover, according to several reports, plasma ET-1 and ET-3 concentrations are increased in patients with cirrhosis [28, 29]. ET is up-regulated by hypoxia, transforming growth factor-beta, IL-1, tumor necrosis factor (TNF)-$\alpha$, and platelet-derived growth factor [30].

NO is also an important regulator of hepatic sinusoidal dilatation. As noted above, rat-cultured HSCs overexpressed iNOS and cGMP and relaxed under IL-1$\beta$ treatment

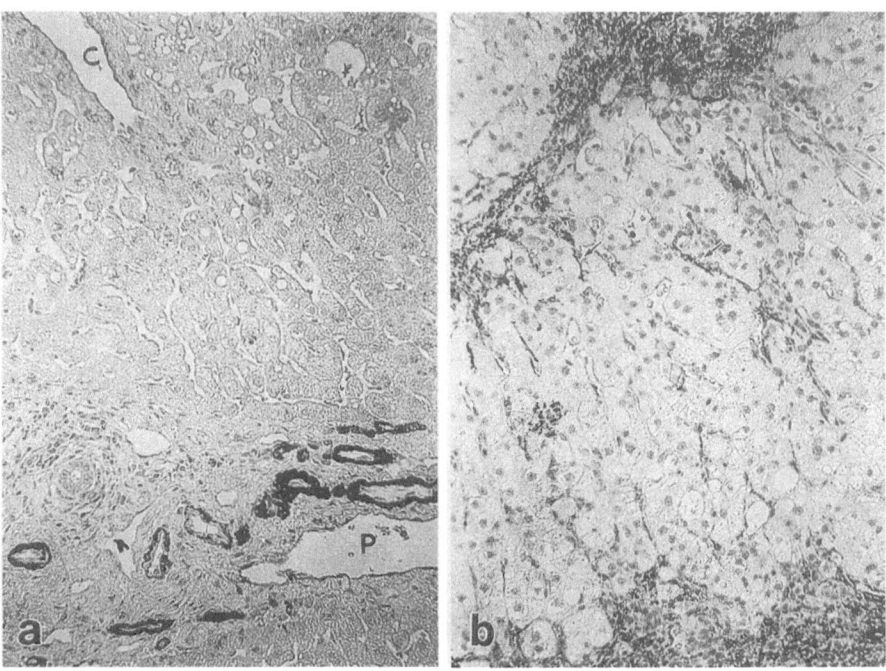

FIG. 5a,b. Immunolocalization of anti-$\alpha$-SMA in normal and cirrhotic livers. Immunoreactive products of anti-$\alpha$-SMA are brightly localized around the hepatic arteries (**a**). Immunoreactive products of anti-$\alpha$-SMA (*arrows*) in the fibrous septa and intralobular spaces are abundant in the cirrhotic liver (**b**) compared with the normal liver (**a**). *P*, portal vein; *C*, central vein. ×300. (From [26], with permission)

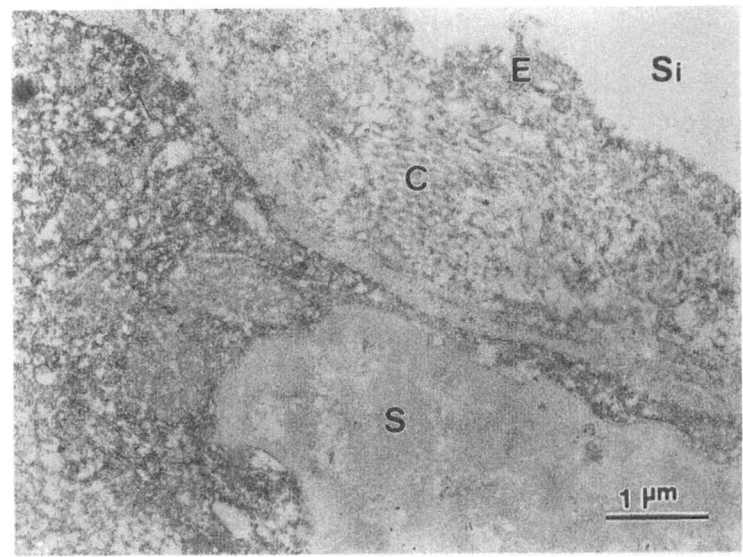

FIG. 6. An electron micrograph showing immunoreactive products of anti-$\alpha$-SMA in the cirrhotic liver. Immunoreactive products of anti-$\alpha$-SMA are observed in the cytoplasm of a HSC (S). Si, sinusoid; E, sinusoidal endothelial cell; C, collagen fiber. (From [26], with permission)

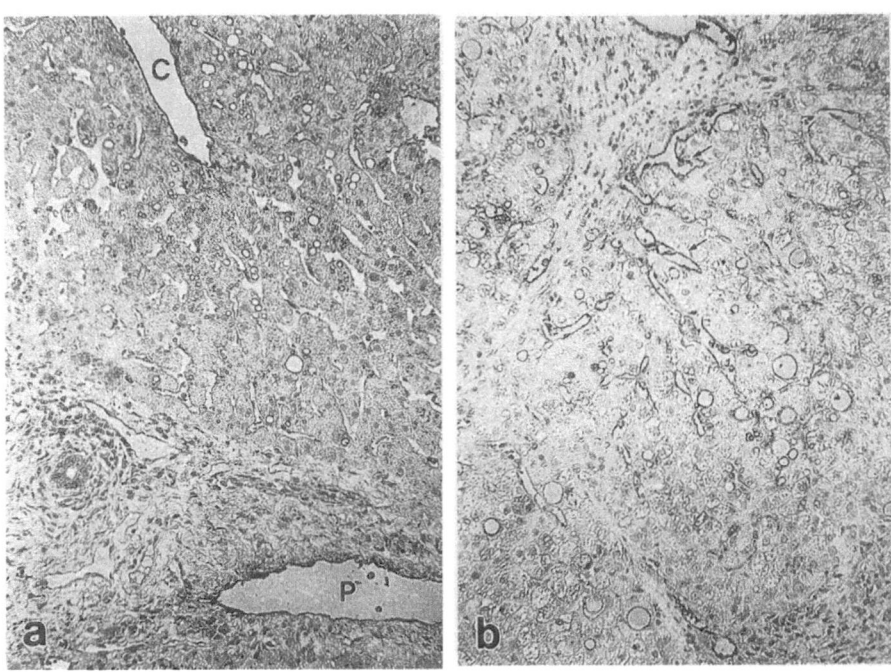

FIG. 7a,b. Immunolocalization of anti-ET receptor (ETR) in normal and cirrhotic livers. Immunoreactive products of anti-ETR (arrows) in the intralobular spaces are abundant in the cirrhotic liver (b) compared with the normal liver (a). In addition, the products are localized along the lumen of the portal veins and central vein. P, portal vein; C, central vein. ×300. (From [26], with permission)

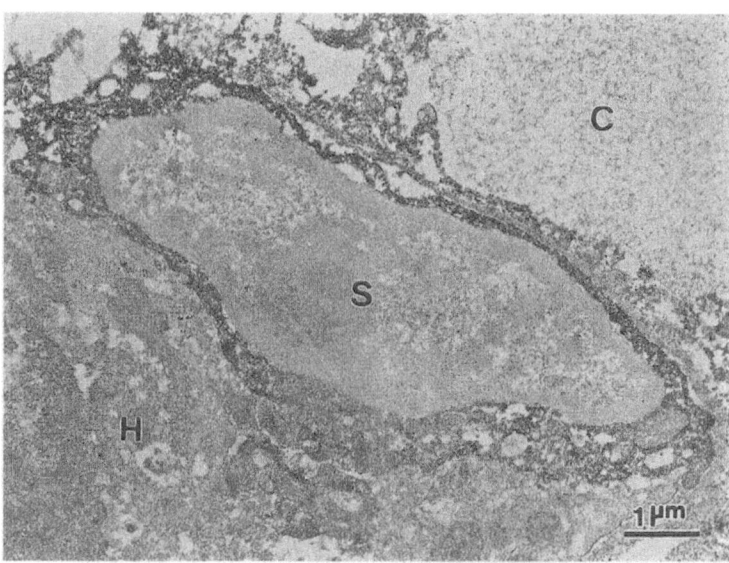

FIG. 8. An electron micrograph showing immunoreactive products of anti-ETR in a cirrhotic liver. Immunoreactive products of anti-ETR are observed in the cytoplasm of a HSC (S). H, hepatocyte; C, collagen fiber. (From [26], with permission)

[25]. Battista et al. suggested that NO is overproduced in human cirrhotic liver [31]. Moreover, in human liver cirrhosis, the concentration of NO as well as ET in blood is increased by endotoxin or cytokines such as IL-1 and -6, and TNF-$\alpha$ [2, 31, 32]. In cirrhosis, NO as well as ET may regulate hepatic vascular tone in response to various stimulants such as IL-1, TNF-$\alpha$, and endotoxin [33]. Hyperdynamic circulation occurs during liver cirrhosis [34], and is involved in systemic cardiovascular complications including clinical hypotension, decreased systemic vascular resistance, increased cardiac output, and the increase of blood flow through the tissues. In cirrhotic animals, the administration of ET-1 did not affect systemic or regional hemodynamics [35]. This phenomenon may indicate the suppression of the pressor response of ET-1 due to NO overproduction in cirrhotic animals. In addition, NO seems to contribute to vascular hypoactivity in the presence of a high level of ET-1 [33].

In conclusion, the regulation of blood flow, resistance, and pressure in the sinusoids of the normal human liver is believed to be performed mainly by neuropeptides such as SP or VIP released from nerve endings. In cirrhotic liver, in contrast, hepatic sinusoidal capillarization is frequently observed [36]. At this stage, resistance in the sinusoidal wall is increased, and the hepatic sinusoidal microcirculation may be limited. With the progression of liver fibrosis, intralobular innervatin becomes scant, whereas the role of HSCs in the hepatic sinusoids may become more prominent. In liver cirrhosis, HSCs are likely to be affected by ET-1 rather than NO [37, 38]. The regulation of microcirculation in the sinusoids of the human cirrhotic liver seems to be regulated by agents such as ET or NO in a paracrine or autocrine manner [39].

# References

1. Lautt WW (1983) Afferent and efferent neural roles in liver function. Prog Neurobiol 21:323–348
2. Ueno T, Tanikawa K (1997) Intralobular innervation and lipocyte contractility in the liver. Nutrition 13:141–148
3. Ueno T, Inuzuka S, Torimura T, et al. (1988) Intrinsic innervation of the human liver. J Clin Electron Microsc 21:481–491
4. Moghimzadeh E, Nobin A, Rosengren E (1983) Fluorescence microscopical and chemical characterization of the adrenergic innervation in mammalian liver. Cell Tissue Res 230:605–613
5. Kyösola K, Penttilä O, Ihamäki T, et al. (1985) Adrenergic innervation of the human liver. A fluorescence histochemical analysis of clinical liver biopsy specimens. Scand J Gastroenterol 20:254–256
6. Amenta F, Cavallotti C, Ferrante F, et al. (1981) Cholinergic nerves in the human liver. Histochem J 13:419–424
7. Miyazawa Y, Fukuda Y, Imoto M, et al. (1988) Immunohistochemical studies on the distribution of nerve fibers in chronic liver diseases. Am J Gastroenterol 83:1108–1114
8. Ueno T, Inuzuka S, Torimura T, et al. (1991) Distribution of substance P and vasoactive intestinal peptide in the human liver: Light and electron immunoperoxidase methods of observation. Am J Gastroenterol 86:1633–1637
9. Lee JA, Ahmed Q, Hines JE, et al. (1992) Disappearance of hepatic parenchymal nerves in human liver cirrhosis. Gut 33:87–91
10. El-Salhy M, Stenling R, Grimelius L (1993) Peptidergic innervation and endocrine cells in the human liver. Scand J Gastroenterol 28:809–815
11. Yanagisawa M, Kurihara H, Kimura S, et al. (1988) A novel potent vasoconstrictor peptide produced by vascular endothelial cells. Nature 332:411–415
12. Furchgott RF (1983) Role of the endothelium in responses of vascular smooth muscle. Circ Res 53:557–573
13. Inoue A, Yanagisawa M, Kimura S, et al. (1989) The human endothelin family: Three structurally and pharmacologically distinct isopeptides predicted by three separate genes. Proc Natl Acad Sci USA 86:2863–2867
14. Muggins JP, Pelton JT, Miller RC (1993) The structure and specificity of endothelin receptors: Their importance in physiology and medicine. Pharmacol Ther 59:55–123
15. Karne S, Jayawickreme CK, Lerner MR (1993) Cloning and characterization of an endothelin-3 specific receptor (ETc receptor) from *Xenopus laevis* dermal melanophores. J Biol Chem 268:19126–19133
16. Jouneaux C, Mallat A, Serradeil-Le Gal C, et al. (1994) Coupling of endothelin B receptors to the calcium pump and phospholipase C via Gs and Gq in rat liver. J Biol Chem 269:1845–1851
17. Eguchi S, Hirata Y, Imai T, et al. (1993) Endothelin receptor subtypes are coupled to adenylate cyclase via different guanyl nucleotide-binding proteins in vasculature. Endocrinology 132:524–529
18. Tsukahara H, Ende H, Magazine HI, et al. (1994) Molecular and functional characterization of the non-isopeptide $ET_B$ receptor in endothelial cells: receptor coupling to nitric oxide synthase. J Biol Chem 269:21778–21785
19. Douglas SA, Meek TD, Ohlstein EH (1994) Novel receptor antagonists welcome a new era in endothelin biology. Trends Biochem Sci 15:313–316
20. Gondo K, Ueno T, Sakamoto M, et al. (1993) The endothelin-1 binding site in rat liver tissue: Light- and electron-microscopic autoradiographic studies. Gastroenterology 104:1745–1749

21. Furuta S, Naruse S, Nakayama T, et al. (1992) Binding of $^{125}$I-endothelin-1 to fat-storing cells in rat liver revealed by electron microscopic radioautography. Anat Embryol 185:97–100
22. Pinzani M, Milani S, De Franco R, et al. (1996) Endothelin 1 is overexpressed in human cirrhotic liver and exerts multiple effects on activated hepatic stellate cells. Gastroenterology 110:534–548
23. Mallat A, Fouassier L, Préaux AM, et al. (1995) Antiproliferative effects of ET-1 in human liver Ito cells: An $ET_B$- and a cyclin AMP-mediated pathway. J Cardiovasc Pharmacol 26:S132–S134
24. Jaffrey SR, Snyder SH (1995) Nitric oxide: A neural messenger. Annu Rev Cell Dev Biol 11:417–440
25. Sakamoto M, Ueno T, Sugawara H, et al. (1997) Relaxing effect of interleukin-1 on rat cultured Ito cells. Hepatology 25:1412–1417
26. Ueno T, Michio S, Ryuichiro S, et al. (1997) Hepatic stellate cells and intralobular innervation in human liver cirrhosis. Hum Pathol 28:953–959
27. Schmitt-Gräff A, Krüger S, Bochard F, et al. (1991) Modulation of alpha smooth muscle actin and desmin expression in perisinusoidal cells of normal and diseased human liver. Am J Pathol 138:1233–1242
28. Asbert M, Ginès A, Ginès P, et al. (1993) Circulating levels of endothelin in cirrhosis. Gastroenterology 104:1485–1491
29. Møller S, Gülberg V, Henriksen JH, et al. (1995) Endothelin-1 and endothelin-3 in cirrhosis: relations to systemic and splanchnic haemodynamics. J Hepatol 23:135–144
30. Mallat A, Lotersztajn S (1996) Multiple hepatic functions of endothelin-1: Physiopathological relevance. J Hepatol 25:405–413
31. Battista S, Bar F, Mengozzi G, et al. (1997) Hyperdynamic circulation in patients with cirrhosis: Direct measurement of nitric oxide levels in hepatic and portal veins. J Hepatol 26:75–80
32. Guarner C, Soriano G, Tomas A, et al. (1993) Increased serum nitrite and nitrate levels in patients with cirrhosis: Relationship to endotoxemia. Hepatology 18:1139–1143
33. Clària J, Jiménez W, Ros J, et al. (1994) Increased nitric oxide-dependent vasorelaxation in aortic rings of cirrhotic rats with ascites. Hepatology 20:1615–1621
34. Bomzon A, Blendis LM (1994) The nitric oxide hypothesis and the hyperdynamic circulation in cirrhosis. Hepatology 20:1343–1350
35. Hartleb M, Moreau R, Cailmail S, et al. (1994) Vascular hyporesponsiveness to endothelin-1 in rats with cirrhosis. Gastroenterology 107:1085–1093
36. Ueno T, Inuzuka S, Torimura T, et al. (1993) Serum hyaluronate reflects hepatic sinusoidal capillarization. Gastroenterology 105:475–481
37. Rockey DC, Fouassier L, Chung JJ, et al. (1998) Cellular localization of endothelin-1 and increased production in liver injury in the rat: Potential for autocrine and paracrine effects on stellate cells. Hepatology 27:472–480
38. Rockey DC, Chung JJ (1998) Reduced nitric oxide production by endothelial cells in cirrhotic rat liver: Endothelial dysfunction in portal hypertension. Gastroenterology 114:344–351
39. Rockey DC (1997) The cellular pathogenesis of portal hypertension: Stellate cell contractility, endothelin and nitric oxide. Hepatology 25:2–5

# Contraction and Relaxation of Ito Cells

Masaharu Sakamoto, Takato Ueno, Takuji Torimura,
Seishu Tamaki, Motoaki Kin, Riko Ogata, Michio Sata,
and Kyuichi Tanikawa

*Summary.* Ito cells (hepatic stellate cells) are localized around liver sinusoidal endothelial cells. The cytoplasm of these cells contains contractile proteins such as actin and myosin, suggesting that microcirculation of liver sinusoids is regulated by the contraction and relaxation of these cells.

Autocrine and paracrine activities of endothelin-1 induce Ito cell contraction, while nitric oxide induces Ito cell relaxation via cyclic-guanosine 3',5'-monophosphate. Therefore, it is considered that Ito cells are deeply involved in the regulation of liver sinusoidal microcirculation.

*Key words.* Ito cells (hepatic stellate cells), Endothelin-1, Nitric oxide, Contraction, Relaxation

## Introduction

Ito cells located in the space of Disse are also called fat-storing cells, hepatic stellate cells, lipocytes, and perisinusoidal cells [1–4]. The cells have many cytoplasmic processes and surround hepatic endothelial cells. The main functions of Ito cells are vitamin A storage [5, 6] and the production of various extracellular matrix components [7–10]. The morphology of the hepatic sinusoidal wall resembles that of a capillary. Ito cells, which correspond to pericytes around capillaries, are localized in the space of Disse around the hepatic sinusoids. Pericytes contain contractile proteins such as actin and myosin, and these cells are deeply involved in the control of capillary blood flow through their contraction and relaxation [11]. Ito cells also contain actin and myosin [12, 13]. The contraction of Ito cells is induced by agents such as substance P, prostaglandin F2 $\alpha$ and a thromboxane A2 analogue [14, 15]. On the other hand, agents such as prostaglandin E2, Iloprost, and adrenomedullin cause the relaxation of Ito cells [16]. It has therefore been suggested that Ito cells play an important role in the regulation of sinusoidal blood flow through contraction and relaxation. In

The Second Department of Internal Medicine, Kurume University School of Medicine, 67 Asahi-machi, Kurume, Fukuoka 830-0011, Japan

this chapter, we discuss the relationship between Ito cells and endothelin (ET)-1 and nitric oxide (NO) in the contraction and relaxation of Ito cells.

## Contraction of Ito Cells

Sinusoid-related cells such as sinusoidal endothelial cells, Ito cells, Kupffer cells, and pit cells have been recognized as very important cell groups in various aspects of the physiology and pathology of the liver. It is also speculated that these cells not only have their own functions, but also control the functions of other cells in the liver. In particular, Ito cells, being mesenchymal cells, are similar to capillary pericytes in location and morphology. These Ito cells have numerous long, slender cytoplasmic processes and surround liver sinusoidal endothelial cells [2]. These morphological characteristics of Ito cells imply that Ito cells are also deeply involved in controlling liver sinusoidal blood flow through contraction and relaxation in conjunction with sinusoid endothelial cells. We have previously reported that ET-1 receptors are present on Ito cells in the rat liver, and that contraction is induced via these receptors [17–21]. Further, Ito cell contraction is induced by ET-1 in a dose-dependent manner and the effect is persistent (Figs. 1 and 2). When changes in desmin immuno-localization in cultured Ito cells were studied, desmin was found to be localized in cytoplasm and along the processes in the absence of ET-1, while in the presence of ET-1, desmin gathered around the nuclei and cytoplasmic desmin decreased (Fig. 3).

ET-1 is a strong and persistent vasoconstrictor peptide derived from vascular endothelial cells. There are three ET isopeptides, ET-1, ET-2, and ET-3 [22], and there are two ET receptors, $ET_A$ and $ET_B$, which are both transmembrane G protein-mediated receptors [23, 24]. $ET_A$ receptors have an affinity to the three ET isopeptides in the order of ET-1 > ET-2 > ET-3, while $ET_B$ receptors have equal affinity to each of the three isopeptides. $ET_A$ receptors, which have high affinity to ET-1 and ET-2, are thought to be present in smooth muscles and mainly involved in contractile activity, while $ET_B$ receptors are thought to be present on endothelial cells and involved in the

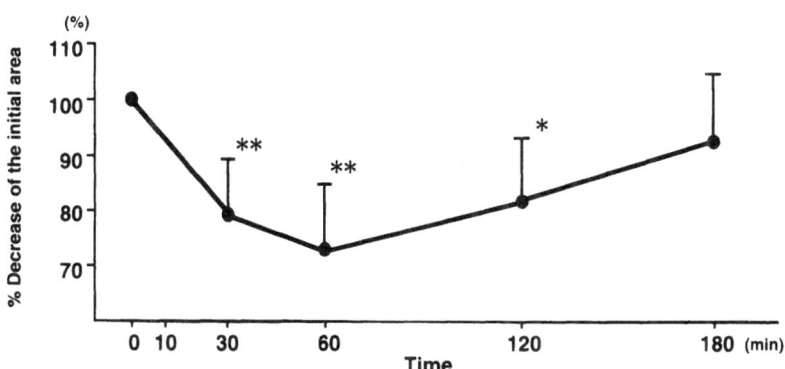

FIG. 1. Serial changes in the area of cultured Ito cells after addition of 200 nM ET-1. The maximal decrease in cell areas occurred 60 min after the addition of ET-1. *$P < 0.05$ and **$P < 0.01$ vs. untreated group. (From [19], with permission)

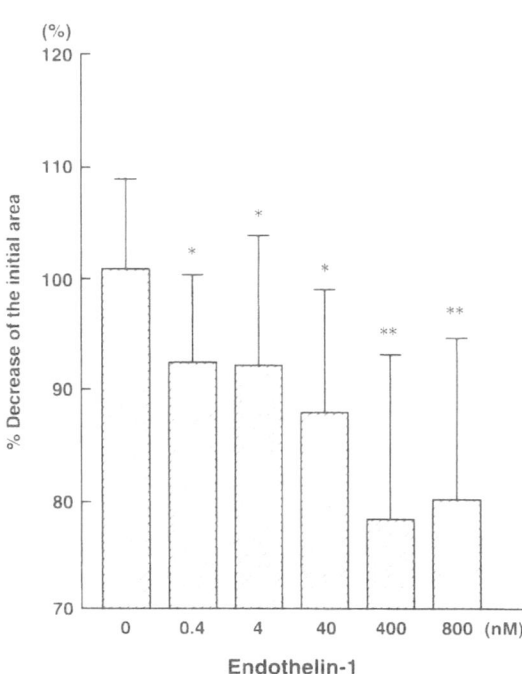

FIG. 2. Changes in cell area after the addition of ET-1 at various concentrations to Ito cells cultured for 24 h. The area of the cultured cells decreased dose-dependently after the addition of ET-1. $*P < 0.05$ and $**P < 0.01$ vs. untreated group. (From [19], with permission)

release of NO, an endothelium-dependent relaxing factor. Regarding the ET-1-induced contraction mechanism, upon binding of ET-1 to $ET_A$ receptors, inositol triphosphate is increased at the cell membrane via phospholipase C and intracellular $Ca^{2+}$ is mobilized, leading to cell contraction [25].

It is currently known that macrophage-derived cytokines interleukin-1 $\beta$ (IL-1$\beta$) and tumor necrosis factor-$\alpha$ (TNF-$\alpha$) act on vascular endothelial cells in inflammatory response, and greatly influence blood coagulation activity and the control of blood vessel tone. It has also been demonstrated that ET-1 is produced by vascular endothelial cells through induction by IL-1 $\beta$ and TNF-$\alpha$ [26]. Furthermore, ET-1 is actually produced in sinusoidal endothelial cells (Fig. 4). These cytokines are considered to accelerate ET-1 production in liver sinusoidal endothelial cells as well as in vascular endothelial cells, suggesting that strong contraction of Ito cells is induced, which considerably affects liver sinusoidal microcirculation.

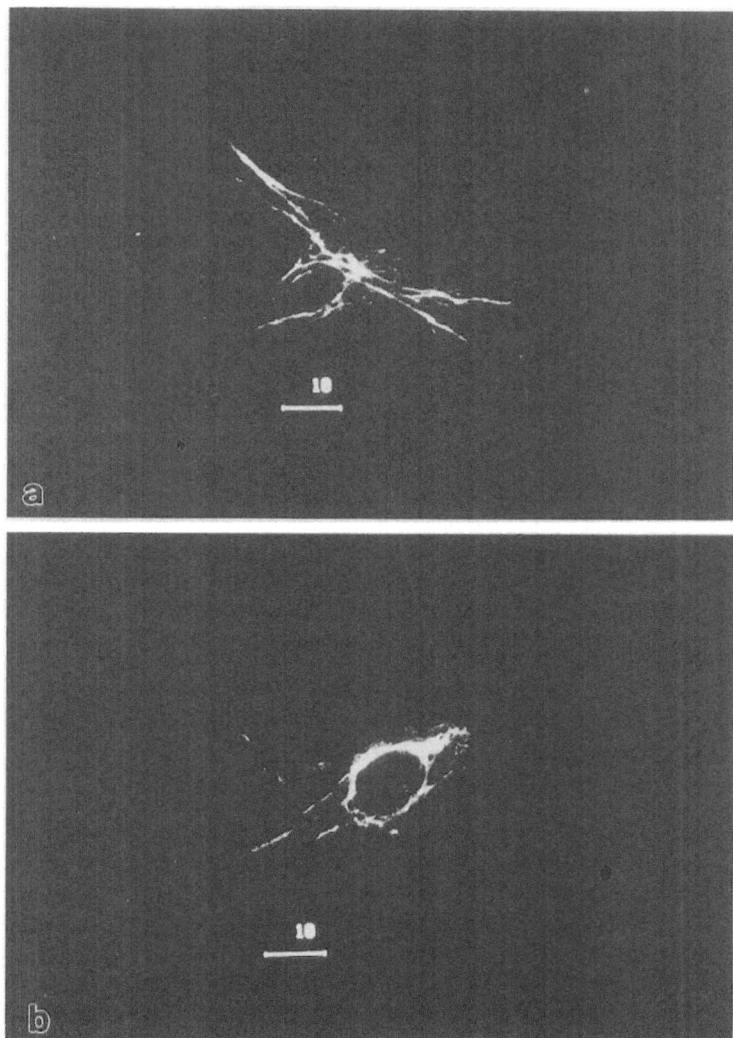

FIG. 3a,b. Ligh micrographs showing FITC-labeled desmin in cultured Ito cells before and after the addition of 200 nmol/L ET-1. **a** Ito cell before ET-1 treatment. (From [19], with permission). **b** Ito cell 60 min after ET-1 treatment. The location of desmin in the Ito cells before ET-1 addition is visible along the slender cytoplasmic processes of the Ito cell. However, the location of desmin after ET-1 treatment changes to a meshlike structure. (From [19], with permission)

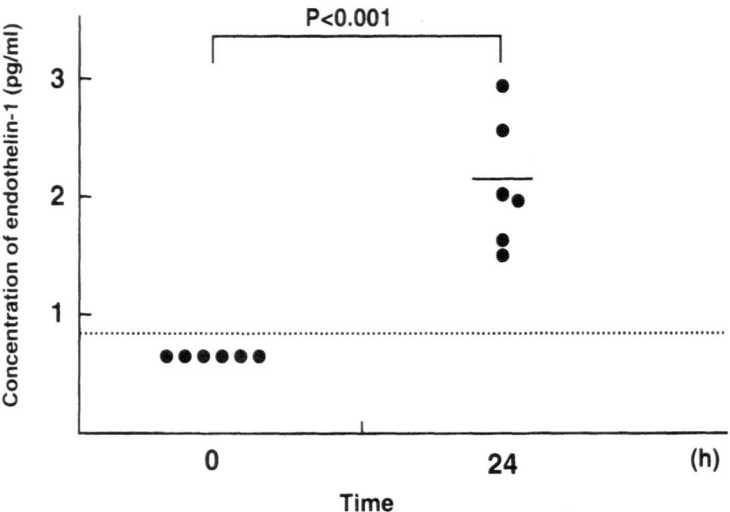

FIG. 4. Concentration of ET-1 in the supernatant of cultured sinusoidal endothelial cells. Significant elevation of ET-1 is noted in the 24-h culture

## Relaxation of Ito Cells

NO, which has a vasodilative effect, is produced by various kinds of cells including vascular endothelial cells [27, 28], macrophages [29], vascular smooth muscle cells [30], sinusoidal endothelial cells [31], Kupffer cells [32], and hepatocytes [33]. NO

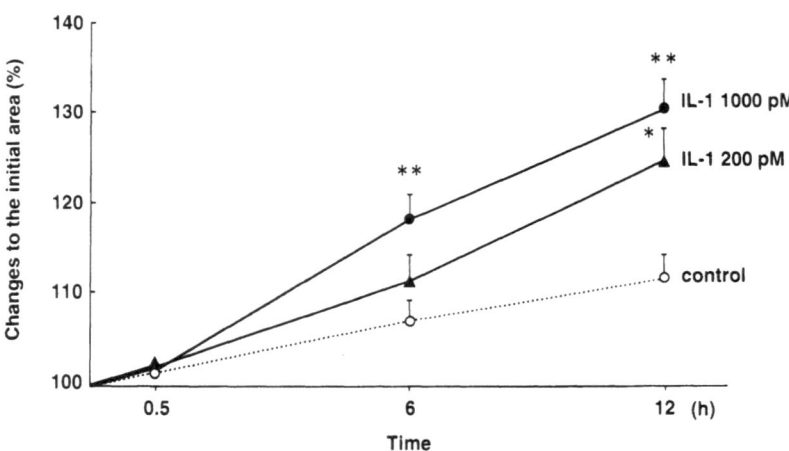

FIG. 5. Serial changes in the area of cultured Ito cells after addition of 0, 200, and 1000 pmol/L IL-1β. Cell areas are significantly greater in the 1000 pmol/L IL-1β-treated group at 6 and 12 h and in the 200 pmol/L IL-1β-treated group at 12 h than in the untreated group. *$P < 0.05$ and **$P < 0.01$ vs. untreated group. (From [45], with permission)

produced by these cells is synthesized by nitric oxide synthase (NOS) using L-arginine as a substrate. There are at least two types of NOS in the vascular system [34]. One is $Ca^{2+}$–calmodulin-dependent constitutive type NOS, and the other is $Ca^{2+}$–calmodulin-independent inducible type NOS (iNOS) which is induced in macrophages and vascular smooth muscle cells. Enzyme activity of iNOS is not normally detected, but once it is induced, NO production persists, resulting in prolonged vasodilation and endothelial cell impairment. In recent years, the association of various shock conditions and NO has been attracting attention, especially the relationship between NO and septic shock, which has now been clarified [35]. After incubating cultured vascular smooth muscle cells with lipopolysaccharide (LPS), IL-1, or TNF-$\alpha$ for several hours, the expression of iNOS mRNA in these cells was observed by Northern blot analysis [36]. It has been suggested that excessive production and release of NO induced by iNOS expressed in these vascular smooth muscle cells cause the relaxation of vascular smooth muscle cells mediated by cyclic guanosine $3',5'$-monophosphate (cGMP), which induces marked vascular dilation, resulting in the development of shock [37].

It has been reported that the blood level of various cytokines including IL-1$\beta$ is increased in patients with liver diseases compared to that in healthy subjects [38]. It is also believed that endotoxins, which are known to show high blood levels in various liver diseases, increase the production of TNF-$\alpha$, IL-1, and interleukin-6 (IL-6) by Kupffer cells and macrophages [39, 40]. Further, it was recently reported that NO is the endogenous mediator responsible for hyperdynamic circulation in liver cirrhosis [41–43]. As described above, in liver diseases, hepatic sinusoidal endothelial cells, and various inflammatory cells mobilized from systemic circulation actively produce various cytokines and are deeply involved in liver pathology, being affected by the cytokines.

In this study, Ito cells were relaxed by administration of IL-1$\beta$ (Fig. 5). It was speculated that IL-1$\beta$ induced the expression of iNOS in Ito cells, which promoted NO synthesis (Fig. 6). The increased NO then induces cGMP elevation, leading to Ito cell relaxation (Fig. 7). Further, since iNOS expression induced in Ito cells started a few hours after the cytokine stimulation and persisted for a long time, the 12-h effect of IL-1$\beta$ on Ito cells observed in this study was also considered to be due to the persistent influence of iNOS on Ito cells [44, 45]. As described above, various cytokines including IL-1$\beta$ are deeply involved in liver pathology. In particular, the contraction and relaxation of Ito cells are deeply involved in liver microcirculation.

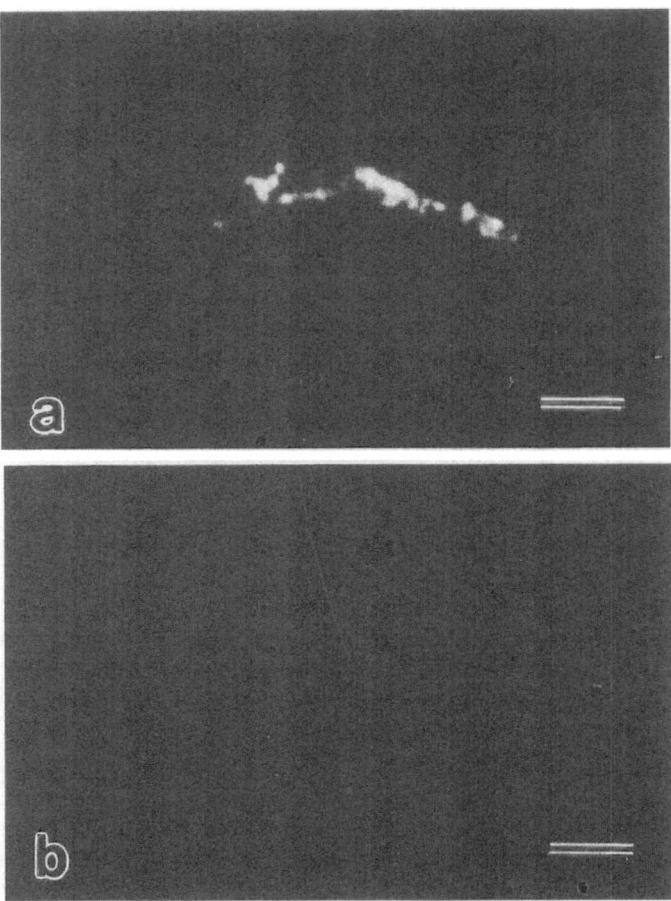

FIG. 6a,b. Light micrographs showing the localization of FITC-labeled iNOS in cultured Ito cells by confocal laser microscopy (bar = 10 μm). a Inducible NOS in the cell body of an Ito cell treated with 1000 pmol/L IL-1β for 12 h. (From [45], with permission). b Negative control showing no fluorescence. (From [45], with permission)

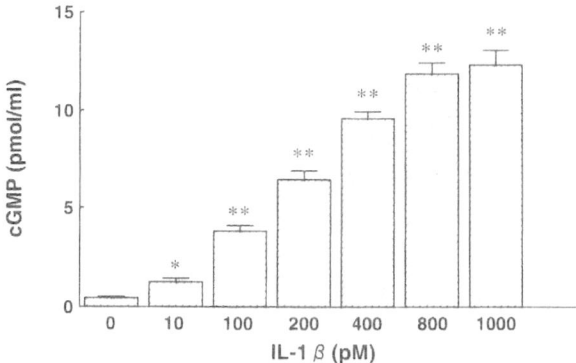

FIG. 7. Cyclic GMP concentration in cultured Ito cells after 12 h treatment with IL-1$\beta$ at various concentrations (0–1000 pmol/L). Cyclic GMP concentration in Ito cells increases significantly in a dose-dependent manner. *$P < 0.05$ and **$P < 0.01$ vs. untreated group. (From [45], with permission)

## Cirrhosis and Portal Hypertension

Two main causes of portal hypertension in cirrhosis have been suggested. The first is an increase in blood flow into the portal vein. This hyperdynamic circulation occurs systemically, but is especially marked in the visceral space. NO is believed to be the cause of the dilation of peripheral arteries, and endotoxins are believed to play the major role in promoting NO production in arterial walls [43]. In cirrhosis, absorption of endotoxins from the intestinal wall is markedly elevated. These endotoxins are very likely to act on the peripheral arteries of the intestinal tract, leading to vasodilation. Generally in cirrhosis, endotoxemia tends to develop due to the decrease in Kupffer cells, which play a central role in dealing with endotoxins, and the formation of collateral circulation [46].

The elevation of vascular resistance in the liver has also been considered as a possible cause of portal hypertension. Although narrowing of the intrahepatic portal vein is initially caused by fibrosis in the liver, shunts are formed inside and outside the liver. It is very possible that the inhibition of sinusoidal blood flow due to sinusoidal wall contraction induced by ET, as described above [19, 47], is the reason for the elevation of vascular resistance in portal hypertension.

Therefore, it is considered that the regulation of both NO and ET production and the prevention of the cellular effects of these substance will lead to developments in the therapy of portal hypertension.

## References

1. Ito T, Nemoto M (1952) Über die Kupfferschen Sternzellen und die "Fettspeicherungszellen" ("fat storing cells") in der Blutkapillarenwand der menschlichen Leber. Okajimas Folia Anat Jpn 24:243–258
2. Wake K (1980) Perisinusoidal stellate cells (fat-storing cells, interstitial cells,

lipocytes), their related structure in and around the liver sinusoids, and vitamin A-storing cells in extrahepatic organs. Int Rev Cytol 66:303-353

3. Blomhoff R, Wake K (1991) Perisinusoidal stellate cells of the liver: Important roles in retinol metabolism and fibrosis. FASEB J 5:271-277
4. Ramadori G (1991) The stellate cell (Ito-cell, fat-storing cell, lipocyte, perisinusoidal cell) of the liver. Virchows Arch B Cell Pathol 61:147-158
5. Hendriks HFJ, Verhoofstad WAMM, Brouwer A, et al. (1985) Perisinusoidal fat-storing cells are the main vitamin A storage sites in rat liver. Exp Cell Res 160:138-149
6. Kent G, Gay S, Inouye T, et al. (1976) Vitamin A containing lipocytes and formation of type III collagen in liver injury. Proc Natl Acad Sci USA 73:3719-3722
7. Clement B, Grimaud JA, Campion JP, et al. (1986) Cell types involved in collagen and fibronectin production in normal and fibrotic human liver. Hepatology 6:225-234
8. Geerts A, Vrijsen R, Rauternberg J, et al. (1989) In vitro differentiation of fat storing cells parallels marked increase of collagen synthesis and secretion. J Hepatol 9:59-68
9. Milani S, Herbst H, Schuppan D, et al. (1989) In situ hybridization for procollagen types I, III and IV mRNA in normal and fibrotic rat liver: Evidence for predominant expression in nonparenchymal liver cells. Hepatology 10:84-92
10. Inuzuka S, Ueno T, Torimura T, et al. (1990) Immunohistochemistry of the hepatic extracellular matrix in acute viral hepatitis. Hepatology 12:249-256
11. Joyce NC, Haire MF, Palade GE (1985) Contractile proteins in pericytes. I. Immunoperoxidase localization of tropomyosin. J Cell Biol 100:1379-1386
12. Tanikawa K, Ueno T (1991) Intrinsic innervation and Ito cells in human liver. In: Tsuchiya M, Nagura H, Hibe T, Moro I (eds) Frontiers of mucosal immunology. vol 2. Excerpta Medica, New York, pp 179-182
13. Rockey DC, Friedman SL (1992) Cytoskeleton of liver perisinusoidal cells (lipocytes) in normal and pathological conditions. Cell Motil Cytoskel 22:227-234
14. Ueno T, Inuzuka S, Torimura T, et al. (1991) Distribution of substance P and vasoactive intestinal peptide in the human liver: Light and electronimmunoperoxidase methods of observation. Am J Gastroenterol 86:1633-1637
15. Kawada N, Tran-thi TA, Klein H, Decker K (1993) The contraction of hepatic stellate (Ito) cells stimulated with vasoactive substances. Possible involvement of endothelin 1 and nitric oxide in the regulation of the sinusoidal tonus. Eur J Biochem 213:815-823
16. Kawada N, Inoue M (1994) Effect of adrenomedullin on hepatic pericytes (stellate cells) of the rat. FEBS Lett 356:109-113
17. Sakamoto M (1991) Effect of endothelin-1 on the contraction of Ito cells (fat-storing cells). Acta Hepatol Jpn 32:1027-1033
18. Sherlock S, Dooley J (1997) Disease of the liver and biliary system. 10th edn. Blackwell Science, Oxford, pp 1-16
19. Sakamoto M, Ueno T, Kin M, et al. (1993) Ito cell contraction in response to endothelin-1 and substance P. Hepatology 18:978-983
20. Ueno T, Tanikawa K (1997) Intralobular innervation and lipocyte contractility in the liver. Nutrition 13:141-148
21. Gondo K, Ueno T, Sakamoto M, et al. (1993) The endothelin-1 binding site in rat liver tissue: Light- and electron-microscopic autoradiographic studies. Gastroenterology 104:1745-1749
22. Yanagisawa M, Kurihara H, Kimura S, et al. (1988) A novel potent vasoconstrictor peptide produced by vascular endothelial cells. Natural 332:411-415
23. Arai H, Hori S, Aramori I, et al. (1990) Cloning and expression of a cDNA encoding an endothelin receptor. Nature 348:730-732
24. Sakurai T, Yanagisawa M, Takuwa Y, et al. (1990) Cloning of a cDNA encoding a non-isopeptide-selective subtype of the endothelin receptor. Nature 348:732-735
25. Marsden PA, Danthuluri NR, Brenner BM, et al. (1989) Endothelin actin on vascular smooth muscle involves inositol trisphosphate and calcium mobilization. Biochem Biophy Res Commun 158:86-93

26. Yoshizumi M, Kurihara H, Morita T, et al. (1990) Interleukin-1 increases the production of endothelin-1 by cultured endothelial cells. Biochem Biophys Res Commun 166:324–329
27. Palmer RMJ, Ashton DS, Moncada S (1988) Vascular endothelial cells synthesize nitric oxide from L-arginine. Nature 333:664–666
28. Sakuma I, Stuehr DJ, Gross SS, et al. (1988) Identification of arginine as a precursor of endothelium-derived relaxing factor. Proc Natl Acad Sci USA 85:8664–8667
29. Xie Q, Cho HJ, Calaycay J, et al. (1992) Cloning and characterization of inducible nitric oxide synthase from mouse macrophages. Science 256:225–228
30. Nunokawa Y, Tanaka S (1992) Interferon-gamma inhibits proliferation of rat vascular smooth muscle cells by nitric oxide generation. Biochem Biophys Res Commun 188:409–415
31. Rocky DC, Chung JJ (1996) Regulation of inducible nitric oxide synthase in hepatic sinusoidal endothelial cells. Am J Physiol 271:G260–G267
32. Billiar TR, Curran RD, Stuehr DJ, et al. (1989) An L-arginine-dependent mechanism mediates Kupffer cell inhibition of hepatocyte protein synthesis in vitro. J Exp Med 169:1467–1472
33. Curran RD, Billiar TR, Stuehr DJ, et al. (1989) Hepatocytes produce nitrogen oxides from L-arginine in response to inflammatory products of Kupffer cells. J Exp Med 170:1769–1774
34. Beasley D, Schwartz JH, Brenner BM (1991) Interleukin 1 induces prolonged L-arginine-dependent cyclic guanosine monophosphate and nitrite production in rat vascular smooth muscle cells. J Clin Invest 87:602–608
35. Stuehr DJ, Marletta MA (1985) Mammalian nitrate biosynthesis: mouse macrophages produce nitrite and nitrate in response to Escherichia coli lipopolysaccharide. Proc Natl Acad Sci USA 82:7738–7742
36. Sirsjö A, Söderkvist P, Sundqvist T, et al. (1994) Different induction mechanisms of mRNA for inducible nitric oxide synthase in rat smooth muscle cells in culture and in aortic strips. FEBS Lett 338:191–196
37. Beasley D (1990) Interleukin 1 and endotoxin activate soluble guanylate cyclase in vascular smooth muscle. Am J Physiol 259:R38–R44
38. Tilg H, Wilmer A, Vogel W, et al. (1992) Serum levels of cytokines in chronic liver diseases. Gastroenterology 103:264–274
39. Knolle P, Schlaak J, Uhrig A, et al. (1995) Human Kupffer cells secrete IL-10 in response to lipopolysaccharide (LPS) challenge. J Hepatol 22:226–229
40. Nain M, Hinder F, Gong JH, et al. (1990) Tumor necrosis factor-$\alpha$ production of influenza A virus infected macrophages and potentiating effect of lipopolysaccharides. J Immunol 145:1921–1928
41. Bomzon A, Blendis LM (1994) The nitric oxide hypothesis and the hyperdynamic circulation in cirrhosis. Hepatology 20:1343–1350
42. Vallance P, Moncada S (1991) Hyperdynamic circulation in cirrhosis: A role for nitric oxide? Lancet 337:776–778
43. Guarner C, Soriano G, Tomas A, et al. (1993) Increased serum nitrite and nitrate levels in patients with cirrhosis: Relationship to endotoxemia. Hepatology 18:1139–1143
44. Rockey DC, Chung JJ (1995) Inducible nitric oxide synthase in rat hepatic lipocytes and the effect of nitric oxide on lipocyte contractility. J Clin Invest 95:1199–1206
45. Sakamoto M, Ueno T, Sugawara H, et al. (1997) Relaxing effect of interleukin-1 on rat cultured Ito cells. Hepatology 25:1412–1417
46. Tomita N, Yamamoto K, Kobayashi H, et al. (1994) Immunohistochemical phenotyping of liver macrophages in normal and diseased human liver. Hepatology 20:317–325
47. Ueno T, Sata M, Sakata R, et al. (1997) Hepatic stellate cells and intralobular innervation in human liver cirrhosis. Hum Pathol 28:953–959

# Portal Hypertension and the Hepatic Sinusoid

DON ROCKEY

*Summary.* Portal hypertension is one of the most important complications of liver cirrhosis, leading to substantial morbidity and mortality. In broad terms, the level of portal hypertension is a function of portal flow and the resistance of blood flow through the liver. Current evidence suggests that both an increase in resistance to blood flow through the liver as well as an increase in portal blood flow contribute to the pathogenesis of portal hypertension. This chapter focuses on the components of increased intrahepatic resistance. The cellular elements that appear to be critical in determining sinusoidal resistance are the hepatic stellate cells and the sinusoidal endothelial cells. Stellate cells are pericyte-like perisinusoidal cells that have been shown to possess contractile properties, and are capable of constricting the sinusoid in vivo. Stellate cell contractility is regulated by endothelin and nitric oxide, which are potent vasoconstricting and relaxing agents, respectively. Importantly, endothelin is overproduced after liver injury by both stellate cells and endothelial cells, setting up an autocrine/paracrine regulatory loop. Recent evidence suggests that after liver injury, endothelial cell nitric oxide synthase, while produced in normal quantities, does not function normally, and leads to decreased production of nitric oxide in the sinusoid. Thus, stellate cells in the injured liver appear to be exposed to increased levels of endothelin and reduced levels of nitric oxide, each contributing to increased resistance to sinusoidal blood flow.

*Key words.* Endothelin, Nitric oxide, Stellate cell, Lipocyte, Cirrhosis

## Introduction

The level of pressure in the portal system is dictated by the resistance and flow in that system: Pressure = Resistance $\times$ Flow. The factors that could result in increased resistance to blood flow through the liver are many, but include those at the microscopic (sinusoid) or macroscopic levels (i.e., regenerating nodules). Further, both fixed and modulable elements appear to participate in the pathogenesis of portal

---

Department of Medicine and Gastroenterology, Duke University Medical Center, Durham, NC 27710, USA

hypertension. At the sinusoidal level, the precise site of increased resistance in patients with liver injury is controversial, but in theory it could be at any of several levels within the liver, including presinusoidal, sinusoidal, or postsinusoidal [1–3]. Recently, it has been demonstrated that sinusoidal flow may be regulated by stellate cells (otherwise known as lipocytes, Ito, or perisinusoidal cells). Moreover, it has been realized that vasoregulatory mediators, including endothelin (ET) and nitric oxide (NO), are important regulators of stellate cell contractility. This review will focus on the role of stellate cells and vasoactive mediators in the pathogenesis of portal hypertension.

## Stellate Cell Contractility and Sinusoidal Blood Flow

Stellate cells are vitamin-A-rich mesenchymal cells which occupy the perisinusoidal space of Disse. In normal liver, they appear to serve largely as a storage site for retinoid esters [4]. During liver injury, they undergo "activation," a process which is a characterized most prominently by production of increased amounts of extracellular matrix [4] (Fig. 1). Culture of normal cells on a plastic matrix in the presence of serum containing growth medium recapitulates many of the features of activation in vivo. From a histological viewpoint, stellate cells are reminiscent of tissue pericytes, a cell type which is thought to regulate blood flow via pericapillary constriction [5]. Because of their anatomic similarity to pericytes and since they express the (smooth) muscle-specific intermediate filament desmin, the possibility was raised that stellate cells may exhibit a contractile phenotype. Further evidence indicating that stellate cells express the putative contractile protein smooth muscle $\alpha$ actin suggested contractile properties for stellate cells [6]. Contraction of stellate cells has been examined directly in a number of systems including on silicone rubber membranes and thick type I collagen lattices in response to serum [7]. Further in vivo

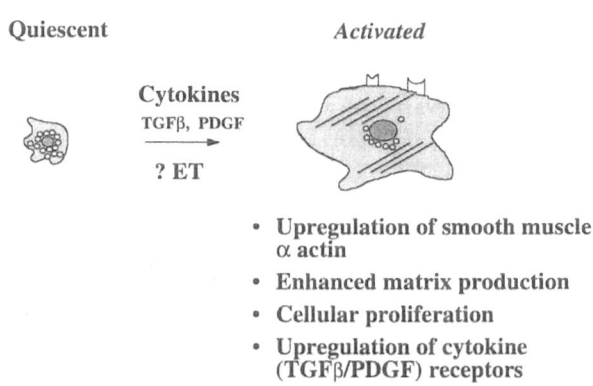

Fig. 1. Stellate cell activation. Stellate cell activation proceeds after liver injury (or during culture in the presence of serum) through a poorly understood cascade of events. The activated phenotype is characterized by the features shown. Similar events occur and result in mesenchymal cell activation in other forms of organ injury

TABLE 1. Mediators of stellate cell contractility

| Contract | Relax |
|---|---|
| Endothelin (1,2,3) | Nitric oxide |
| Angiotensin II | Carbon monoxide |
| Thrombin | |
| Prostaglandin $F_{2\alpha}$ | |
| U46619 (Thromboxane $A_2$) | |
| Substance P | |
| Serum | |

microscopic studies have co-localized sinusoidal constriction to the autofluorescence of stellate cells, providing further evidence that stellate cells are responsible for sinusoidal constriction. In aggregate, the data provide compelling evidence that stellate cells function as perisinusoidal contractile cells in the hepatic sinusoid. Moreover, evidence suggests that this cellular compartment within the sinusoid contributes to the elevated intrahepatic resistance typical of portal hypertension. A number of compounds have been identified as potential mediators of stellate cell contraction [7–13] (Table 1); the most prominent modulators are the endothelins and nitric oxide, and these are reviewed in the next section.

# Regulators of Stellate Cell Contractility

## Endothelin (ET)

The endothelins are a group of potent vasoconstrictors with three unique members: ET-1, ET-2, and ET-3 [14]. The mature peptides, each composed of 21 amino acid residues, are cleavage products of large precursor proteins, termed preproendothelin [15]. Current models suggest that endothelins are produced by primarily by endothelial cells and exert paracrine effects on adjacent smooth muscle cells. However, other data, including our own (see below) on the liver, indicate that endothelins may have autocrine or intracrine effects. Although the major function of endothelins appears to be in the control of vascular tone [14], they also have promitogenic effects. In addition, the production of ET-1/ET-3-deficient mice has implicated the endothelins as regulatory components of mammalian neural crest development [16–18]. The effects of the endothelins depend in part on the ET receptors to which they bind. Two types of G-protein-coupled receptors have been identified, including ET A ($ET_A$) and ET B ($ET_B$) receptors [19]. $ET_A$ receptors are found predominantly on the vasculature and are activated largely by ET-1. Rank order affinities are ET-1 > ET-2 >>> ET-3; the affinity of ET-1 for the $ET_A$ receptor is more than 100-fold that of ET-3 [19]. $ET_B$ receptors are widely distributed and have equal affinity for all endothelin peptides [19]. $ET_B$ receptor stimulation appears to bring about divergent responses and depends in part on the cell type expressing the receptor. For example, stimulation of $ET_B$ receptors on endothelial cells results in the release of nitric oxide (NO) and subsequent relaxation of vascular smooth muscle via activation of cyclic guanosine monophosphate (cGMP) [20]. Conversely, stimulation of $ET_B$ receptors on smooth muscle cells may induce vasoconstriction. It has been proposed that endothelium-dependent relaxation and smooth muscle vasoconstriction mediated by the $ET_B$ receptor are brought about by two related but distinct $ET_B$ receptors, termed "$ET_{B1}$" and "$ET_{B2}$," respectively [20].

Endothelin receptors have been identified on all types of liver cells (stellate, endothelial, Kupffer cells, and hepatocytes) [9, 21–25]. However, the number of receptors on stellate cells far outnumbers that for other hepatic cells [9], implying that stellate cells are the major target of endothelins in the liver. Competitive binding studies indicate that stellate cells express both $ET_A$ and $ET_B$ receptors, but the latter to a greater degree than the former (unpublished observation), which coincides with expression of specific $ET_A$ and $ET_B$ mRNAs [9]. Both receptors mediate stellate cell contraction and do so with equal effectiveness [23]. The $ET_B$ receptor may also regulate growth of human myofibroblast-like stellate cells [26]. Data relating to modulation of receptor subtype are conflicting. While some studies have failed to find changes in receptor expression during liver injury or in culture [9], others report that with repeated passage of cultured cells, the relative abundance of $ET_A$ receptors on stellate cells decreases markedly [22]. Other studies examining endothelin receptors in whole liver after injury further imply that there is up-regulation of endothelin receptors on stellate cells [27].

Recent studies showing that endothelins are produced in the liver are critical given the abundance of ET receptors on stellate cells [22, 28]. Further, circulating ET-1 and ET-3 are increased [29–33], probably representing a spillover of endothelins from the liver. The cellular source of endothelins in liver injury is an active area of investigation. In human and experimental liver injury, preproET-1 mRNA and/or immunoreactive ET-1 appear to be localized to stellate and endothelial cells [22, 28]. Endothelin in stellate cells appears to be stimulated by TGF-$\beta$ [34], implying that cytokines present in the injured liver may be important regulators of endothelin synthesis during liver injury. During liver injury, preproET-1 mRNA and immunoreactive peptide are up-regulated in whole liver (Fig. 2) and specifically in sinusoidal endothelial and stellate cells, although the relative increase is greater for stellate cells than endothelial cells [22, 28, 34] (Figs. 2 and 3). Further, ET-1 has important effects on stellate cells themselves, including stimulation of proliferation and smooth muscle $\alpha$ actin expression. These data imply that during liver injury (since endothelin receptors are most abundant on stellate cells and endothelins

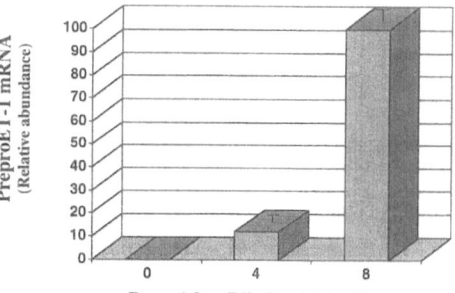

FIG. 2. Preproendothelin(ET)-1 mRNA expression in whole liver after liver injury. Liver injury was induced by bile duct ligation and whole liver total RNA was isolated and subjected to RNase protection assay (10 μg total RNA). The relative abundance of preproendothelin-1 mRNA is shown. $*p < 0.05$ compared to "0". (Adapted from [28])

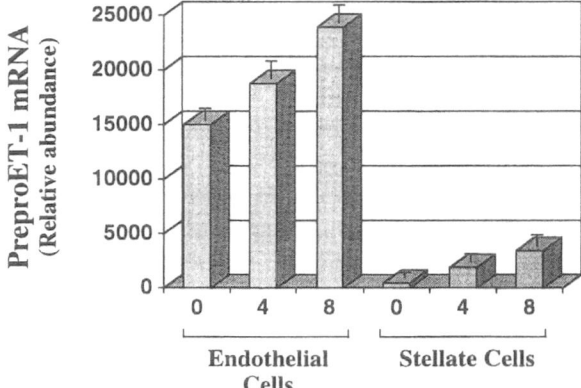

Days After Bile Duct Ligation

FIG. 3. Preproendothelin-1 mRNA abundance in hepatic cells after liver injury. Liver injury was induced by bile duct ligation. After 0, 4, or 8 days, sinusoidal endothelial or stellate cells were isolated and RNase protection assay was performed. The relative abundance of pre-proendothelin-1 mRNA is shown. (Adapted from [28])

appear to act in a paracrine (or autocrine) manner), locally produced endothelin serves as an important component of the activating milieu. Such data have relevance for other forms of tissue injury in which endothelin is overproduced and in which target cells expressing endothelin receptors are prominent. This possibility is supported by the finding that bosentan, a mixed $ET_A$ and $ET_B$ receptor antagonist, inhibited features of stellate cell activation in an in vivo model of fibrogenic liver injury [35].

The finding that ET-1 is overproduced in liver injury has important implications for the pathogenesis of portal hypertension given the perisinusoidal location of stellate cells and their potential for contractile phenotype. While a number of compounds have been advanced as potential regulators of stellate cell contractility, including substance P, angiotensin II, thrombin, and prostaglandins, the endothelins are the most potent [7–12]. ET-1 induces intracellular calcium flux and transient cell rounding in human myofibroblast-like stellate cells [8]. It is also the most potent inducer of silicone rubber membrane wrinkling [11] and contraction of collagen lattices by rat stellate cells [7]. In contrast to many smooth muscle cells, stellate cell contraction proceeds readily via the $ET_B$ receptor [23]. Intravital microscopy has helped to clarify the contractile effects of endothelins on stellate cells [2, 36–39]. For example, Zhang et al. [36] demonstrated dynamic modulation of sinusoidal width in response to ET-1 that co-localized to autofluorescent stellate cells, thus implicating stellate cells as the cellular element responsible for sinusoidal constriction.

An area of controversy surrounds the contractility of stellate cells in normal liver. In vivo microscopy studies indicate that normal cells are contractile and respond endothelins to by contraction [2, 36–39]. However, culture studies indicate that freshly isolated normal stellate cells exhibit little or no contractile behavior. While it is difficult entirely to reconcile these two observations, both the culture-based experiments and the in vivo microscopy studies are subject to potential artifact. For example, freshly isolated stellate cells could be contractile, but all known methods to detect this contractility are not actually sensitive enough to detect it. In contrast, with regard to in vivo studies, it is important to acknowledge that infused endothelins (used to stimulate contractility) are likely to have extrasinusoidal effects (i.e., on smooth muscle cells in the portal venous system) which may be difficult to distinguish from intrasinusoidal effects. Resolution of the controversy awaits alternative methods of detecting stellate cell contractility, or methods which allow the differentiation of stellate cell contraction from other components of the portal system.

## Nitric Oxide

Nitric oxide (NO) has received considerable attention as an important vasoregulator, in particular as an agent that counters the contractile activity of endothelin. The half-life of NO is short, and the diffusion capacity is of the order of microns, emphasizing the autocrine or paracrine nature of its biological actions. Furthermore, the interation of NO with reactive oxygen intermediates (e.g., NO plus superoxide, yielding peroxynitrite) results in products with longer half-lives that may also exert important local effects. NO is produced by one of three isoforms of NO synthase (NOS). Endothelial cells and neurons produce NO from L-arginine via two distinct constitutive NOS enzymes, while a wide variety of cells express inducible NOS [40]. The constitutive isoforms typically produce small amounts of NO and are regulated by intracellular changes in calcium. In contrast, iNOS produces large amounts of NO and functions independently of intracellular calcium [40].

The amount and duration of NO production in a biological system depends in large part on its enzymatic source. While the term constitutive implies that these isoforms are not regulated, their mRNA and protein levels may be altered by changes in the environment such as hypoxia, cytokines, or stretch [41]. The inducible isoform is stimulated by a wide array of compounds/stimuli, including cytokines and lipopolysaccharide (LPS), which have been emphasized as prominent inducers of iNOS. Cytokines and/or LPS initiate dissociation of the NF$\kappa$–B/I$\kappa$–B$\alpha$ complex, releasing NF$\kappa$–B/rel which stimulates iNOS transcription in the nucleus. iNOS regulation is particularly complex, as recent studies indicate that iNOS enzymatic activity is itself inhibited by NO [42].

The potential role of NO in the modulation of sinusoidal blood flow and the pathogenesis of portal hypertension has been emphasized in several recent studies. The NO inhibitor NNA ($N^w$-nitro-L-arginine) increased portal pressure in normal rat livers, while L-NAME ($N^w$-nitro-L-arginine methyl ester), another NO inhibitor, had no effects [43, 44]. Although NO levels in the normal liver appear to be quite low (implying a minor role for NO), perfusion of cirrhotic livers with L-arginine reduced portal reactivity to norepinephrine, suggesting a defect in endogenous NO production in this state [45]. Nitrite levels are elevated in patients with cirrhosis, and iNOS mRNA is up-regulated in the peripheral vasculature of these patients. Such data have implied a role for NO in causing the vasodilation which is typical in cirrhotics with portal hypertension.

At a cellular level, the effects of NO on stellate cells are pronounced. Current data indicate that exogenous NO is capable of preventing endothelin-induced contraction, as well as inducing relaxation in cells that have already undergone contraction [11, 46]. Stellate cells themselves produce NO in response to interferon $\gamma$ and other cytokines with or without LPS [46, 47]. Further, NO produced in an autocrine fashion has a strong relaxing effect on stellate cells [13, 46].

Because essentially all liver cell types are capable of producing NO, signals which stimulate NO are theoretically important paracrine or autocrine mediators of stellate cell relaxation. Therefore, regulation of NOS has been studied in experimental liver injury and portal hypertension. Immediately after toxin-induced liver injury, iNOS is induced. However, this response is transient and iNOS is not detectable with long-standing injury, including in animals after the development of cirrhosis and portal hypertension. These data are consistent with the possibility that a lack of NO may be important in the perpetuation of intrahepatic portal hypertension, particularly in the setting of overproduced endothelin [28].

Recent data have also examined endothelial-cell-dependent production of NO in injured liver. While some studies report an overall increase in ecNOS after liver injury, the majority have not borne this finding out; it has recently been reported that NOS enzymatic activity is reduced in cirrhosis or in endothelial cells from cirrhotic animals [48, 49]. While ecNOS mRNA and protein quantity appeared to be unchanged after two forms of experimental liver injury, production of NO by this isoform was found be reduced compared with normal levels. These data raise the possibility that with liver injury, reduced NO contributes to increased intrasinusoidal resistance to blood flow and therefore to portal hypertension.

## Carbon Monoxide

While NO has received a great deal of attention as a mediator of stellate cell relaxation, Suematsu et al. [44] have recently raised the possibility that locally produced carbon monoxide (CO) might also control stellate cell contractility and thus sinusoidal blood flow. These authors demonstrated that inhibition of CO production (CO is produced by the oxidative destruction of heme via heme oxygenase) caused an increase in portal vascular resistance. While these data are potentially important, it is important to emphasize that CO is much less potent than NO in stimulating guanylate cyclase and thus cGMP-induced smooth muscle cell (i.e., stellate cell) relaxation.

# Liver Injury, and Stellate Cell Contractility and Activation

The liver responds to chronic injury by scarring, which is analogous to the response of other organs. It has been well established that the primary effector cells in hepatic wounding are stellate cells [4]. During liver injury, stellate cells undergo a striking morphologic and functional transition so that they develop stress fibers and produce abundant amounts of extracellular matrix. Importantly, this process is also character-ized by the acquisition of the smooth-muscle-specific protein, i.e., smooth muscle $\alpha$ actin (see Fig. 1). These data have helped establish that during liver injury, stellate cells transform into myofibroblasts, a cell type prominent in healing wounds. Localization of liver myofibroblasts to fibrous bands in the context of the enhanced contractility of the entire liver (personal observation and [50]) raises the possibility that endothelin-mediated contraction of large fibrous bands may lead to an alteration of the hepatic structural architecture and contribute to abnormal blood flow patterns with increased resistance to blood flow. This possibility is emphasized by the demonstration of integrins mediating binding to type I collagen ($\alpha 1\beta 1$ and $\alpha 2\beta 1$) on stellate cells, and by the finding that the blocking function of these integrins inhibits stellate-mediated contraction of type I collagen lattices [51].

While the relative contractility of stellate cells in normal liver is an area of some controversy, available evidence indicates that the conversion of stellate cells to myofibroblasts is associated with substantially enhanced contractility. Culture-based contraction assays have demonstrated that stellate cells expressing smooth muscle $\alpha$ actin were much more contractile than those which did not [52]. Further, Bauer et al. [53] have shown that smooth muscle $\alpha$ actin up-regulation in vivo is associated with increased sinusoidal responsiveness to the constrictor effect of ET-1. Since it is known that liver injury and cirrhosis are associated with a striking up-regulation of smooth muscle $\alpha$ actin and stellate cell contractility, these data have very important implications for the pathogenesis of portal hypertension. Specifically, highly activated (contractile) stellate cells undoubtedly contribute to the increased resistance to sinusoidal blood flow in the injured liver.

The link between stellate cell activation and contractility has important biological implications for the function of cells expressing smooth muscle $\alpha$ actin. Further, acquisition of smooth muscle $\alpha$ actin by stellate cells during activation (Fig. 1) may result in functional changes beyond enhanced contractility. Smooth muscle $\alpha$ actin appears to retard fibroblast motility and may be important for the immobilization of cells [54]. In addition, inhibition of smooth muscle $\alpha$ actin expression by antisense oligonucleotides inhibits stellate cell contractility [55]. These data imply that immobile cells expressing smooth muscle $\alpha$ actin, such as stellate cells, may serve as contractile "anchors" in the wound-healing environment.

# Conclusion

The regulation of sinusoidal blood flow in normal and injured liver is complex and involves structural, cellular, and humoral components. Recent evidence indicates that stellate cells, i.e., resident mesenchymal cells with a histologic orientation in the sinusoid analogous to vasoregulatory pericytes, help modulate sinusoidal blood flow via perisinusoidal constriction. While available data indicate that normal stellate cells regulate sinusoidal blood flow, the contractile potential of stellate cells after injury is markedly enhanced. Endothelin and NO appear to play an important role in modulating stellate cell contractility (Fig. 4), and their interplay is likely to be an important determinant of local sinusoidal blood flow, especially in the injured liver. Moreover, since stellate cell contractility appears to be a dynamic process, manipulation of either or both of these factors may benefit patients with portal hypertension.

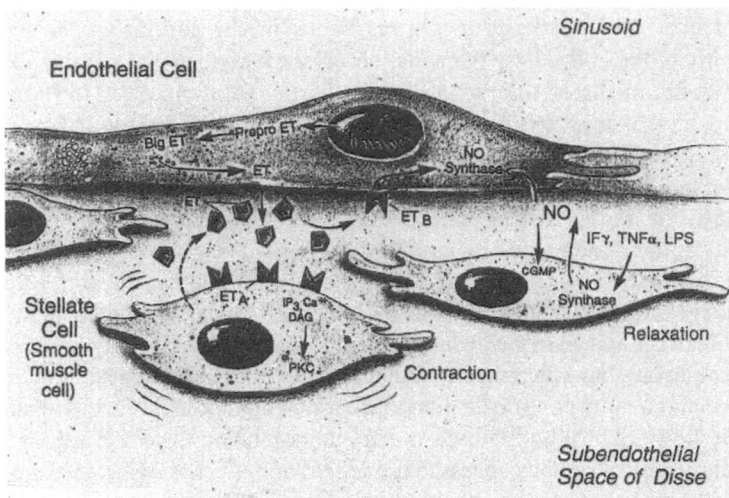

Fig. 4. Stellate cell contractility, endothelin (ET), and nitric oxide (NO). In the normal liver, endothelins are produced primarily by endothelial cells. The mature peptides act in either a paracrine or an autocrine manner on either stellate or endothelial cells, each of which possess endothelin receptors. During liver injury, stellate cells become activated and become an important source of endothelins. Recent evidence indicates that injured endothelial cells underproduce NO, further disrupting the normal homeostatic balance of endothelin-mediated stellate cell contraction and NO-mediated relaxation. Abbreviations: *TNFα*, tumor necrosis alpha; *IFγ*, interferon gamma; *LPS*, lipopolysaccharide; *PKC*, protein kinase C; *DAG*, diacylglycerol; *IP3*, inositol triphosphate. (From [56], with permission)

*Acknowledgments.* This work was supported by grants from the NIH (DK 02124 and DK 50574).

## References

1. Lautt WW, Greenway CV, Legare DJ, et al. (1986) Localization of intrahepatic portal vascular resistance. Am J Physiol 251:G375–G381
2. Zhang JX, Bauer M, Clemens MG (1995) Vessel- and target-cell-specific actions of endothelin-1 and endothelin-3 in rat liver. Am J Physiol 269:G269–G277
3. McCuskey RS (1966) A dynamic and static study of hepatic arterioles and hepatic sphincters. Am J Anat 119:455–478
4. Friedman SL (1993) Seminars in medicine of the Beth Israel Hospital, Boston. The cellular basis of hepatic fibrosis. Mechanisms and treatment strategies. N Engl J Med 328:1828–1835
5. Sims DE (1986) The pericyte—a review. Tissue Cell 18:153–174
6. Rockey DC, Boyles JK, Gabbiani G, et al. (1992) Rat hepatic lipocytes express smooth muscle actin upon activation in vivo and in culture. J Submicrosc Cytol Pathol 24: 193–203
7. Rockey DC, Housset CN, Friedman SL (1993) Activation-dependent contractility of rat hepatic lipocytes in culture and in vivo. J Clin Invest 92:1795–1804

8. Pinzani M, Failli P, Ruocco C, et al. (1992) Fat-storing cells as liver-specific pericytes. Spatial dynamics of agonist-stimulated intracellular calcium transients. J Clin Invest 90:642–646
9. Housset C, Rockey DC, Bissell DM (1993) Endothelin receptors in rat liver: Lipocytes as a contractile target for endothelin 1. Proc Natl Acad Sci USA 90:9266–9270
10. Kawada N, Klein H, Decker K (1992) Eicosanoid-mediated contractility of hepatic stellate cells. Biochem J 285:367–371
11. Kawada N, Tran-Thi TA, Klein H, et al. (1993) The contraction of hepatic stellate (Ito) cells stimulated with vasoactive substances. Possible involvement of endothelin 1 and nitric oxide in the regulation of the sinusoidal tonus. Eur J Biochem 213:815–823
12. Sakamoto M, Ueno T, Kin M, et al. (1993) Ito cell contraction in response to endothelin-1 and substance P. Hepatology 18:978–983
13. Sakamoto M, Ueno T, Sugawara H, et al. (1997) Relaxing effect of interleukin-1 on rat cultured Ito cells. Hepatology 25(6):1412–1417
14. Yanagisawa M (1994) The endothelin system. A new target for therapeutic intervention (editorial; comment). Circulation 89:1320–1322
15. Xu D, Emoto N, Giaid A, et al. (1994) ECE-1: a membrane-bound metalloprotease that catalyzes the proteolytic activation of big endothelin-1. Cell 78:473–485
16. Hosoda K, Hammer RE, Richardson JA, et al. (1994) Targeted and natural (piebald-lethal) mutations of endothelin-B receptor gene produce megacolon associated with spotted coat color in mice. Cell 79(7):1267–1276
17. Baynash AG, Hosoda K, Giaid A, et al. (1994) Interaction of endothelin-3 with endothelin-B receptor is essential for development of epidermal melanocytes and enteric neurons. Cell 79(7):1277–1285
18. Kurihara Y, Kurihara H, Suzuki H, et al. (1994) Elevated blood pressure and craniofacial abnormalities in mice deficient in endothelin-1 (see comments). Nature 368:703–710
19. Sakurai T, Yanagisawa M, Masaki T (1992) Molecular characterization of endothelin receptors. Trends Pharmacol Sci 13:103–108
20. Clozel M, Gray GA, Breu V, et al. (1992) The endothelin ETB receptor mediates both vasodilation and vasoconstriction in vivo. Biochem Biophys Res Commun 186:867–873
21. Stephenson K, Harvey SA, Mustafa SB, et al. (1995) Endothelin association with the cultured rat Kupffer cell: Characterization and regulation. Hepatology 22:896–905
22. Pinzani M, Milani S, De Franco R, et al. (1996) Endothelin 1 is overexpressed in human cirrhotic liver and exerts multiple effects on activated hepatic stellate cells. Gastroenterology 110(2):534–548
23. Rockey DC (1995) Characterization of endothelin receptors mediating rat hepatic stellate cell contraction. Biochem Biophys Res Commun 207:725–731
24. Gondo K, Ueno T, Sakamoto M, et al. (1993) The endothelin-1 binding site in rat liver tissue: Light- and electron-microscopic autoradiographic studies. Gastroenterology 104:1745–1749
25. Serradeil-Le Gal C, Jouneaux C, Sanchez-Bueno A, et al. (1991) Endothelin action in rat liver. Receptors, free $Ca^{2+}$ oscillations, and activation of glycogenolysis. J Clin Invest 87:133–138
26. Mallat A, Fouassier L, Preaux AM, et al. (1995) Growth inhibitory properties of endothelin-1 in human hepatic myofibroblastic Ito cells. An endothelin B receptor-mediated pathway. J Clin Invest 96:42–49
27. Ueno T, Sata M, Sakata R, et al. (1997) Hepatic stellate cells and intralobular innervation in human liver cirrhosis. Hum Pathol 28(8):953–959
28. Rockey D, Fouassier L, Chung JJ, et al. (1998) Cellular localization of endothelin-1 and increased production in liver injury in the rat: Potential for autocrine and paracrine effects on stellate cells. Hepatology 27:472–480

29. Moller S, Emmeluth C, Henriksen JH (1993) Elevated circulating plasma endothelin-1 concentrations in cirrhosis. J Hepatol 19:285–290
30. Nakamuta M, Ohashi M, Tabata S, et al. (1993) High plasma concentrations of endothelin-like immunoreactivities in patients with hepatocellular carcinoma. Am J Gastroenterol 88:248–252
31. Isobe H, Satoh M, Sakai H, et al. (1993) Increased plasma endothelin-1 levels in patients with cirrhosis and esophageal varices. J Clin Gastroenterol 17:227–230
32. Uchida Y, Watanabe M (1993) Plasma endothelin-1 concentrations are elevated in acute hepatitis and liver cirrhosis but not in chronic hepatitis. Gastroenterol Jpn 28:666–672
33. Uchihara M, Izumi N, Sato C, et al. (1992) Clinical significance of elevated plasma endothelin concentration in patients with cirrhosis. Hepatology 16:95–99
34. Gandhi CR, Sproat LA, Subbotin VM (1996) Increased hepatic endothelin-1 levels and endothelin receptor density in cirrhotic rats. Life Sci 58(1):55–62
35. Rockey DC, Chung JJ (1996) Endothelin antagonism in experimental hepatic fibrosis. Implications for endothelin in the pathogenesis of wound healing. J Clin Invest 98(6):1381–1388
36. Zhang JX, Pegoli WJ, Clemens MG (1994) Endothelin-1 induces direct constriction of hepatic sinusoids. Am J Physiol 266:G624–G632
37. Okumura S, Takei Y, Kawano S, et al. (1994) Vasoactive effect of endothelin-1 on rat liver in vivo. Hepatology 19:155–161
38. Bauer M, Zhang JX, Bauer I, et al. (1994) ET-1 induced alterations of hepatic microcirculation: Sinusoidal and extrasinusoidal sites of action. Am J Physiol 267:G143–G149
39. Bauer M, Zhang JX, Bauer I, et al. (1994) Endothelin-1 as a regulator of hepatic microcirculation: Sublobular distribution of effects and impact on hepatocellular secretory function. Shock 1:457–465
40. Moncada S, Higgs A (1993) The L-arginine–nitric oxide pathway. N Engl J Med 329:2002–2012
41. Sessa WC (1994) The nitric oxide synthase family of proteins. J Vasc Res 31:131–143
42. Vodovotz Y, Kwon NS, Pospischil M, et al. (1994) Inactivation of nitric oxide synthase after prolonged incubation of mouse macrophages with IFN-gamma and bacterial lipopolysaccharide. J Immunol 152:4110–4118
43. Mittal MK, Gupta TK, Lee FY, et al. (1994) Nitric oxide modulates hepatic vascular tone in normal rat liver. Am J Physiol 267:G416–G422
44. Suematsu M, Goda N, Sano T, et al. (1995) Carbon monoxide: An endogenous modulator of sinusoidal tone in the perfused rat liver. J Clin Invest 96(5):2431–2437
45. Gupta TK, Chung MK, Sessa WC, et al. (1995) Impaired endothelial function in the intrahepatic microcirculation of cirrhotic livers. Hepatology 22:156
46. Rockey DC, Chung JJ (1995) Inducible nitric oxide synthase in rat hepatic lipocytes and the effect of nitric oxide on lipocyte contractility. J Clin Invest 95(3):1199–1206
47. Helyar L, Bundschuh DS, Laskin JD, et al. (1994) Induction of hepatic Ito cell nitric oxide production after acute endotoxemia. Hepatology 20:1509–1515
48. Rockey DC, Chung JJ (1998) Reduced nitric oxide production by endothelial cells in cirrhotic rat liver: Endothelial dysfunction in portal hypertension. Gastroenterology 114:344–351
49. Van de Casteele M, Reichen J (1997) Hepatic NO synthase (NOS) is decreased in cirrhotic rats and correlates with hepatic functional impairment. Hepatology 26:280A
50. Irle C, Kocher O, Gabbiani G (1980) Contractility of myofibroblasts during experimental liver cirrhosis. J Submicrosc Cytol 12:209–217
51. Racine-Samson L, Rockey DC, Bissell DM (1997) The role of alpha 1–beta 1 integrin in wound contraction. J Biol Chem 272(49):30911–30917

52. Rockey DC, Weisiger RA (1996) Endothelin induced contractility of stellate cells from normal and cirrhotic rat liver: Implications for regulation of portal pressure and resistance. Hepatology 24(1):233–240
53. Bauer M, Paquette NC, Zhang JX, et al. (1995) Chronic ethanol consumption increases hepatic sinusoidal contractile response to endothelin-1 in the rat. Hepatology 22(5):1565–1576
54. Ronnov-Jessen L, Petersen OW (1996) A function for filamentous alpha-smooth muscle actin: Retardation of motility in fibroblasts. J Cell Biol 134:67–80
55. Chung JJ, Rockey DC (1996) Inhibition of stellate cell contraction by smooth muscle alpha actin antisense oligonucleotides. Hepatology 24:461A
56. Rockey DC (1997) The cellular pathogenesis of portal hypertension: stellate cell contractility, endothelin and nitric oxide, Hepatology 25:2–5

# Role of Sinusoidal Endothelial Cells in Alcoholic Liver Disease

Takeshi Okanoue, Shinichi Sakamoto, Takashi Mori, Yoshihiko Sawa, Hikoharu Kanaoka, Kenichi Nishioji, and Yoshito Itoh

*Summary.* We investigated the role of sinusoidal endothelial cells (SECs) in alcoholic liver disease (ALD) using cases of ALD and experimental rat models. In ALD, ballooning of hepatocytes was noted, and in alcoholic liver fibrosis sinusoidal endothelial fenestrae (SEFs) had decreased in size and in number. In chronic ethanol-fed rats (E-rats), ballooned hepatocytes compressed sinusoids, especially in zone 3. However, the porosity of SEFs in zone 3 significantly increased, and hepatic blood flow also increased, resulting in compensating hypoxia of hepatocytes in zone 3 in E-rats. Thioacetoamide-administrated-rats demonstrated that defenestration developed in proportion to the progress of hepatic fibrosis, resulting in liver injury by hypoxia. The present studies using an in vitro flow system demonstrated that adhesion molecules on SECs and their ligands were very important in the adhesion and migration of polymorphonuclear leukocytes (PMNs). Dexamethasone inhibited the adhesion and migration of PMNs.

*Key words.* Alcoholic liver disease, Ballooning of hepatocyte, Sinusoidal endothelial cell, Hypoxia, Adhesion molecule

In alcoholic liver disease (ALD) there are many morphological characteristics such as ballooning of hepatocytes, fatty changes, polymorphonuclear leukocyte (PMN) infiltration, alcoholic hyalin (Mallory body), giant mitochondria, hemosiderin deposit, pericellular fibrosis, perivenular fibrosis, and stellate fibrosis extending from the portal area. It has been considered that the disturbance of hepatic microcirculation plays an important role in the development of ALD [1, 2]. PMN infiltration is also very important in the development of alcoholic hepatitis. Corticosteroids have been used for the treatment of alcoholic hepatitis.

We attempted to clarify the developmental mechanism of disturbances in the hepatic microcirculation in ALD, focusing on the relationship between ballooning of hepatocytes and its effect on sinusoidal endothelial cells (SECs) and hepatic sinusoids.

---

Third Department of Internal Medicine, Kyoto Prefectural University of Medicine, Kawaramachi-Hirokoji, Kamigyo-ku, Kyoto 602-0841, Japan

We also investigated the mechanism of PMN infiltration via the SEC barrier, and the significance of corticosteroid therapy for alcoholic hepatitis.

# Materials and Methods

## Study of Hepatic Microcirculation

Wistar male rats were used to study portal pressure and hepatic blood flow, ballooning of hepatocytes induced by alcohol, its effect on sinusoidal caliber and sinusoidal endothelial fenestrae (SEFs), basement membrane formation and its effect on SEFs, and isolation of SECs. SECs were isolated using an elutriation rotor according to methods previously reported [3, 4]. Rats fed Lieber's liquid diet for 6 weeks were used as chronic ethanol-fed rats (E-rats), and the control rats (C-rats) were fed a standard diet. Sinusoidal casts were made using resin, and these were used to study the changes in sinusoids by scanning electron microscopy.

Portal pressures in C- and E-rats were measured with a manometer, and portal and hepatic blood flows were estimated using the microsphere method reported previously [5]. Rats' livers were perfused using saline via the portal vein, and this served to observe SEFs by transmission and scanning electron microscopy.

To investigate the effect of hepatic fibrosis on SEF, we used rats which had hepatic fibrosis induced by thioacetoamide (TAA) administration (an intraperitoneal injection of 200 mg/kg body weight three times a week for 12 weeks) according to the method reported previously [6].

Sinusoidal caliber, the diameter of SEFs, the number of SEFs per mm$^2$, and their porosity were investigated morphometrically in C-, E-, and TAA-rats using scanning electron micrographs.

## Polymorphonuclear Leukocyte Infiltration

Isolated rat SECs were cultured confluently and used to study the mechanism of PMN infiltration via the SEC barrier using an in vitro flow system attached to a phase-contrast microscope (Olympus, Tokyo, Japan). PMNs of rats were isolated from the peritoneal fluid. Suspensions of PMNs were passed through the chamber at a wall shear stress of 0.5 dyne/cm$^2$.

The roles of adhesion molecules and tumor necrosis factor-α (TNF-α) and the effect of corticosteroids on the adhesion and migration of PMNs were studied. The details of the adhesion assay for PMNs, the expression of ICAM-1 on SECs, and the assay for injury to SECs have been reported previously [7]. CD-18 is a component of Mac-1, which belongs to the integrin family and is an adhesion molecule on PMN.

# Results

## Sinusoid and Sinusoidal Endothelial Cells

In ALD, especially in alcoholic foamy degeneration, ballooning of hepatocytes was conspicuous but disappeared within 3 weeks after abstinence. In E-rats, portal pres-

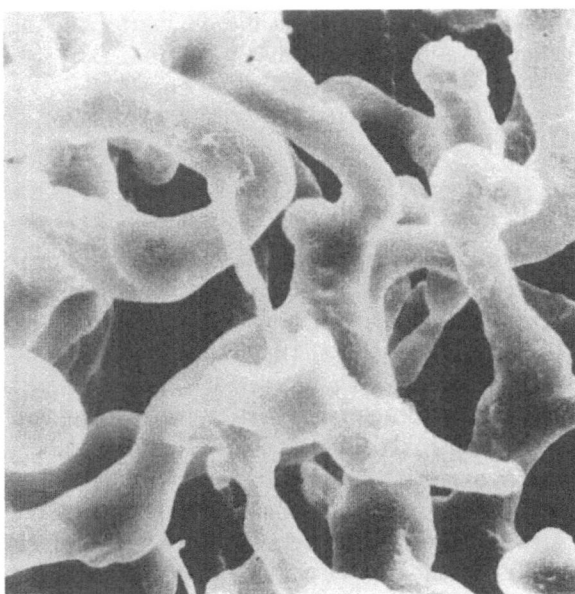

FIG. 1. Scanning electron micrograph of sinusoidal casts in zone 3 (pericentral area) in chronic ethanol-fed rat. Many sinusoids are tortuous and narrowed. ×1500

sure rose to 16.7 cm in $H_2O$ (11.8 cm $H_2O$ in C-rats). The microsphere method demonstrated that both portal and hepatic arterial blood flows were significantly increased by ethanol administration [8].

In E-rats, sinusoidal casts observed by scanning electron microscopy demonstrated that sinusoids in zone 3 became narrow and tortuous as a result of compression by ballooned hepatocytes (Fig. 1). Scanning electron microscopy also showed many pores in the cytoplasm of SECs of around 100 nm in diameter [9, 10] which are called SEFs (Fig. 2A). In C-rats there were heterogenities in the diameter, number, and porosity of SEFs between the pericentral area (zone 3) and the periportal area (zone 1), as shown in Fig. 3. The porosity of SEFs in zone 3 is originally larger than that of SEFs in zone 1, resulting in compensating hypoxia in zone 3.

In E-rats, the diameter, number, and porosity of SEFs were changed. The diameter of SEFs increased considerably in zone 3 (Fig. 2B), and the porosity of SEFs was also significantly increased, especially in zone 3, resulting in compensating hypoxia of hepatocytes in zone 3 (Fig. 3).

In fibrotic liver, the number and porosity of SEFs significantly decreased in ALD (Fig. 4) and in TAA rats. In TAA rats, the number and porosity of SEFs decreased in proportion to the progress of the hepatic fibrosis (Table 1). Defenestration was noted in association with basement membrane formation in the Disse space, and this has been called sinusoidal capillarization [11]. In this condition the exchange of blood flow between the sinusoids and the Disse spaces might be inhibited, resulting in hypoxia of hepatocytes.

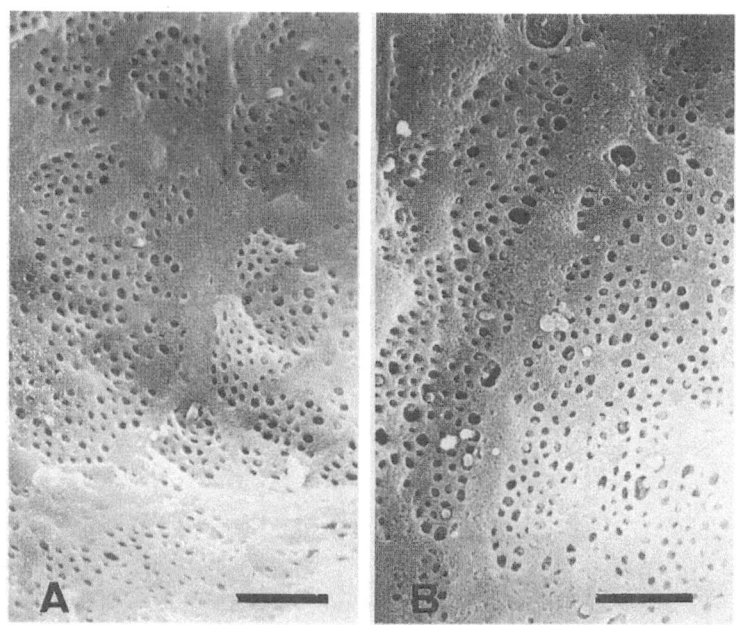

FIG. 2. A Scanning electron micrograph of sinusoidal endothelial cells in zone 3 in a control rat. There are many pores (sinusoidal endothelial fenestrae, SEF) with diameter around 100 nm in the cytoplasm of the sinusoidal endothelial cell, some of which form a sieve plate. In chronic ethanol-fed rats, SEFs in zone 3 were significantly increased (**B**) compared with controls (**A**). The bar indicates 1 micron. ×15 000

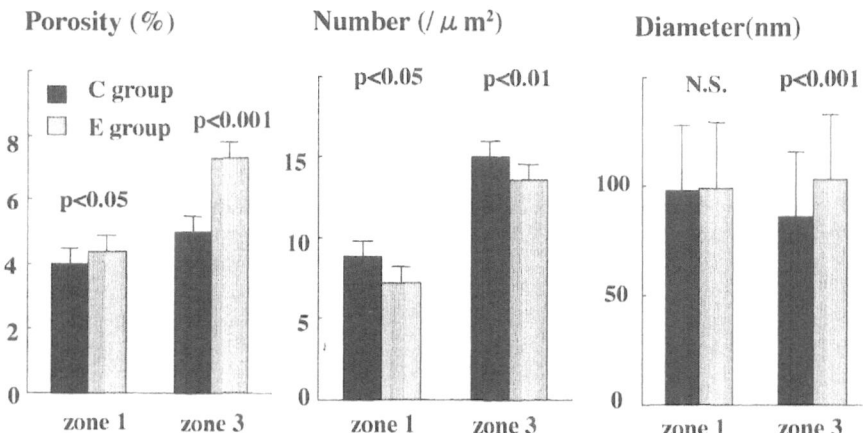

FIG. 3. Morphometric analysis of sinusoidal endothelial fenestrae in zone 1 (periportal area) and zone 3 (pericentral area) in control (C group) and chronic ethanol-fed (E group) rats. There are heterogenities in the diameter, number, and porosity of SEFs in the C group. In the E group, the diameter and porosity of SEFs in zone 3 are significantly increased compared with those in C group. Number is the number of SEFs per square micron of the endothelial surface. Porosity is the ratio of the total area of SEFs per square micron of the endothelial surface

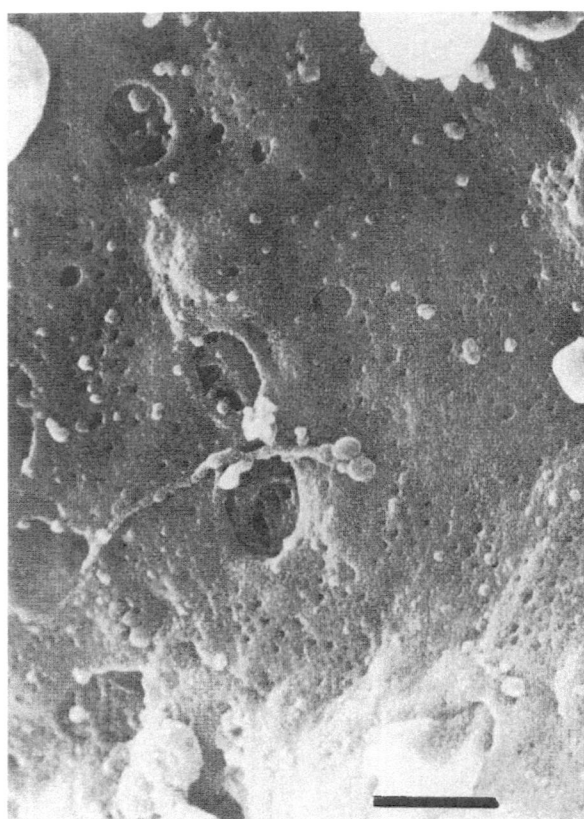

FIG. 4. Scanning electron micrograph of sinusoidal endothelial cells in the case of alcoholic liver fibrosis with basement membrane formation. The diameter and the number of SEFs have significantly decreased, resulting in defenestration. The bar indicates 1 micron. ×17 000

TABLE 1. Morphometric quantitation of the porosity of SEFs in TAA-treated Rats ($\times 10^4 \, mm^2/\mu m^2$)

| Rats | Zone 1 | Zone 3 |
|---|---|---|
| Control ($n = 5$) | 2.48 ± 0.41 (a) | 3.34 ± 0.98 |
| TAA treatment | | |
| 2 weeks ($n = 5$) | 2.30 ± 0.58 | 3.37 ± 1.60 |
| 4 weeks ($n = 5$) | 1.32 ± 0.40 (b) | 1.59 ± 0.31 (b) |
| 6 weeks ($n = 5$) | 0.43 ± 0.28 (b) | 0.60 ± 0.51 (b) |

(a) Data are expressed as mean ± S.D.
(b) $P < 0.01$.

## Polymorphonuclear Leukocyte Infiltration and Sinusoidal Endothelial Cells

The number of PMNs adhering to the monolayer of SECs was increased significantly by stimulation with 100 U/ml rhTNF-α (Fig. 5). To determine whether the increase in PMN adherence induced by rhTNF-α was related to the increase in the expression of ICAM-1 on SECs, the expression of ICAM-1 on SECs was measured by cellular ELISA. TNF-α enhances the expression of ICAM-1 on SECs in a dose-dependent manner [7]. Dexamethasone also inhibited the adhesion and migration of PMNs to SECs in a dose-dependent manner (Fig. 5).

We then studied SEC injury by phorbol 12-myristate 13-acetate (PMA) or N-formyl-methionyl-leucyl-phenylalanine (fMLP). $^{51}$Cr release assay demonstrated that a reduction in the number of co-cultured PMNs resulted in a decrease in endothelial cytotoxicity. Anti-ICAM-1 and anti-CD-18 antibodies and catalase suppressed PMA-induced injury to SEC (Fig. 6A). fMLP (protease generator)-stimulated PMNs also induced SEC injuries, which were also inhibited by anti-ICAM-1, anti-CD-18, and also aprotinin (radical scavenger) (Fig. 6B).

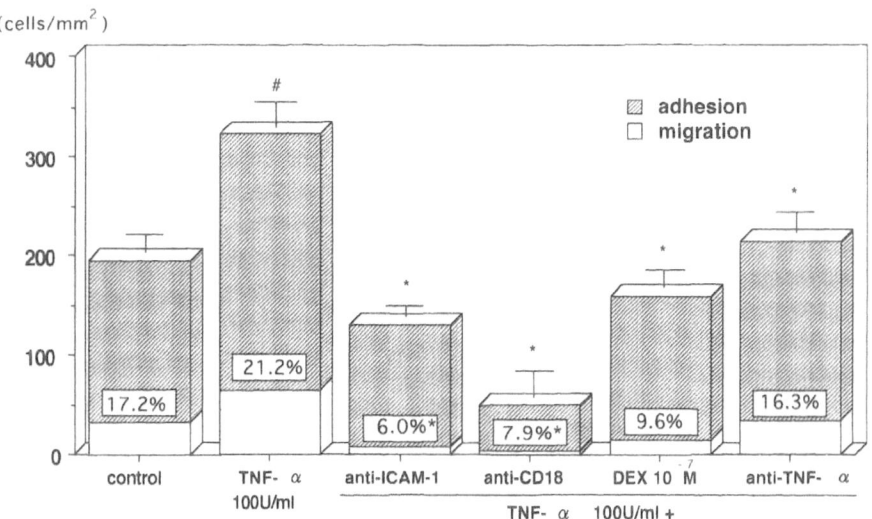

Fig. 5. Effects of monoclonal antibodies to ICAM-1 or CD-18 and dexamethasone (DEX, $1 \times 10^{-7}$ mol/l) and anti-TNF-α on neutrophil adhesion and migration to SECs induced by rhTNF-α (100 U/ml for 4 h). Monoclonal antibodies were added at a final concentration of 5 μg/ml. Each value represents means ± SEM of three experiments performed in duplicate. The percentage shows the migration rate of neutrophils determined by the following equation: Migration rate (%) × Migrated PMNs × 100 − (Adhered PMNs + Migrated PMNs). #$P < 0.05$ compared with controls. *$P < 0.05$ compared with the 100 U/ml TNF-α group without monoclonal antibody or dexamethasone

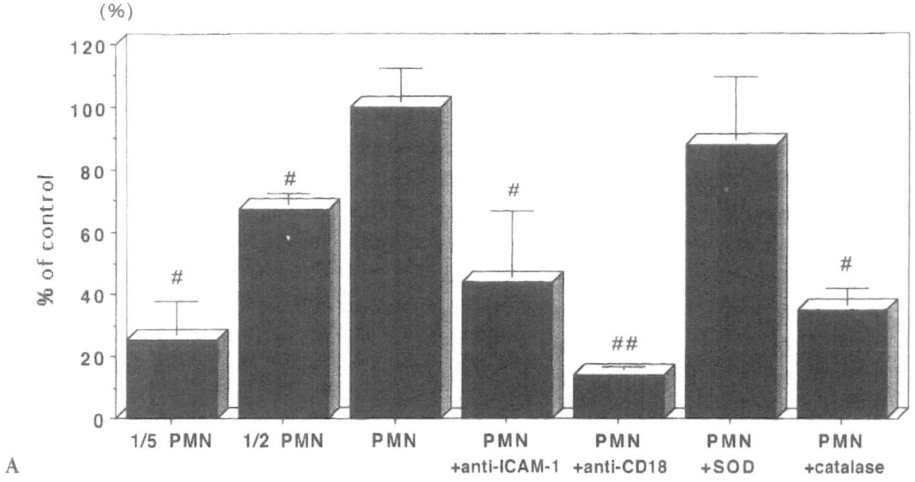

A

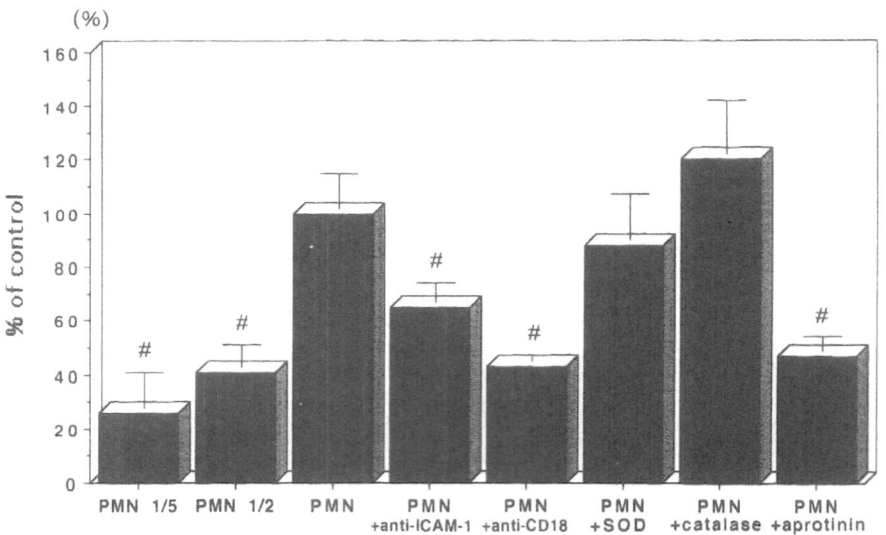

B

Fig. 6. Role of adhesion and neutrophil-derived oxidants in SEC injury induced by PMNs. [51]Cr release was assessed 6 h after incubation. Each value represents means ± SEM of three experiments performed in triplicate, and is expressed as a percentage of the control. The control represents cytotoxicity induced by $1 \times 10^5$ cells of rat PMNs. The 1/5 PMN and the 1/2 PMN represent cytotoxicity induced by $2 \times 10^4$ cells and $5 \times 10^4$ cells of PMNs, respectively. #$P < 0.05$ compared with PMN group (control); ##$P < 0.01$ compared with PMN group

## Discussion

We have described the compensatory mechanism of hypoxia of hepatocytes in zone 3 in chronic ethanol-fed rats, the mechanism of defenestration of SEF in fibrotic liver, the role of adhesion molecules in the adhesion and migration of PMN, and the effect of dexamethasone on the inhibition of PMN infiltration.

Alcohol dehydrogenase (ADH) and acetaldehyde dehydrogenase (ALDH) are abundant in zone 3, which needs oxygen when they metabolize ethanol and acetaldehyde. In chronic ethanol-fed rats, sinusoids in zone 3 were made narrow and tortuous by ballooned hepatocytes, resulting in the disturbance of hepatic micro-circulation and then in hypoxia of hepatocytes in zone 3. However, the porosity of SEFs significantly increased in zone 3 and hepatic blood flow also significantly increased, which might compensate for the hypoxia of hepatocytes in zone 3.

Defenestration was noted in fibrotic liver associated with basement membrane formation at the subendothelial level. In ALD, pericellular fibrosis and pericentral fibrosis are characteristic morphological features. In such conditions, oxygen and nutrients cannot reach enough hepatocytes in zone 3, resulting in liver injury.

In alcoholic hepatitis, the infiltration of many PMNs is noted, and corticosteroids have been used in the treatment. However, the mechanism of their infiltration is not well understood. To clarify the mechanism of liver injury mediated by PMNs, we focused on the interaction between ICAM-1 and CD-18 using an in vitro flow system. Our studies showed that the interaction between ICAM-1 and CD-18 was involved in PMN adhesion to and migration through SECs, and that this interaction was important for the injury to SECs induced by PMA- and fMLP-activated PMNs.

It has been reported that ICAM-1 is important in the migration and adhesion of PMNs [12, 13]. CD-11b/CD-18 monoclonal antibody is reported to prevent the hepatic infiltration of PMNs and the necrosis of hepatocytes induced by intraperitoneal injection of endotoxin [14].

We investigated the role of ICAM-1 and CD-18 in the adhesion of PMNs to SECs, and the migration of PMNs through SECs by means of an in vitro flow system. Our results indicated that both ICAM-1 and CD-18 play a key role in the adhesion and migration of PMNs in hepatic sinusoids. Our cellular ELISA showed that ICAM-1 was expressed on SECs in basal conditions in vitro, and that rhTNF-$\alpha$ increased its expression in a dose-dependent manner [7]. Ohira et al. [15] reported that serum levels of TNF-$\alpha$ and ICAM-1 expression on SECs were increased in rats treated with lipopolysaccharide, and these are also increased in alcoholic hepatitis.

The injury to the endothelial cells elicited by activated leukocytes is the initial event in various forms of inflammation. It is mainly caused by the active oxygen species or by several proteases released by activated PMNs [16, 17]. We showed that both PMA- and fMLP-activated PMNs induced SEC injury in a PMN/SEC ratio-dependent manner. This shows that PMNs infiltrating hepatic sinusoids could induce the endothelial cell damage that causes the disturbance of sinusoidal microcirculation.

The involvement of leukocyte adhesion in the pathogenesis of hepatic injury related to alcoholism has clinical relevance. It is reported that corticosteroids improve survival in patients with severe alcoholic hepatitis [18], but its mechanism has not yet been clarified. We investigated the effects of dexamethasone on TNF-$\alpha$-induced overexpression of ICAM-1 on SECs, and on the interaction between PMNs and SECs, to clarify the mechanism of the antiinflammatory effects of dexamethasone in PMN-mediated liver injury. Dexamethasone inhibited the expression of ICAM-1 on SECs in a dose-dependent manner.

To summarize the early stage of ALD hypoxia of hepatocytes in zone 3 was compensated for in part by the increased porosity of SEFs and increased hepatic blood flow. However, liver injury might be induced by defenestration in the fibrotic liver associated with basement membrane formation. The interaction between ICAM-1 and

CD-18 was involved in the adhesion and migration of PMNs in hepatic sinusoids mediated by TNF-α. This interaction was the key to the SEC injury induced by activated PMNs. Dexamethasone inhibited the adhesion of PMNs to SECs by reducing the expression of ICAM-1 on SECs. Blocking the interaction of ICAM-1–CD-18 might be a reasonable treatment for alcoholic hepatitis.

## References

1. Oshita M, Sato N, Yoshihara H, et al. (1992) Ethanol-induced vasoconstriction causes focal hepatocellular injury in the isolated perfused rat liver. Hepatology 16:1007–1013
2. Okanoue T, Mori T, Sakamoto S, et al. (1995) The role of sinusoidal endothelial cells in alcoholic liver disease. J Gastroenterol Hepatol 10:S35–S37
3. Itoh Y, Okanoue T, Morimoto M, et al. (1992) Functional heterogenity of rat liver macrophages: Interleukin-1 secretion and Ia antigen expression in contrast with phagocytic activity. Liver 12:26–33
4. Mori T, Okanoue T, Sawa Y, et al. (1993) Defenestration of the sinusoidal endothelial cell in a rat model of cirrhosis. Hepatology 17:891–897
5. Sawa Y, Okanoue T, Itoh Y, et al. (1990) Systemic and hepatic hemodynamics in the experimental liver cirrhosis induced by thioacetoamide administration. Acta Hepatol Jpn 31:1064–1069
6. Hori N, Okanoue T, Sawa Y, et al. (1993) Hemodynamic characterization in experimental liver cirrhosis induced by thioacetoamide administration. Dig Dis Sci 38:2195–2202
7. Sakamoto S, Okanoue T, Itoh Y, et al. (1997) Intercellular adhesion molecule-1 and CD18 are involved in neutrophil adhesion and its cytotoxicity to cultured sinusoidal endothelial cells in rats. Hepatology 26:658–663
8. Sawa Y, Okanoue T, Kanaoka H, et al. (1990) The study of acute effects of ethanol on hepatic blood flow using radioactive microsphere method. Acta Hepatol Jpn 31:302–308
9. Wisse E, De Zanger RB, Chareles K, et al. (1985) The liver sieve: Considerations concerning the structure and function of endothelial fenestrae. The sinusoidal wall and the space of Disse. Hepatology 5:683–692
10. Kanaoka H, Okanoue T, Sawa Y, et al. (1988) Morphometric quantitation of rat liver sinusoidal endothelial fenestration in various degrees of perfusion pressure. Acta Hepatol Jpn 28:578–586
11. Schaffner F, Popper H (1963) Capillarization of hepatic sinusoids in man. Gastroenterology 44:239–242
12. Laurence MB, McIntire LV, Eskin SG, et al. (1987) Effect of flow on polymorphonuclear leukocyte/endothelial cell adhesion. Blood 70:1284–1290
13. Lawrence MB, Smith CW, Eskin SG, et al. (1990) Effect of venous shear stress on CD-18-mediated neutrophil adhesion to cultured endothelium. Blood 75:227–237
14. Jaeschke H, Farhood A, Smith CW, et al. (1991) Neutrophil-induced liver injury in endotoxin shock is a CD11b/CD-18-dependent mechanism. Am J Physiol 261:G1051–G1056
15. Ohira H, Ueno T, Torimura T, et al. (1995) Leukocyte adhesion molecules in the liver and plasma cytokine levels in endotoxin-induced rat liver injury. Scand J Gastroenterol 30:1027–1035
16. Harlan JM, Schwartz BR, Reidy MA, et al. (1985) Activated neutrophils disrupt endothelial monolayer integrity by an oxygen radical-independent mechanism. Lab Invest 52:141–150
17. Weiss SJ (1989) Tissue destruction by neutrophils. N Engl J Med 320:365–376
18. Ramond MJ, Poynard T, Rueff B, et al. (1992) A randomized trial of prednisolone in patients with severe alcoholic hepatitis. N Engl J Med 326:507–512

# The Role of Neutrophils in Liver Cell Injury in Alcoholic Hepatitis

Ryukichi Kumashiro, Kazunori Noguchi, Shotaro Sakisaka, Kazuya Sato, Kunihide Ishii, Michio Sata, and Kyuichi Tanikawa

*Summary.* We describe the role of neutrophils in the pathogenesis of alcoholic hepatitis (AH). Endotoxemia, leukocytosis in the peripheral blood, and infiltration of the liver by neutrophils are common features in patients with AH.

We observed increased serum levels of tumor necrosis factor (TNF)-$\alpha$, interleukin (IL)-8, soluble intercellular adhesion molecule (ICAM)-1, and neutrophil counts in the liver of patients with AH. Neutrophil counts in the liver correlated positively with serum IL-8 concentration. Lipopolysaccharide (LPS) uptake by Kupffer cells evaluated by anti-LPS antibody staining was reduced in severe alcoholic hepatitis. The numbers of apoptotic bodies in the liver were proportional to the severity of the alcoholic liver disease. In experimental studies, we observed increased absorption of endotoxins from the intestine and decreased phagocytosis of endotoxins by the Kupffer cells. The splenic macrophages were more potent in generating TNF-$\alpha$ than the Kupffer cells, and splenectomy reduced the elevation of serum IL-8 following liver injury after LPS injection in ethanol-fed rats.

These findings suggested that increased absorption and decreased uptake of endogenous endotoxins lead to neutrophil infiltration of the liver via the activated cytokine cascade and increased adhesion molecules, and that splenic macrophages are important as the origin of TNF-$\alpha$.

*Key words.* Alcoholic hepatitis, Leukocyte, Interleukin-8, Tumor necrosis factor-$\alpha$, Endotoxin

## Introduction

There are several hypotheses about the pathogenesis of alcoholic hepatitis (AH). The hypoxic theory is based on the lower oxygen tension in zone 3 of the hepatic lobule. Recently, vasoconstriction under higher ethanol concentration was shown to be responsible for hypoxia [1]. Acetaldehyde-induced liver injury is related to

The Second Department of Internal Medicine, Kurume University, School of Medicine, 67 Asahi-machi, Kurume, Fukuoka 830-0011, Japan

polymorphism of ALDH2 [2] and cytochrome P-450 2E1(CYP2E1) [3]. Acetaldehyde becomes neo-antigen if it forms an acetaldehyde adduct and provokes an immune reaction [4, 5]. Free radicals facilitate lipid peroxidation by the acetaldehyde originating from ethanol oxidation by CYP2E1. Oxygen radicals liberated in the xanthine oxidase pathway also trigger lipid peroxidation.

Patients with AH frequently have fever, leukocytosis, and endotoxemia. However, there are few reports on the pathological role of neutrophils in AH. In this report, we evaluate the role of neutrophils in the pathogenesis of AH.

## Leukocytosis and Endotoxemia in AH

Leukocytosis is common in patients with AH, and on admission the mean number of leukocytes in the peripheral blood is greater than that in fulminant hepatitis (Table 1) [6]. The peripheral leukocyte count is proportional to the severity of the AH. We showed by logistic analysis that peripheral leukocyte count on admission, together with age, serum creatinine, and hepaplastin time, was of prognostic value in patients with AH (Table 2) [7].

TABLE 1. Results of routine laboratory admission tests in patients with alcoholic hepatitis and fulminant hepatitis

|  | Alcoholic hepatitis ($n = 50$) | Severe alcoholic hepatitis ($n = 24$) | Fulminant hepatitis ($n = 50$) |
|---|---|---|---|
| White blood cells (/microliter) | $7210 \pm 3000$ | $18\,425 \pm 9125$ | $12\,692 \pm 5971$ |
| Red blood cells (million/microliter) | $4.03 \pm 0.63$ | $3.03 \pm 0.68$ | $4.12 \pm 0.62$ |
| Platelets ($\times 10\,000$/microliter) | $13.6 \pm 1.9$ | $12.8 \pm 8.4$ | $13.1 \pm 11.8$ |
| Total bilirubin (mg/dl) | $3.4 \pm 3.5$ | $15.5 \pm 9.4$ | $11.3 \pm 5.4$ |
| Aspartate aminotransferase (IU/l) | $267 \pm 146$ | $403 \pm 1022$ | $1\,665 \pm 1594$ |
| Alanine aminotransferase (IU/l) | $118 \pm 143$ | $75 \pm 150$ | $2\,092 \pm 1584$ |
| AST/ALT | $2.8 \pm 1.4$ | $4.7 \pm 2.4$ | $0.83 \pm 0.44$ |
| $\gamma$-glutamyl transpeptidase (IU/l) | $723 \pm 506$ | $324 \pm 318$ | $62 \pm 52$ |
| Albumin (g/dl) | $4.2 \pm 0.6$ | $2.6 \pm 0.5$ | $3.1 \pm 0.6$ |
| Prothrombin time (%) | $77 \pm 25$ | $32.7 \pm 13.6$ | $18.4 \pm 9.0$ |
| Total cholesterol (mg/dl) | $203 \pm 86$ | $125 \pm 60$ | $102 \pm 30$ |
| Blood urea nitrogen (mg/dl) | $13.0 \pm 7.7$ | $33.3 \pm 27.8$ | $16.3 \pm 14.0$ |
| Creatinine (mg/dl) | $0.95 \pm 0.31$ | $3.1 \pm 2.9$ | $1.6 \pm 1.3$ |

TABLE 2. Prognostic indices in patients with alcoholic hepatitis analyzed by logistic regression

| Variable | Regression coefficient | $P$ | Odds | 95% confidence interval | |
|---|---|---|---|---|---|
| Hepaplastin test (HPT) | $-0.0703$ | 0.009 | 0.93 | 0.89 | – 0.97 |
| Leukocytes (WBC) | 0.000092 | 0.0523 | 1.00 | 1.00 | – 1.00 |
| Age (AGE)[a] | 2.2479 | 0.0063 | 9.47 | 1.89 | – 47.45 |
| Creatinine (CR)[b] | 1.5508 | 0.0356 | 4.72 | 1.08 | – 20.60 |

[a] If age is under 40 or over 60, then AGE is 1, otherwise 0.
[b] If serum creatinine is over 1.4 mg/dl, then CR is 1, otherwise 0.
Logit $= 0.4564 + 2.2479 \times$ AGE $+ 0.000092 \times$ WBC $+ 1.5508 \times$ CR $- 0.0703 \times$ HPT.

FIG. 1. Positive rate for a plasma endotoxin (>5 pg/ml) and b serum levels of tumor necrosis factor (TNF)-α in patients with alcoholic liver diseases. *FL*, fatty liver; *HF*, hepatic fibrosis; *LC*, liver cirrhosis; *AH*, alcoholic hepatitis; *AH + LC*, alcoholic hepatitis on liver cirrhosis; *SAH*, severe alcoholic hepatitis. (From [6], with permission)

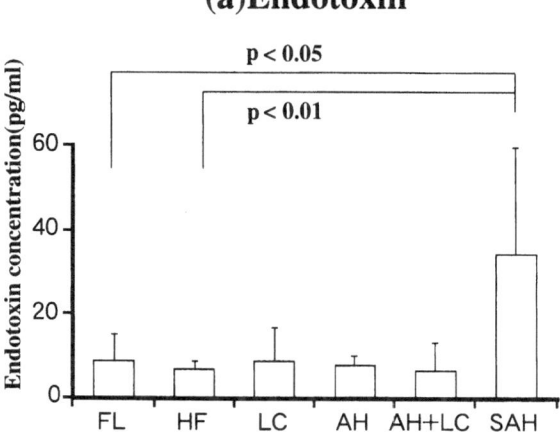

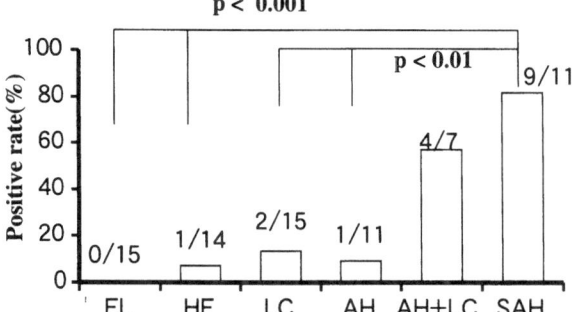

The positive rate for plasma endotoxins (>5 pg/ml) determined by chromogenic endotoxin-specific assay (Endospec SP Test, Seikagakukogyou Co., Tokyo) [8] was 33% in severe AH, and was much higher than that in other forms of alcoholic liver disease (Fig. 1a). Serum tumor necrosis factor (TNF)-α (Fig. 1b) was also high in AH.

These data show that certain mechanisms are involved in the severity of AH in relation to leukocytosis, endotoxemia, and TNF-α.

## Histological Findings

Histological studies revealed neutrophil infiltration in the liver, and neutrophils were often associated with a focal necrosis. In severe AH, Mallory bodies were observed within hepatocyte which infiltrated by neutrophil (Fig. 2). Electron microscope studies showed a neutrophils directly attached to a hepatocyte (Fig. 3). The hepatocyte with the neutrophil showed changes suggestive of the early stages

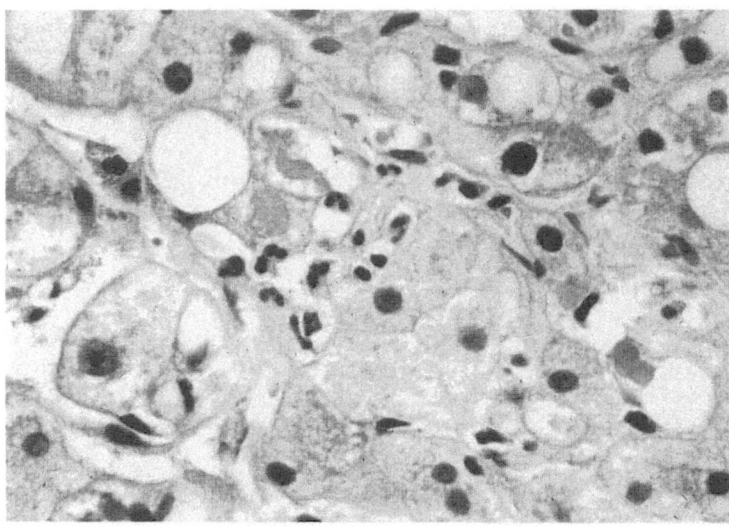

FIG. 2. Light micrograph of the liver from a patient with alcoholic hepatitis. Neutrophil infiltration was observed around a hepatocyte containing a Mallory body. (From [6], with permission.) Hematoxilin–eosin staining. Original magnification 200×

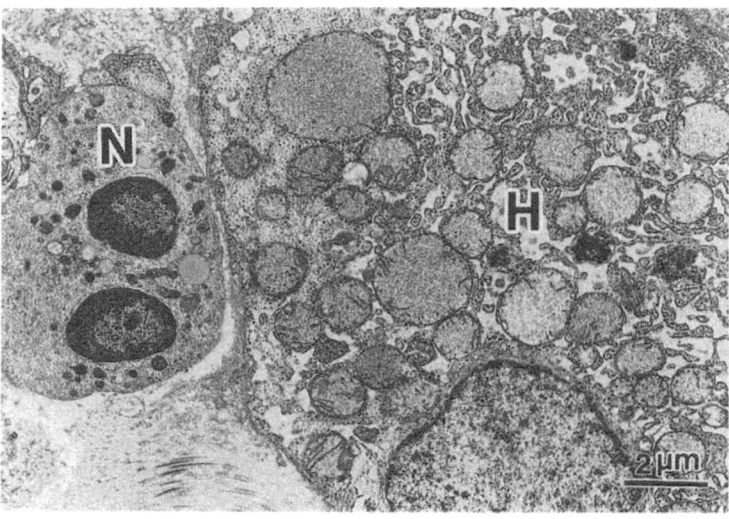

FIG. 3. Electron micrograph of the liver from a patient with alcoholic hepatitis. A neutrophil (N) directly attached to a hepatocyte (H) with the early stage of necrosis. (From [6], with permission.) Original magnification 200×

of necrosis, such as vacuoles and the disappearance of mitochondrial cristae. Disruption of the plasma membrane of hepatocytes was observed in more advanced forms of necrosis, and subcellular organellae were flowing out into the sinusoid.

These findings lead us to consider a relationship between endotoxemia and neutrophil-mediated liver cell injury.

## Cause of Endotoxemia in AH

There are two possible reasons for endotoxemia in AH. One is the increased absorption of endotoxins from the intestine, and the other is the decreased clearance by the Kupffer cells. We studied the effect of ethanol on the intestinal absorption of lipopolysaccharide (LPS). LPS was administered into the ascending colon at a dose of 0.5 mg/body, and its concentration in the portal blood was determined in chronic ethanol-fed rats. LPS concentration was significantly elevated in ethanol-fed rats, suggesting that endotoxin absorption is increased by ethanol ingestion (Fig. 4).

We also assessed the phagocytotic activity of Kupffer cells in patients with AH. LPS in Kupffer cells was stained immunohistochemically on a liver specimen obtained by biopsy using fluorescein isothiocyamate (FITC)-bound antilipid A (gift from Pfeizer Pharmaceutical Inc., USA). Figure 5 shows phagocytosis of FITC-bound LPS in a patient with AH (Fig. 5a) and a control subject (Fig. 5b). There was less LPS uptake in the patient than in the control, suggesting that endotoxin clearance is impaired.

From these results, the increased level of circulating endotoxin in AH may have resulted from both increased absorption of endotoxin from the intestine and decreased phagocytosis of endotoxin by the Kupffer cells.

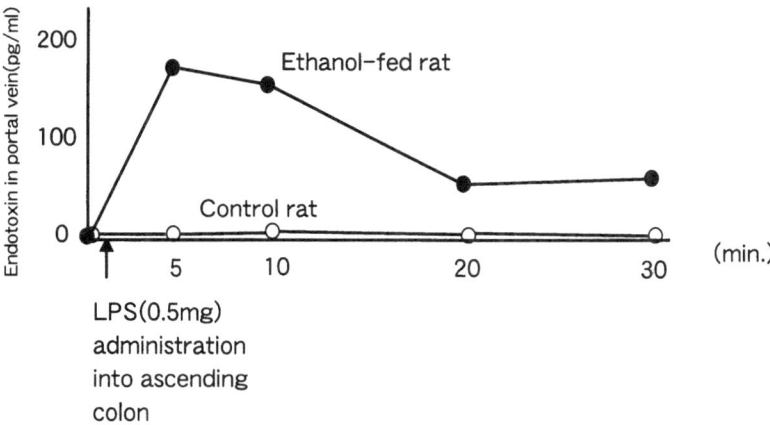

FIG. 4. Endotoxin concentration in the portal blood after administration of lipopolysaccharide into the ascending colon in a chronic ethanol-fed rat. Lipopolysaccharide (LPS) concentration was significantly high in ethanol-fed rats, suggesting that endotoxin absorption is increased by ethanol feeding. (From [6], with permission)

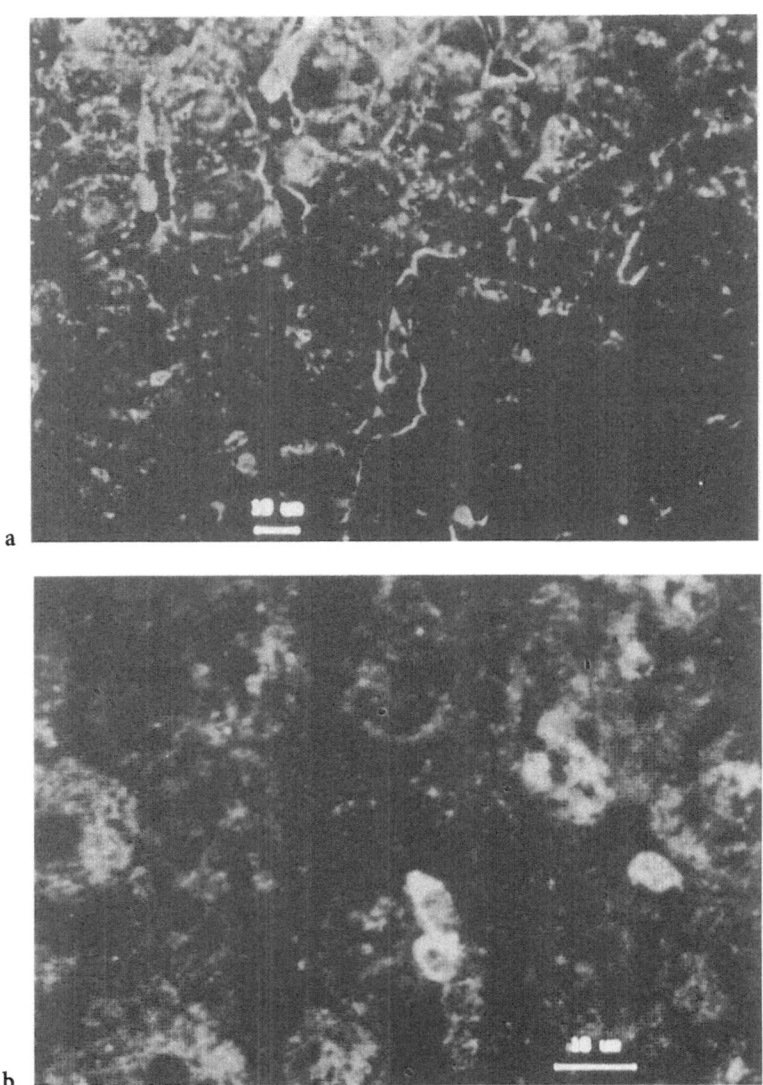

Fig. 5. **a** A confocal LASER microgram of the liver of a patient with alcoholic hepatitis. Distribution of FITC-labeled anti-lipopolysaccharide was sparse in patients with alcoholic hepatitis compared with the control (**b**)

## Origin of Circulating TNF-$\alpha$

In order to clarify the origin of the additional TNF-$\alpha$ in serum, we compared the abilities of Kupffer cells and splenic macrophages to generate TNF-$\alpha$. Differences in TNF-$\alpha$-mRNA were assessed by the reverse transcription-polymerase chain reaction

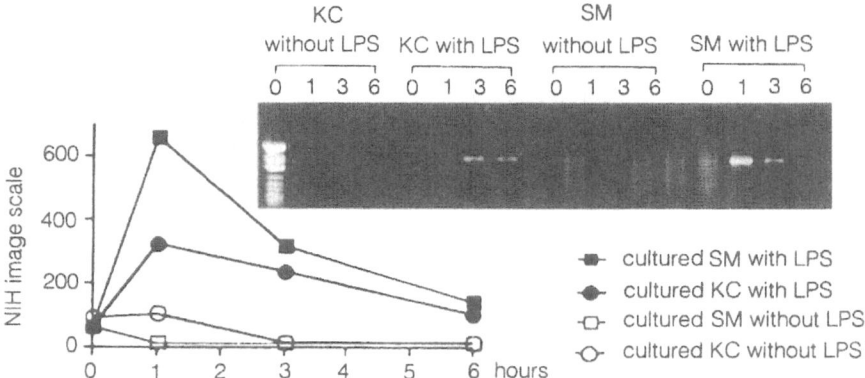

SM and KC were incubated for various periods in 1 ml RPMI/10% FBS
with and without 1 μg/ml of LPS and isolated total RNA was used for PCR

FIG. 6. Tumor necrosis factor-α-mRNA expression by reverse transcription-polymerase chain reaction in splenic macrophages (*SM*) and Kupffer cells (*KC*). Splenic macrophages and Kupffer cells were incubated with LPS (1 μg/ml) and total RNA was applied for the polymerase chain reaction. Splenic macrophages were more potent at generating TNF-α than Kupffer cells. (From [6], with permission)

FIG. 7. Rats underwent sham splenectomy (*squares*) or actual splenectomy (*circles*) 1 week before LPS (2 mg/kg BW, i.v.) injection. Plasma TNF-α level was significantly lower in the splenectomized rats than in those which had the sham operation 1 h after LPS injection

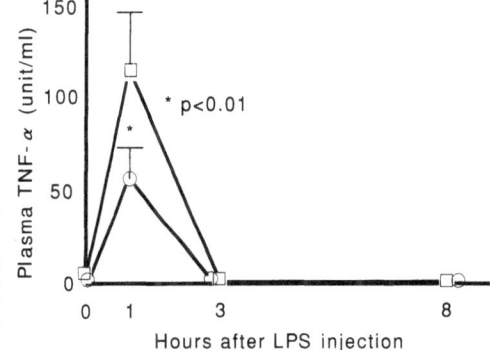

(RT-PCR). Splenic macrophages and Kupffer cells were incubated with LPS (1 μg/ml) and total RNA was applied for a PCR. It was found that splenic macrophages were more potent at generating TNF-α than Kupffer cells (Fig. 6). It is known that there is a functional difference between Kupffer cells and splenic macrophages, i.e., Kupffer cells are phagocytotic in nature, whereas splenic macrophages are potential cytokine generators [9].

We also observed the effect of splenectomy on TNF-α level in LPS-induced liver injury in rats fed ethanol for 6 weeks. Serum levels of TNF-α were significantly reduced by the splenectomy, suggesting that one source of TNF-α was the spleen (Fig. 7).

These findings show that the main source of TNF-α in this model is the spleen.

# Mechanisms by which Neutrophils Infiltrate the Liver

A chemotactic factor is necessary for neutrophil infiltration. IL-8 is a cytokine produced by hepatocytes, macrophages, and fibroblasts in response to LPS and TNF-$\alpha$. To clarify the relationship between LPS and IL-8, the hepatic concentration of IL-8 was determined in ethanol-fed rats. IL-8 in liver homogenate increased from 1 h after LPS injection (2 mg/kg BW, i.v.). Hepatic IL-8 level 3 h after LPS injection was significantly lower in rats with a splenectomy than in sham-operated rats (Fig. 8). In patients with AH, serum levels of IL-8 were higher than those in any other form of alcoholic liver disease (Fig. 9), and there was a significant correlation between neutrophil counts in the liver tissue and serum levels of IL-8 (Fig. 10).

Another condition for neutrophil infiltration is the expression of ICAM-1 on sinusoidal endothelial cells (SEC) [10, 11]. Immunohistochemical studies showed ICAM-1 expression on the surface of SEC (figure not shown), and serum sICAM-1 levels were high in AH (Fig. 11).

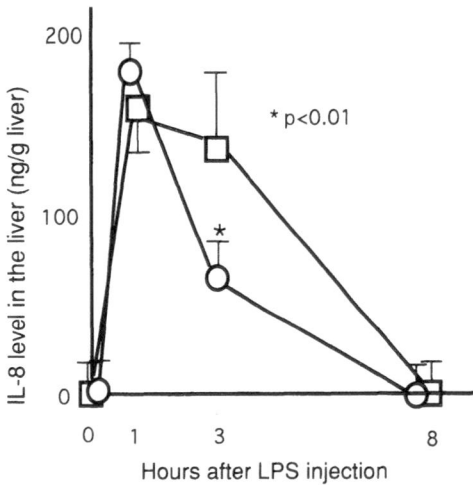

FIG. 8. Interleukin-8 levels in liver homogenate after lipopolysaccharide injection in chronic ethanol-fed rats with (*circles*) and without (*squares*) splenectomy. In rats with splenectomy, the hepatic interleukin-8 level at 3 h was significantly ($P < 0.01$) lower than that of sham-operated rats

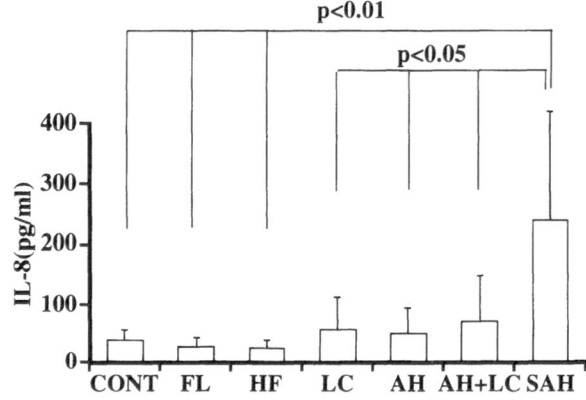

FIG. 9. Serum levels of interleukin-8 in alcoholic liver diseases. (From [6], with permission)

FIG. 10. Correlation between neutrophil counts in the liver tissue and serum levels of interleukin (*IL*)-8 in patients with alcoholic hepatitis. (From [6], with permission)

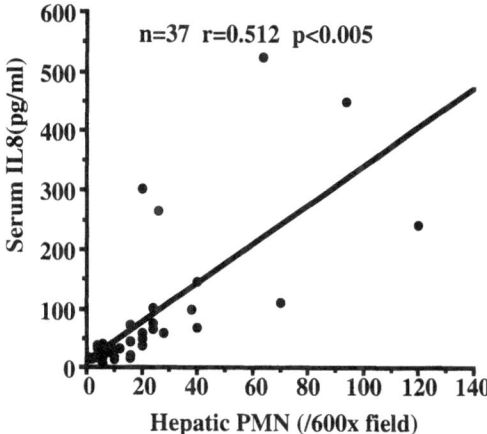

FIG. 11. Serum soluble intercellular adhesion molecule-1 (*ICAM-1*) levels in various alcoholic liver diseases. *CONT*, control. (From [6], with permission)

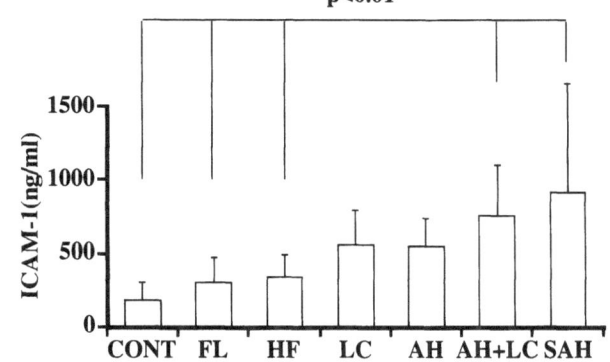

## Participation of Apoptosis in AH

The frequency of TUNEL-positive cells [12] in liver tissue was assessed. Their frequency was as low as 12.3 per gross (600×) in alcoholic hepatitis. However, there was a significant correlation between the numbers of TUNEL-positive cells and serum TNF-$\alpha$ levels. As apoptotic cells are readily phagocytosed by neighboring cells within a few hours, they are not usually observed in conventional histology. However, if phagocytotic activity is impaired in the presence of severe hepatitis, as in severe AH, the number of visible TUNEL-positive cells will increase.

## Conclusion

The cytokine cascade is activated by endotoxemia, finally resulting in leukocytes infiltrating the liver in AH. As one of the pathogeneses of AH, mechanisms suggested from this study may be summarized as follows. Endotoxemia due to impaired Kupffer cell function and increased absorption from the intestine activates macrophages to release TNF-$\alpha$. TNF-$\alpha$ then increases the production of IL-8 and up-regulates ICAM-1 on hepatic sinusoidal endothelia. These two factors provide suitable conditions for neutrophils to accumulate in the liver and result in neutrophil-mediated liver injury in AH.

## References

1. Oshita M, Sato N, Yoshihara H, et al. (1992) Ethanol-induced vasoconstriction causes focal hepatocellular injury in isolated perfused rat liver. Hepatology 16:1007–1013
2. Enomoto N, Takase S, Takada N, et al. (1991) Alcoholic liver diseases in heterozygotes of mutant and normal aldehyde dehydrogenase-2 gene. Hepatology 13:1071–1075
3. Tsutsumi M, Lasker JM, Shimizu M, et al. (1989) The intralobular distribution of ethanol-inducible P450IIE1 in rat and human liver. Hepatology 10:437–446
4. Israel Y, Hurwitz E, Niemela O, et al. (1986) Monoclonal and polyclonal antibodies against acetaldehyde-containing epitopes in acetaldehyde–protein adducts. Proc Natl Acad Sci USA 83:7923–7927
5. Yokoyama H, Ishii H, Nagata S, et al. (1996) Experimental hepatitis induced by ethanol after immunization with acetaldehyde adducts. Hepatology 17:14–19
6. Kumashiro R, Sakisaka S, Noguchi K, et al. (1997). Liver cell death in alcoholic hepatitis. In: Okita K (ed) Yamaguchi symposium on liver cell death. Axel Springer Japan, Tokyo, pp 67–79
7. Kumashiro R, Sata M, Ishii K, et al. (1996) Prognostic factors for short-term survival in alcoholic hepatitis in Japan: Analysis by logistic regression. Alcoholism: Clin Exp Res 20:383A–386A
8. Obayashi T, Tamura H, Tanaka S, et al. (1985) A new chromogenic endotoxin-specific assay using recombined limulus coagration enzymes and its clinical applications. Clin Chim Acta 149:55–65
9. Shimauchi Y (1992) Functional differences between rat Kupffer cells and splenic macrophages. Acta Hepatol Jpn 33:779–786
10. Ohira M, Ueno T, Shakado S, et al. (1994) Cultured rat hepatic sinusoidal endothelial cells express intercellular adhesion molecule-1 (ICAM-1) by tumor necrosis factor-$\alpha$ or interleukin-1 stimulation. J Hepatol 20:729–734
11. Fujita H, Morita I, Murota S (1991) Involvement of adhesion molecules (CD 11a-ICAM-1) intravascular endothelial cell injury elicited by PMA-stimulated neutrophils. Biochem Biophys Res Commun 177:664–672
12. Iseki S (1986) DNA strand breaks in rat tissues as detected by in situ nick translation. Exp Cell Res 167:311–326

# Ethanol-Induced Perturbation of Hepatic Microcirculation: Roles of Endothelin-1 and Nitric Oxide in Regulation of Sinusoidal Tone

YOSHIYUKI TAKEI[1,2], SUNAO KAWANO[2], MASAHIDE OSHITA[2], TAIZO HIJIOKA[2], TAKENOBU KAMADA[2], and NOBUHIRO SATO[1]

*Summary.* The role of microcirculation in the pathogenesis of alcoholic liver injury was investigated in isolated perfused rat liver. Upon initiation of ethanol infusion into the portal vein at concentrations ranging from 25 to 100 mM, portal pressure began to increase in a concentration-dependent manner and reached maximal levels in 2–5 min (initial phase), followed by a gradual decrease over the period of ethanol infusion (escape phenomenon). Sodium nitroprusside, a known vasodilator, diminished the ethanol-induced increase in portal pressure, increased oxygen consumption leading to inhibition of the reduction of the respiratory cytochromes of the liver, and diminished liver injury. The data indicate that ethanol-induced hepatic vasoconstriction disturbs hepatic microcirculation, resulting in hepatic hypoxia and hepatocellular injury. Endothelin-1 antiserum significantly inhibited hepatic vasoconstriction induced by ethanol by 45–80%. Cessation of infusion of endothelin-1 antiserum was followed by a subsequent increase in portal pressure. On the other hand, when a nitric oxide synthesis inhibitor, $N^G$-monomethyl-L-arginine (L-NMMA), was infused into the portal vein simultaneously with ethanol, the initial phase of the response of portal pressure to ethanol was not altered, and the peak values of portal pressure remained unchanged. However, following the peak increase in portal pressure, the rate of decrease was less than in the absence of L-NMMA. Thus, L-NMMA diminished the escape phenomenon and sustained the vasoconstriction. The data suggest that two endothelium-derived vasoactive factors, endothelin-1 and nitric oxide, regulate the sinusoidal tone in the presence of ethanol.

*Key words.* Ethanol, Vasoconstriction, Liver, Endothelin-1, Nitric oxide

[1] Department of Gastroenterology, Juntendo University School of Medicine, 2-1-1 Hongo, Bunkyo-ku, Tokyo 113-8421, Japan
[2] First Department of Medicine, Osaka University School of Medicine, 2-2 Yamadaoka, Suita, Osaka 565-0871, Japan

# Introduction

Alcoholic liver injury predominates in the pericentral region, in which oxygen tension is physiologically lowest. It is well documented that ethanol increases hepatic oxygen consumption. The enhanced injurious effect of ethanol at this site is postulated to be due to hypoxia, resulting from an enhanced oxygen demand of hepatocytes for the oxidative metabolism of ethanol [1, 2].

It has also been reported that ethanol consumption leads to an increase in portal vein blood flow, and that this phenomenon is possibly a compensatory mechanism for the ethanol-induced increase in oxygen demand [3]. However, this view has been refuted by data showing that the ethanol-induced increase in portal blood flow was not sufficient to compensate for elevated oxygen consumption [4]. Indeed, there have been conflicting reports concerning the action of ethanol on hepatic hemodynamics, with some showing a decreased hepatic blood flow, and with others reporting either no effect or an increase [5–7].

The reason for this discrepancy is not clear; however, differences in experimental conditions such as species of animal used, methods of ethanol administration, and ethanol concentration could explain the discrepancy. In particular, ethanol concentrations in the portal blood vary widely in those studies, and in general, relatively low ethanol concentrations were used [3, 8]. We found that ethanol at higher concentrations induces hepatocellular injury by causing microcirculatory disturbance and impaired oxygen supply to the tissue because of hepatic vasoconstriction.

A potent vasoactive peptide, endothelin-1 [9], was shown to produce sustained vasoconstriction in the liver [10–12]. Moreover, interaction between endothelin-1 and nitric oxide has been reported to be of importance in the regulation of vascular tone [13–16]. These data led us to hypothesize that these endothelium-derived vasoactive factors, endothelin-1 and nitric oxide, participate in the regulation of the microvascular tone of the liver in the presence of ethanol [17].

# Materials and Methods

## *Nonrecirculating Liver Perfusion*

To evaluate the effect of ethanol on hepatic hemodynamics, fed rats were anesthetized with sodium pentobarbital (45 mg per kg i.p.). Livers were isolated and perfused with Krebs–Henseleit bicarbonate buffer (pH 7.4, 37°C) saturated with $95\%O_2/5\%CO_2$ in a hemoglobin-free, nonrecirculating system at a constant flow rate (36 ml/min) [18]. Perfusate was pumped with a rotor pump into the liver via a cannula inserted in the portal vein. The effluent perfusate was collected with a cannula placed in the vena cava. Ethanol was mixed with the perfusate at the final concentrations just prior to the start of continuous infusion. Various dilutions of endothelin-1 antiserum (Peptide Institute, Osaka, Japan) were infused with ethanol for 10 min following the initiation of ethanol infusion. An inhibitor of nitric oxide synthesis, $N^G$-monomethyl-L-arginine (L-NMMA), was infused from 10 min before the initiation of ethanol infusion to the end of the infusion.

## Spectrophotometric Analysis

The hepatic absorption spectrum was analyzed by a reflection method using organ reflectance spectrophotometry, as described previously [19]. For spectral analysis of hepatic tissue hemoglobin, a rinsed erythrocyte preparation was infused into perfused liver (final hematocrit of perfusate: 1%), and the difference spectrum of regional hepatic tissue was obtained between the livers perfused with and without erythrocyte suspensions [20].

## Portal Pressure

Portal pressure was monitored continuously by measuring the height of perfusate in an open vertical capillary column (ID = 2 mm) attached to the perfusion system just before the inflow cannula [17, 20, 21]. The column was calibrated for baseline pressure at the end of each experiment by the fluid level in the capillary when perfusate was pumped through the influent cannula in the absence of liver at the same flow rate as was used with tissue.

# Results

## Effect of Acute Ethanol Load on Hepatic Microcirculation

Upon the initiation of ethanol infusion into the liver at concentrations higher than 25 mM, portal pressure began to increase in a concentration-dependent manner and reached maximal levels in 2–5 min (initial phase), followed by a gradual decrease over the period of ethanol infusion (escape phenomenon) [17] (Fig. 1). However, portal pressure remained at levels higher than the basal value throughout the period of ethanol infusion (Fig. 1). The maximal value of change in portal pressure increased in a dose-dependent fashion. The degree of vasoconstriction was represented by the change in portal pressure averaged over 10 min (the 10-min period following initiation of ethanol infusion). Higher concentrations of ethanol (>25 mM) increased the

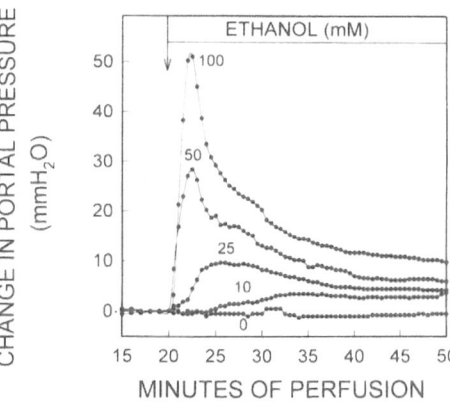

FIG. 1. Time-course of ethanol-induced change in portal pressure in the isolated perfused rat liver. Livers from fed rats were isolated and perfused with Krebs–Henseleit bicarbonate buffer saturated with 95%$O_2$/5%$CO_2$ in a hemoglobin-free, nonrecirculating system at a constant flow rate (36 ml/min). Ethanol was infused into the influent at a concentration of 0, 10, 25, 50, or 100 mM. (From [17], with permission)

change in portal pressure averaged over 10 min in a concentration-dependent manner, but 10 mM ethanol did not cause any change in portal pressure [17].

The regional hepatic tissue hemoglobin concentration after perfusion with added erythrocyte suspension (hematocrit 1%), measured by tissue-reflectance spectrophotometry, was significantly diminished by the infusion of ethanol at $\geq$ 50 mM, suggesting vasoconstriction of hepatic microvasculature and impairment of the microcirculation of the liver [20]. When the absorption spectrum of the liver was examined by reflectance spectrophotometry, infusion of ethanol caused a parallel reduction of all the mitochondrial respiratory cytochromes in a concentration-dependent fashion, concomitant with the increase of portal pressure, indicating a marked reduction of oxygen concentration in superficial liver tissue. The reduction in respiratory cytochromes was also associated with the decrease in oxygen consumption by the liver, indicating that the hepatic hypoxia was due to the reduction of oxygen delivery to hepatocytes rather than the increased oxygen consumption of the liver.

Lactate dehydrogenase (LDH) appeared in the perfusate 20–40 min after the onset of ethanol. The LDH level in the effluent perfusate at 60 min was dependent on the ethanol concentration and was significantly higher than in the control (no ethanol infusion) group. In histological examinations, focal hepatocellular necrosis, evidenced by trypan blue staining of cell nuclei, was detected predominantly in midzonal and pericentral areas of the liver lobule after 60 min of ethanol infusion. Change in portal pressure during 60 min of ethanol infusion correlated with levels of LDH after ethanol infusion [21].

Simultaneous infusion of sodium nitroprusside (100 μM), a known vasodilator, with ethanol (at 25–200 mM) significantly diminished ethanol-induced increase in portal pressure by 30–70% and LDH release by 30–60%. Moreover, nitroprusside increased oxygen consumption during infusion of ethanol and inhibited the reduction of the respiratory cytochromes.

## Role of Endothelin-1 Antiserum on Ethanol-Induced Hepatic Vasoconstriction

When ethanol (100 mM) was infused into the liver simultaneously with various dilutions of endothelin-1, the increase in portal pressure was attenuated, and was significantly smaller than in the absence of endothelin-1 antiserum (Fig. 2): $1:3.6 \times 10^3$ or $1:7.2 \times 10^3$ diluted endothelin-1 antiserum decreased the peak value of portal pressure significantly [17]. Furthermore, infusion of antiserum significantly inhibited the change in portal pressure averaged over 10 min of ethanol infusion by 45–80%. On the other hand, endothelin-1 antiserum did not affect portal pressure in the absence of ethanol.

## Role of Endogenous NO in Ethanol-Induced Hepatic Vasoconstriction and Liver Injury

When a nitric oxide synthesis inhibitor, L-NMMA, was infused into the portal vein simultaneously with ethanol (100 mM), the initial phase of the response of portal pressure to ethanol was not altered and the peak values of portal pressure remained

FIG. 2. Time-course of change in portal pressure during ethanol (100 mM) infusion in the presence and absence of endothelin-1 antiserum. Conditions as described in Fig. 1. Various dilutions of endothelin-1 antiserum infused with ethanol for 10 min, as indicated at the top of the figure. (From [17], with permission)

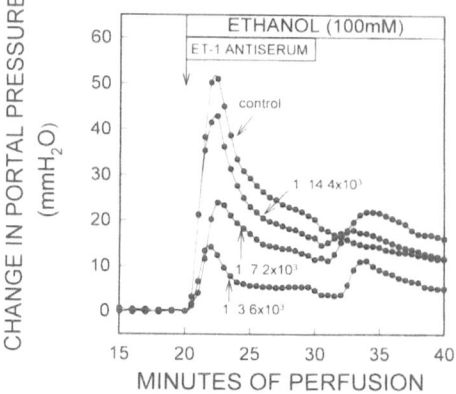

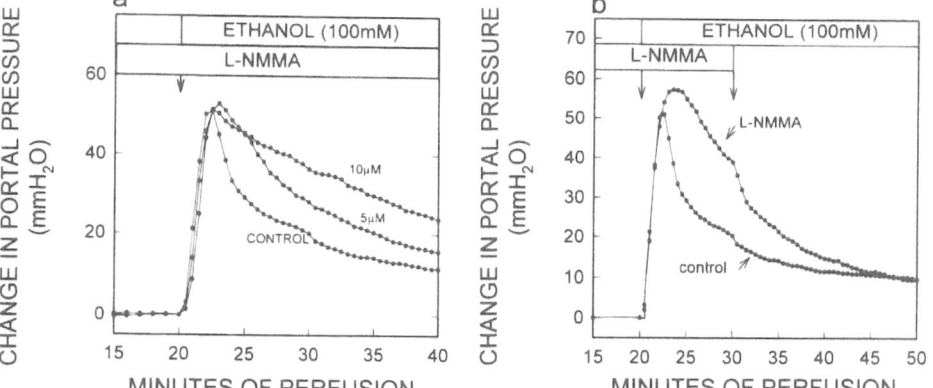

FIG. 3. Effect of L-NMMA on change in portal pressure during ethanol infusion. Conditions as described in Fig. 1. **a** L-NMMA (5 or 10 µM) was infused with ethanol (100 mM) from 10 min before the initiation to the end of ethanol infusion. **b** L-NMMA (100 µM) was infused for 20 min beginning 10 min before the initiation of ethanol (100 mM) infusion. L-NMMA infusion was discontinued at 10 min after the initiation of ethanol infusion. (From [17], with permission)

unchanged (Fig. 3a). However, following the peak increase in portal pressure, the rate of decrease was less than in the absence of L-NMMA, i.e., L-NMMA diminished the escape phenomenon and sustained the vasoconstriction [17] (Fig. 3a). Furthermore, when L-NMMA infusion was discontinued after 10 min of ethanol infusion, portal pressure began to decrease at a greater rate than the control, and approached the basal level (Fig. 3b).

Changes in portal pressure after 30 min of ethanol infusion at concentrations >10 mM were about twice as high in the presence of L-NMMA than in its absence. Furthermore, L-NMMA increased LDH release from the liver following ethanol load by 40–80% [22]. These effects of L-NMMA on the ethanol-induced increase in portal

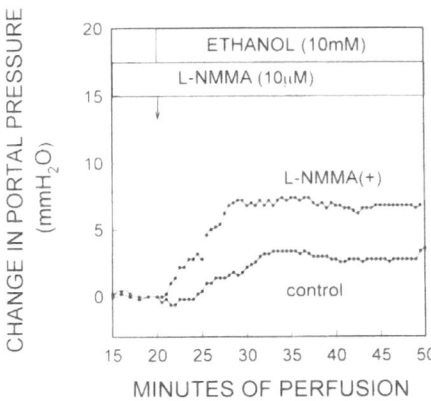

FIG. 4. Time-course of change in portal pressure during ethanol (10 mM) infusion in the presence and absence of L-NMMA. L-NMMA (10 μM) was infused with 10 mM ethanol from 10 min before the initiation to the end of ethanol infusion. (From [17], with permission)

pressure and hepatocellular injury were completely reversed by co-infusion of an excess dose of L-arginine.

It is notable that L-NMMA elicited an increase in portal pressure when ethanol was present at 10 mM, a concentration at which ethanol alone caused no visible change in portal pressure (Fig. 4). On the other hand, L-NMMA did not affect portal pressure in the absence of ethanol (Fig. 4).

## Discussion

Ethanol at concentrations of 25 mM or higher elevated portal pressure in a concentration-dependent fashion (Fig. 1), with the peak increase occurring 2–5 min after the onset of ethanol infusion. This increase in portal pressure was due to vasoconstriction, as evidenced by decreased tissue hemoglobin concentration. Nitroprusside reduced the ethanol-induced increase in portal pressure, increased oxygen consumption leading to inhibition of the reduction of the respiratory cytochromes, and diminished liver injury. Collectively, the data indicate that the ethanol-induced hepatic vasoconstriction disturbs hepatic microcirculation, resulting in hepatic hypoxia and reduction of mitochondrial respiratory cytochromes and culminating in hepatocellular injury (Fig. 5). In addition, increased hepatic vascular resistance may lead to exacerbation of portal hypertension (Fig. 5). This concept has been supported by recent clinical studies in which acute ethanol administration in noncirrhotic [23] and cirrhotic [24] alcoholic patients was shown to exert a vasoconstrictive effect on the hepatic circulation.

When ethanol was infused into the liver simultaneously with endothelin-1 antiserum, the increase in portal pressure in the presence of endothelin-1 antiserum was significantly smaller than in its absence (Fig. 2). Moreover, cessation of infusion of endothelin-1 antiserum was followed by a subsequent increase in portal pressure (Fig. 2). These data indicate that the vasoconstrictive effect of ethanol on the liver was predominantly mediated by endothelin-1.

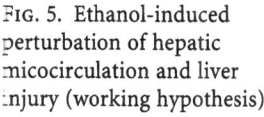

Fig. 5. Ethanol-induced
perturbation of hepatic
micocirculation and liver
injury (working hypothesis)

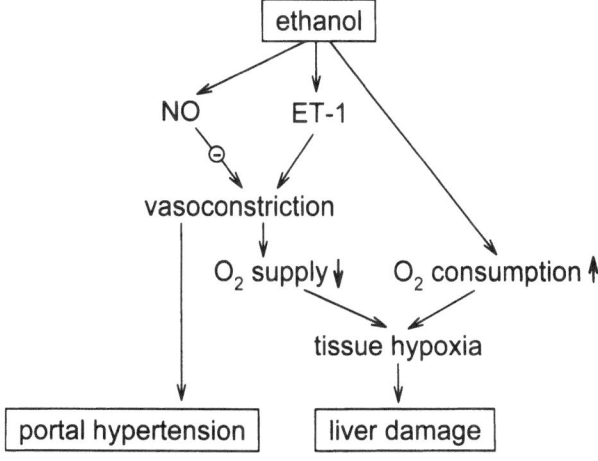

In contrast to the effect of antiendothelin-1 treatment, L-NMMA, which blocks
synthesis of nitric oxide from L-arginine [25], did not affect the initial phase of portal
pressure in response to ethanol infusion, and the peak values of portal pressure
remained unchanged. L-NMMA, however, sustained vasoconstriction, resulting in a
weakened "escape phenomenon" (Fig. 3a), evidenced by the fact that the change in
portal pressure averaged over 10 min of ethanol infusion was significantly higher in
the presence of L-NMMA than in its absence. These data suggest that endogenous
nitric oxide participates in the "escape phenomenon" during ethanol load by acting as
a vasodilator following the peak increase of portal pressure.

Interestingly, simultaneous infusion of L-NMMA and ethanol (10 mM) significantly
elevated the portal pressure (Fig. 4); however, L-NMMA or endothelin-1 antiserum
alone did not affect portal pressure in the absence of ethanol. The data suggest
the possibility that, even with lower ethanol concentrations ($\leqq$10 mM) which do not
cause a visible change in portal pressure, nitric oxide is involved in the regulation
of portal pressure: the vasodilating action of nitric oxide completely offsets the
vasoconstrictive effect of ethanol at lower ethanol concentrations. In addition, inhibition of the action of endogenous nitric oxide was associated with an increase in
hepatocellular damage. Taken together, endogenous nitric oxide is likely to contribute to the prevention of ethanol-induced liver injury by improving perturbations of
microcirculation caused by ethanol [22].

Based on the above observations, a likely sequence of events following ethanol
administration into the portal vein is as follows [17]: upon initiation of ethanol
infusion at concentrations higher than 25 mM, endothelin-1 elicits vasoconstriction in
the hepatic vasculature resulting in a rapid increase in portal pressure (initial phase).
After the portal pressure has reached its maximal level, nitric oxide acts as a
vasodilator and causes portal pressure to decrease gradually and reach a new steady
state in 20–30 min of ethanol infusion (escape phenomenon). This new steady state
appears to be determined by the balance between the degree of vasoconstriction
induced by ethanol and the action of nitric oxide.

The origin of endothelin-1 was not determined in this study. However, it seems
reasonable to postulate that sinusoidal endothelial cells are responsible for synthesis

of endothelin-1 since it has been shown that ethanol stimulates immunoreactive endothelin-1 release from cultured human umbilical vein endothelial cells [26]. In addition, hepatic sinusoidal endothelial cells release endothelin in response to transforming growth factor $\beta$ [27]. On the other hand, the site(s) at which ET-1 exerts vasoconstrictive action remains uncertain. The sinusoidal endothelium and stellate (Ito) cells might be possible candidates responsible for the endothelin-1-induced constriction of the sinusoids because both cell types contain contractile proteins [28, 29]. In particular, stellate cells were shown recently to contract when endothelin-1 was added in vitro [30, 31], suggesting a role for the stellate cell in the regulation of hepatic microcirculation. On the other hand, nitric oxide has been reported to be synthesized by hepatocytes [32]. However, the precise mechanism by which ethanol causes nitric oxide release and the site(s) on which nitric oxide acts in the presence of ethanol remain to be elucidated.

The endothelium-derived vasoactive substances endothelin-1 and nitric oxide have been reported to play an important role in the regulation of vascular tone [13–16], but very little is known about whether exogenous substances exert vasoactive effects via the same mechanism. Based on the current results, we propose that the sinusoidal tone in the presence of ethanol is regulated predominantly by the actions of endothelin-1 and nitric oxide [17, 22]. The data from this study provide evidence that portal venous flow is regulated by the liver, although it has long been believed that in the presence of ethanol the liver cannot regulate portal venous blood flow, and that any change which occurs is entirely passive [3, 7].

## References

1. Israel Y, Kalant H, Orrego H, et al. (1975) Experimental alcohol-induced hepatic necrosis: Suppression by propylthiouracil. Proc Natl Acad Sci USA 72:1137–1141
2. Ji S, Lemasters JJ, Christensen V, et al. (1982) Periportal and pericentral pyridine nucleotide fluorescence from the surface of the perfused liver: Evaluation of the hypothesis that treatment with ethanol produces pericentral hypoxia. Proc Natl Acad Sci USA 79:5415–5419
3. Bredfeldt JE, Riley EM, Groszmann RJ (1985) Compensatory mechanism in response to an elevated hepatic oxygen consumption in chronically ethanol-fed rats. Am J Physiol 248:G507–G511
4. Tsukamoto H, Xi X (1989) Incomplete compensation of enhanced hepatic oxygen consumption in rats with alcoholic centrilobular liver necrosis. Hepatology 9:302–306
5. Bravo IR, Acevdo CG, Callards V (1980) Acute effects of ethanol on liver blood circulation in anesthetized dog. Alcohol Clin Exp Res 4:248–253
6. Castenfors H, Hultman E, Josephson B (1960) Effect of intravenous infusions of ethyl alcohol on estimated hepatic blood flow in man. J Clin Invest 39:776–781
7. Verma-Ansil B, Carmichael FJ, Saldivia V, et al. (1989) Effect of ethanol on splanchnic hemodynamics in awake and unrestrained rats with portal hypertension. Hepatology 10:946–952
8. Oshita M, Takei Y, Kawano S, et al. (1993) The effect of ethanol on intrahepatic vasoconstriction (Correspondence). Hepatology 18:467–469
9. Yanagisawa M, Kurihara H, Kimura S, et al. (1988) A novel vasoconstrictor peptide produced by vascular endothelial cells. Nature 332:411–415
10. Withrington PG, Nucci G, Vane JR (1989) Endothelin-1 causes vasoconstriction and vasodilation in the blood perfused liver of the dog. J Cardiovasc Pharmacol 13(Suppl.5):S209–S210

11. Gandhi CR, Stephenson K, Olson MS (1990) Endothelin, a potent peptide agonist in the liver. J Biol Chem 265:17432–17435
12. Okumura S, Takei Y, Kawano S, et al. (1994) Effect of endothelin-1 on hepatic microcirculation in rat in vivo. Hepatology 19:155–161
13. Rubanyi GM (1991) Endothelium-derived relaxing and contracting factors. J Cell Biochem 46:27–36
14. Furchgott RF, Vanhoutte PM (1989) Endothelium-derived relaxing and contracting factors. FASEB J 3:2007–2018
15. Luscher TF (1989) Endothelium-derived relaxing and contracting factors: Potential role in coronary artery disease. Eur Heart J 10:847–857
16. Luscher TF, Yang Z, Tschudi M, et al. (1990) Interaction between endothelin-1 and endothelium-derived relaxing factor in human arteries and vein. Circ Res 66:1088–1094
17. Oshita M, Takei Y, Kawano S, et al. (1993) Roles of endothelin-1 and nitric oxide in the mechanism for ethanol-induced vasoconstriction in rat liver. J Clin Invest 91:1337–1342
18. Sholz R, Hausen W, Thurman RG (1973) Interaction of mixed-function oxidation with biosynthetic processes. I. Inhibition of gluconeogenesis by aminopyrine in perfused rat liver. Eur J Biochem 38:64–72
19. Sato N, Matsumura T, Shichiri M, et al. (1981) Hemoperfusion, rate of oxygen consumption and redox levels of mitochondrial cytochrome $c(+c_1)$ in livers in situ of anesthetized rat measured by refelectance spectrophotometry. Biochim Biophys Acta 634:1–10
20. Hijioka T, Sato N, Matsumura T, et al. (1991) Ethanol-induced disturbance of hepatic microcirculation and hepatic hypoxia. Biochem Pharmacol 41:1551–1557
21. Oshita M, Sato N, Yoshihara H, et al. (1992) Ethanol-induced vasoconstriction causes focal hepatocellular injury in the isolated perfused rat liver. Hepatology 16:1007–1013
22. Oshita M, Takei Y, Kawano S, et al. (1994) Endogenous nitric oxide attenuates ethanol-induced perturbation of hepatic circulation in the isolated perfused liver. Hepatology 20:961–965
23. Silva G, Fluxa F, Bresky G, et al. (1994) Splanchnic and systemic hemodynamics in early abstinence and after ethanol administration in non-cirrhotic alcoholic patients. J Hepatol 20:494–499
24. Luca A, Garcia-Pagan JC, Bosch J, et al. (1997) Effects of ethanol consumption on hepatic hemodynamics in patients with alcoholic cirrhosis. Gastroenterology 112:1284–1289
25. Palmer RMJ, Rees DD, Ashton DS, et al. (1988) L-arginine is the physiological precursor for the formation of nitric oxide in endothelium-dependent relaxation. Biochem Biophys Res Commun 153:1251–1256
26. Tsuji S, Kawano S, Michida T, et al. (1992) Ethanol stimulates immunoreactive endothelin-1 and -2 release from cultured human umbilical vein endothelial cells. Alcoholism: Clin Exp Res 16:347–349
27. Rieder H, Ramadori G, Meyer zum Buschenfelde KH (1991) Sinusoidal endothelial liver cells in vitro release endothelin-augmentation by transforming growth factor b and Kupffer cell-conditioned media. Klin Wochenschr 69:387–391
28. Oda M, Tsukada N, Watanabe N, et al. (1984) Functional implication of the sinusoidal endothelial fenestrae in the regulation of the hepatic microcirculation (abstract). Hepatology 4:754
29. Friedman SL, Rockey DC, McGuire RF, et al. (1992) Isolated hepatic lipocytes and Kupffer cells from normal human liver: Morphological and functional characteristics in primary culture. Hepatology 15:234–243
30. Kawada N, Tran-Thi TA, Klein H, et al. (1993) The contraction of hepatic stellate (Ito) cells stimulated with vasoactive substances: Possible involvement of endothelin-1 and nitric oxide in the regulation of the sinusoidal tonus. Eur J Biochem 213:815–823

31. Sakamoto M, Ueno T, Kin M, et al. (1993) Ito cell contraction in response to endothelin-1 and substance P. Hepatology 18:978–983
32. Curran RD, Billiar TR, Steur DJ, et al. (1989) Hepatocytes produce nitrogen oxides from L-arginine in response to inflammatory products of Kupffer cells. J Exp Med 170:1769–1774

# Morphological Aspects of Hepatic Fibrosis and Ito Cells (Hepatic Stellate Cells), with Special Reference to Their Myofibroblastic Transformation

Hideaki Enzan[1], Yoshihiro Hayashi[1], Eriko Miyazaki[1], Keishi Naruse[1], Rikka Tao[1], Naoto Kuroda[1], Hirofumi Nakayama[1], Hiroshi Kiyoku[1], Makoto Hiroi[1], and Toshiji Saibara[2]

*Summary.* Ito cells play a major role in various types of liver fibrosis in humans and experimental animals through initial myofibroblastic transformation. In granulation tissue following liver cell necrosis, the transformed Ito cells are large and star-shaped, and are easily identified by strong immunoreactivity for α-smooth muscle actin (ASMA), and characteristic electron-microscopic findings such as a well-developed rough endoplasmic reticulum, a large Golgi complex, bundles of numerous microfilaments with dense bodies beneath the cell membrane, and irregular cytoplasmic processes. These cells are closely associated with activated Kupffer cells, macrophages, lymphocytes, and neutrophils. In the fully developed stage they actively synthesize and secrete components of the extracellular matrix, resulting in the formation of the loose young fibrous tissue. With the progression of fibrosis, the transformed Ito cells become spindle-shaped and are arranged in parallel with dense collagen fibers. They lose both the well-developed rough endoplasmic reticulum and the large Golgi complex, but there is a more significant increase in subplasmalemmal microfilaments. This type of transformed cell, positive for ASMA, may not participate in the production of extracellular matrix components, but does participate in the contraction of old fibrotic tissue. On the other hand, portal fibroblasts show no significant changes in any type of fibrosis. The myofibroblastic transformation of Ito cells is seen not only in fibrosis, but also in the late stage of fetal liver development, when the perisinusoidal reticular fibers are more abundant than in normal adult livers. These findings suggest that the myofibroblastic transformation of Ito cells, the most important event in fibrosis, is a recapitulation of a normal developmental process.

*Key words.* Ito cell, Hepatic stellate cell, Myofibroblastic transformation, Hepatic fibrosis, α-Smooth muscle actin

[1]Department of Pathology and [2]Department of Internal Medicine, Kochi Medical School, Nankoku, Kochi 783-8505, Japan

# Introduction

Ito cells (hepatic stellate cells) [1] in normal livers, like pericytes, bring sinusoidal endothelial cells from outside and compose the sinusoidal cellular wall, together with endothelial cells, Kupffer cells, and pit cells. Ito cells have three major physiological functions: the deposition of vitamin A in their intracytoplasmic fat droplets; the secretion and degradation of extracellular matrix components in the space of Disse; the control of sinusoidal blood flow owing to their contractile activity. Almost all of them are in the resting stage and do not show any mitotic activity. However, when the liver cells are damaged, the Ito cells within or adjacent to necrotic areas are promptly activated by various cytokines secreted by infiltrated inflammatory cells or platelets, and by the alteration of the extracellular matrix around the Ito cells. They proliferate and change their phenotype to myofibroblasts [2, 3]. If the injuries are mild and transient, liver cells regenerate, resulting in complete recovery, and the transformed Ito cells return to a state of rest. However, both a continuous injury, like that which occurs in chronic viral hepatitis, and more extensive necrosis disturb this complete regeneration. Subsequently, the necrotic areas are first replaced by granulation tissue and then by fibrotic tissue. In the formation of granulation tissue and liver fibrosis following liver cell necrosis, the myofibroblastic transformation of Ito cells is an initial and key event [4]. The transformed Ito cells can actively synthesize type III and type I collagen and also other components of the extracellular matrix. After that, with the progression of fibrosis, they change morphology and function and appear to decrease in number.

This chapter summarizes the morphological criteria of the myofibroblastic transformation of Ito cells, and demonstrates the sequential morphological changes from resting to activated (transformed) in association with various types of liver fibrosis. We also discuss the functional significance of the myofibroblastic transformation of Ito cells, and compare the transformation of Ito cells in liver fibrosis with that of livers in the late fetal stage.

# Morphological Criteria of Myofibroblastic Transformation of Ito Cells

Ito cells are located in the space of Disse of all vertebrate livers and extend slender cytoplasmic processes along the abluminal surface of sinusoidal endothelial cells. The Ito cells have a few intracytoplasmic fat droplets containing vitamin A, a moderately developed rough-surfaced endoplasmic reticulum, and a juxtanuclear small Golgi complex. Microtubules and microfilaments are also present, but in small numbers. Around the cells, collagen fibrils are rarely observed. The immunoreactivity of the resting Ito cells with the antibody against $\alpha$-smooth muscle actin (ASMA) is preferentially positive in the periphery of the cell and the slender cytoplasmic processes (Fig. 1a). Other types of sinusoidal lining cells, and also liver cells, are negative for ASMA [4]. Correspondingly, immunohistochemistry reveals an interrupted linear ASMA-reactivity along the sinusoidal wall (Fig. 1b). When the Ito cells are activated, they become large in size and irregularly extend cytoplasmic processes. Moreover, they

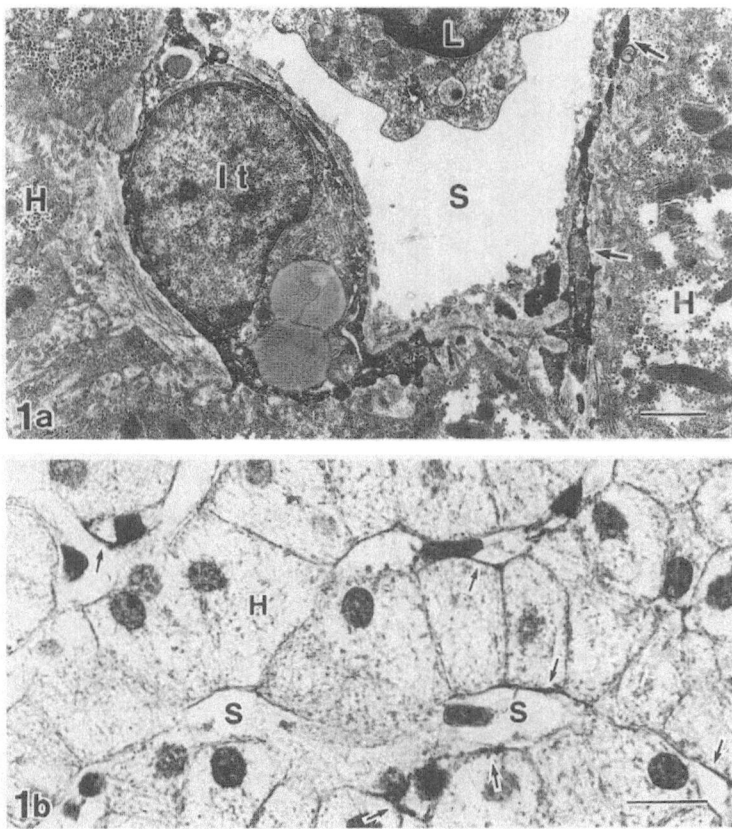

FIG. 1. α-smooth muscle actin expression of Ito cell (*It*) in adult human liver with no significant abnormalities. **a** Immunoelectron micrograph. The Ito cell contains three fat droplets. The cell periphery and cytoplasmic processes (*arrows*) are positive for ASMA. Bar = 2 μm, ×5100. **b** The linear immunoreaction for ASMA (*arrows*) is scattered along the sinusoidal wall. Bar = 20 μm, ×570. *H*, liver cell; *L*, lymphocyte; *S*, sinusoid

lose their characteristic fat droplets and concomitantly show a more well-developed rough endoplasmic reticulum and a larger Golgi complex. Beneath the cell membrane, bundles of numerous microfilaments appear. They run in parallel with the long axis of the cell. A few dense bodies are present on the bundles of filaments. The transformed Ito cells with these features are closely associated with newly formed collagen fibrils (Fig. 2a) and show a strong immunoreaction (Fig. 2b).

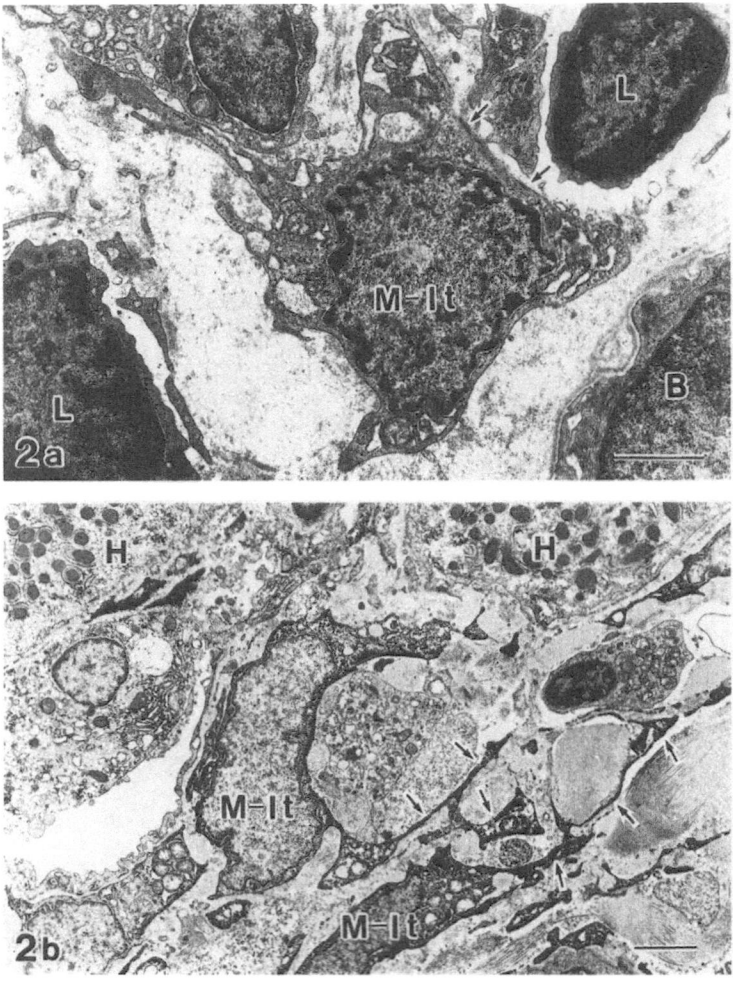

FIG. 2. Myofibroblast-like transformed Ito cell (*M-It*) in an area of piecemeal necrosis. **a** The enlarged cell extends cytoplasmic processes, resulting in irregularity of cell shape, and contains well-developed rough endoplasmic reticulum. Beneath the cell membrane there are bundles of microfilaments with dense bodies (*arrows*). Bar = 2 μm, ×6500. **b** Immunoelectron micrograph of an ASMA-positive myofibroblast-like Ito cell with irregularly formed cytoplasmic processes (*arrows*). Bar = 3 μm, ×2600. *B*, bile duct; *H*, liver cell; *L*, lymphocyte

FIG. 3. ASMA expression in massive and submassive hepatic necrosis. **a** Strong immunoreaction for ASMA is diffusely seen in panlobular necrotic areas on the 7th day of illness. Edematously enlarged portal tracts (*P*) show mild lymphocytic infiltration and ductular proliferation. Bar = 100 μm, ×80. **b** Immunoreaction for ASMA in submassive hepatic necrosis on the 50th day of illness. The area of central-to-central bridging necrosis has been replaced by newly formed fibrous tissue containing numerous ASMA-positive myofibroblast-like Ito cells. *C*, central vein. Bar = 300 μm, ×30

# Sequential Morphological Changes of the Transformed Ito Cells From the Stage of Granulation Formation to the Fibrotic Stage in Various Types of Liver Fibrosis

## Postnecrotic Liver Fibrosis

When panlobular liver cell necrosis is caused by any etiologies, almost all Ito cells within the necrotic areas swell and show strong immunoreactivity for ASMA (Fig. 3a). Kupffer cells are also activated. In submassive hepatic necrosis the change is roughly limited to the cells in necrotic areas. These changes indicate that the myofibroblastic transformation of Ito cells is a local reaction closely associated with liver cell necrosis

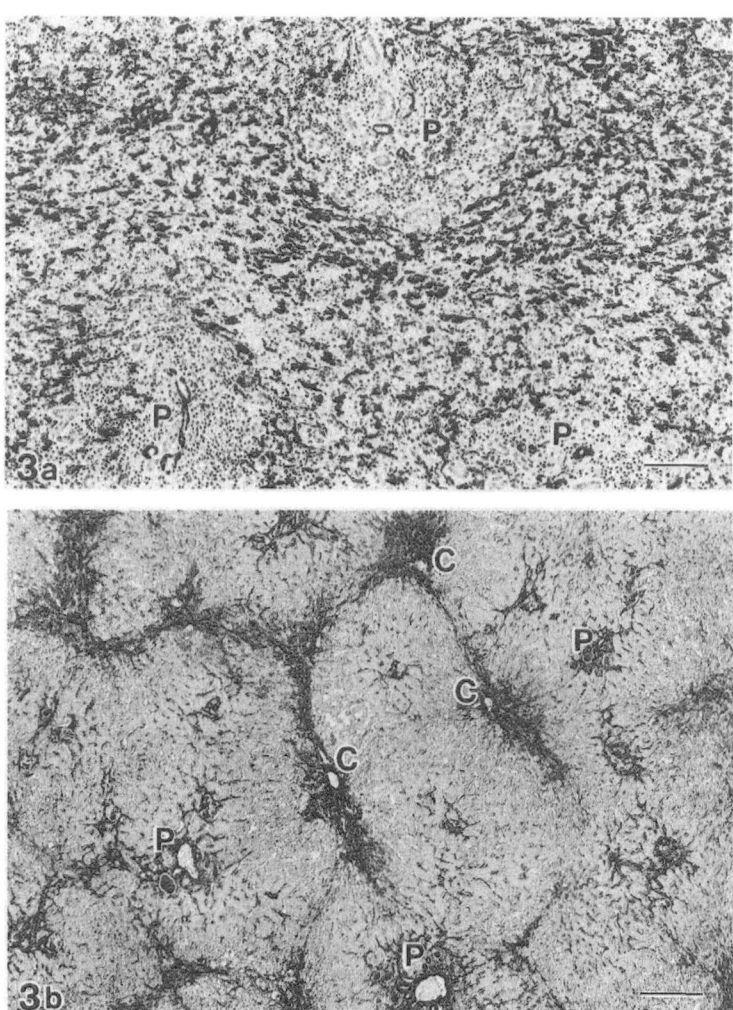

224     H. Enzan et al.

and stromal changes in the space of Disse in necrotic areas [5]. Monocytes and lymphocytes are mainly infiltrated in the case of viral hepatitis, but neutrophils are predominant in hypoxic hepatitis. In time, the necrotic tissue is removed and the sinusoids are collapsed. In this area, ASMA-positive myofibroblast-like Ito cells markedly increase in number and form a new fibrotic zone (Fig. 3b). About 1 month after massive or submassive liver cell necrosis, pseudolobules are formed. Between the pseudolobules, the fibrous stroma is composed of a dense cellular network of ASMA-positive transformed Ito cells and newly formed fibrous tissue (Fig. 4a). In spite of these significant changes within liver lobules, the basic structure of portal tracts is well preserved. This fact indicates that portal fibroblasts do not play any significant role in this type of fibrosis [5]. In old fibrosis, the ASMA-positive stromal cells originating from Ito cells become spindle-shaped and are arranged in parallel with dense collagen fibers (Fig. 4b).

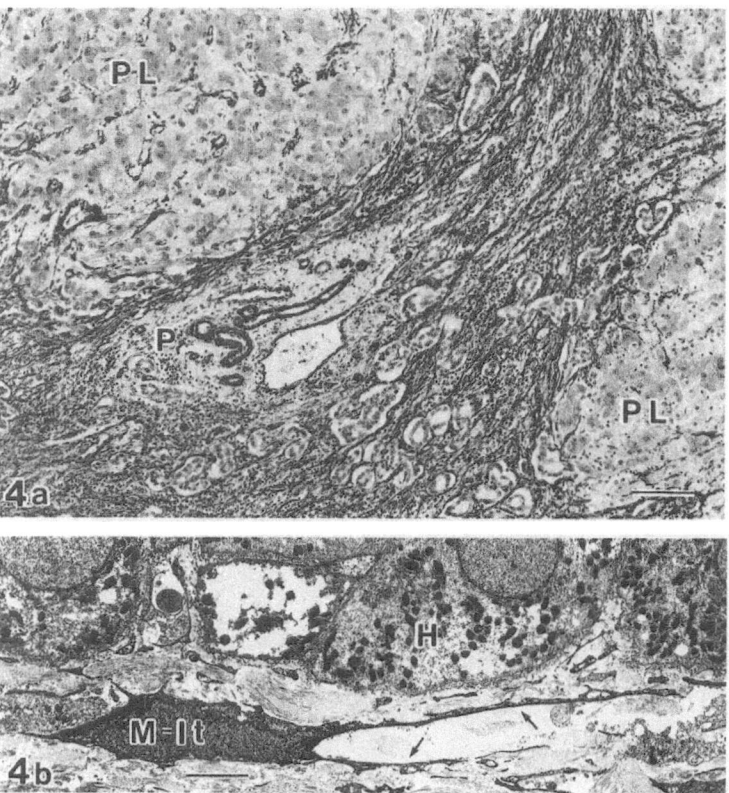

FIG. 4. Immunoreaction for ASMA in postnecrotic liver cirrhosis. **a** The fibrous stroma between pseudolobules (*PL*) contains a dense network of ASMA-positive stromal cells and proliferating bile ductules. The portal tract (*P*) keeps its proper structure. Bar = 100 μm, ×80. **b** ASMA-positive spindle-shaped myofibroblast-like cells (*M-It*) with long slender cytoplasmic processes (*arrows*). *H*, liver cell. Bar = 5 μm, ×1540

## Posthepatitic (Hepatitic) Liver Fibrosis

The myofibroblastic transformation of Ito cells is always seen in areas of piecemeal necrosis of chronic active hepatitis. In fibrotic areas, they irregularly extend ASMA-positive cytoplasmic processes (Fig. 5). Figure 6 shows the transition from the perilobular Ito cells containing very few fat droplets to myofibroblast-like stromal cells in the periportal fibrotic tissue. As the fibrotic changes progress, the ASMA-

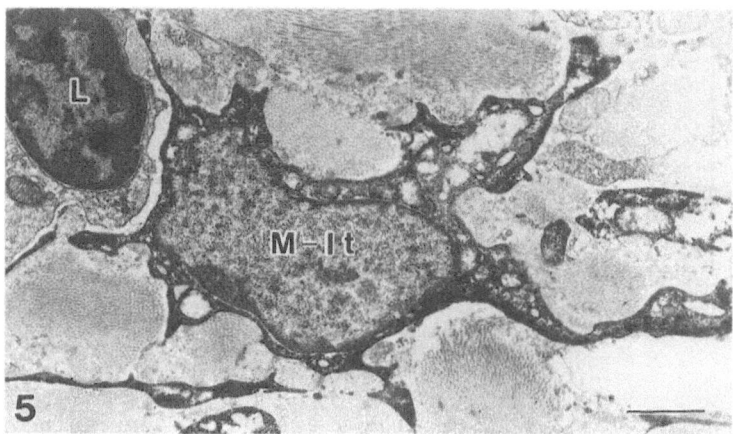

FIG. 5. ASMA expression of a dendritic myofibroblast-like cell (*M-It*) in a fibrotic area. *L*, lymphocyte. Bar = 2 μm, ×4900

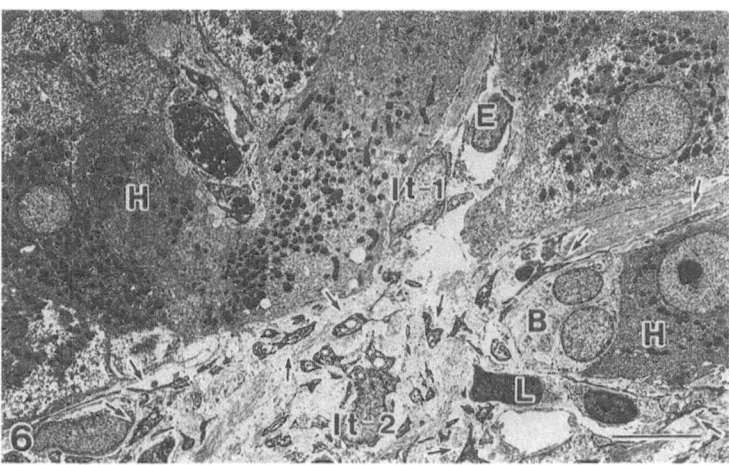

FIG. 6. The transition from a perilobular Ito cell (*It-1*) to a myofibroblast-like stromal cell (*It-2*) in the periportal fibrotic area. *Arrows* indicate cytoplasmic processes of ASMA-positive myofibroblast-like stromal cells. Immunoelectron micrograph for ASMA. *B*, bile duct; *E*, sinusoidal endothelial cell; *H*, liver cell; *L*, lymphocyte. Bar = 10 μm, ×1240

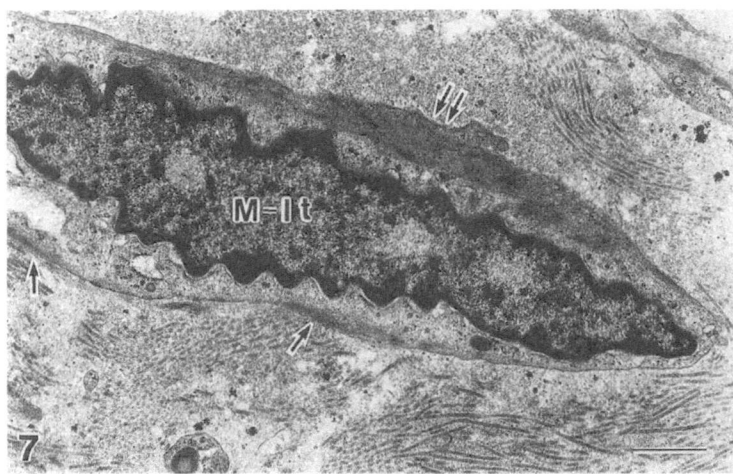

FIG. 7. Myofibroblast-like cell (*M-It*) in an old fibrotic area. The nucleus shows irregular and mild indentation. Beneath the cell membrane there are thick bundles of microfilaments (*double arrows*). *Single arrows* show dense bodies in the bundles of microfilaments. Bar = 1 μm, ×9900

positive myofibroblast-like cells gradually lose their rough-surfaced endoplasmic reticulum and Golgi complex. On the other hand, the increase in subplasmalemmal microfilaments is significant (Fig. 7). Judging from a morphological standpoint, the formation of a wide circumferential zone of increased filaments appears to be a barrier in the secretion of synthesized protein from the cell.

## Alcoholic Liver Fibrosis

The myofibroblastic transformation of Ito cells is particularly seen around the ballooned hepatocytes and in the pericellular fibrosis (Fig. 8a). In general, the transformation occurs in the Ito cells within, or immediately adjacent to, necrotic areas of liver cells. However, in alcoholic liver diseases even Ito cells distant from necrotic areas show myofibroblastic transformation. It is easily identified by the strong im-munoreactivity for ASMA of the Ito cells in nonnecroinflammatory regions (Fig. 8b). This suggests that the metabolites of alcohol directly activate Ito cells, and then the transformed Ito cells cause perisinusoidal fibrosis, irrespective of liver cell necrosis.

## Cardiogenic Liver Fibrosis

Acute myocardial infarction occasionally causes severe hypoxic hepatitis, resulting in irregularly formed zonal necrosis, predominantly involving zones 3 and 2. In the necrotic areas (Fig. 9), the Ito cells are activated and transformed into myofibroblasts in the same way as those in massive and submassive liver cell necrosis due to viral hepatitis, but in hypoxic hepatitis most of the infiltrated inflammatory cells are neutrophils. Cardiogenic liver fibrosis shows a typical central-to-central bridging

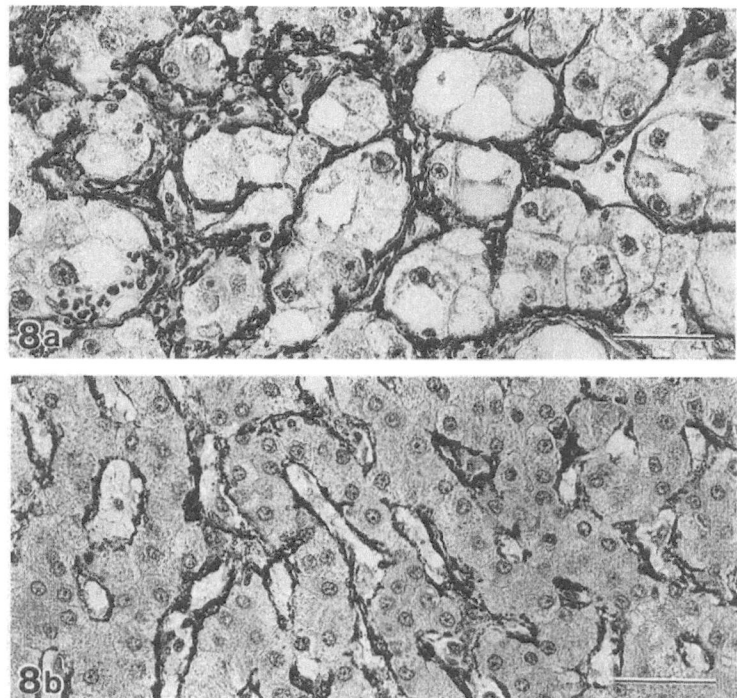

FIG. 8. ASMA expression in a liver with alcoholic hepatitis. **a** Numerous myofibroblast-like Ito cells, strongly positive for ASMA, are seen around ballooned hepatocytes containing alcoholic hyalin. **b** Myofibroblast-like Ito cells, strongly positive for ASMA, are also seen in the nonnecroinflammatory area of liver tissue in alcoholic hepatitis. Bars = 50 μm, ×310

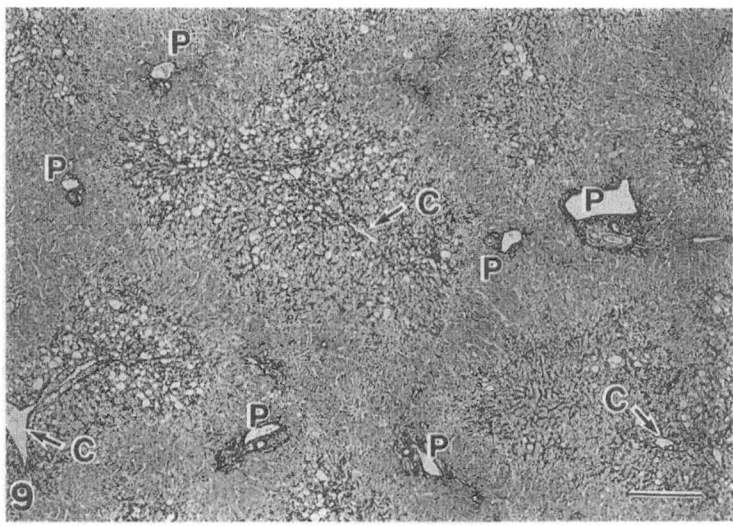

FIG. 9. Immunoreaction for ASMA in severe hypoxic hepatitis. The positive reaction is strictly localized to Ito cells in necrotic areas of liver cells (*arrows*). *C*, central vein; *P*, portal tract. Bar = 300 μm, ×30

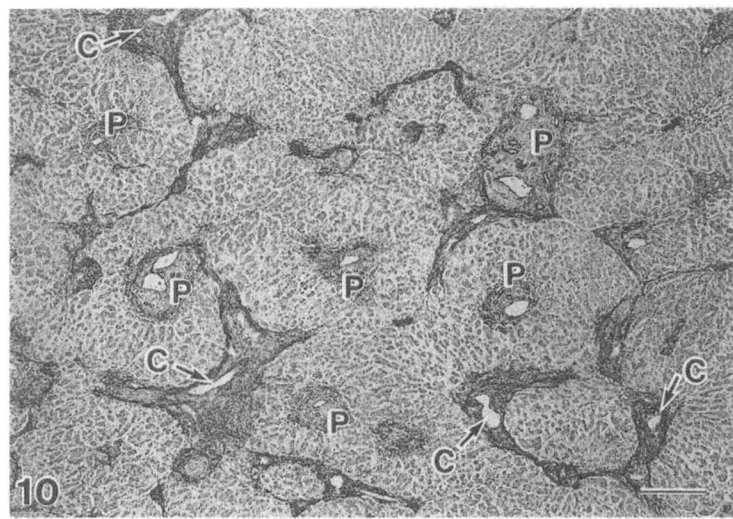

F1G. 10. ASMA expression in cardiogenic liver fibrosis. In central-to-central bridging fibrosis there are numerous spindle-shaped ASMA-positive stromal cells (*arrows*). P, portal tract; C, central vein. Bar = 300 μm, ×30

fibrosis made of bundles of dense collagen fibers and spindle-formed, ASMA-positive stromal cells originating from Ito cells. The portal tracts keep their basic structure and show no significant abnormalities (Fig. 10).

## Experimental Liver Fibrosis

*Carbon Tetrachloride (CCl₄)-Induced Intralobular Liver Fibrosis.* After a single intraperitoneal injection of $CCl_4$, Ito cells within or adjacent to necrotic areas of liver cells increase in cell size, proliferate [6], and show a significant increase in protein synthesis [7]. They are strongly positive for ASMA. If the injection is repeated, the area of central-to-central bridging necrosis is replaced by fibrous tissue. This tissue is composed of ASMA-positive myofibroblast-like cells and newly formed collagen fibers (Fig. 11).

*Fibrosis Following Ligation of Common Bile Ducts.* In the early acute phase of bile duct ligation, the portal and periductal stromal cells proliferate and transform the phenotype [9], but with the extension of periportal fibrosis the myofibroblastic transformation of perilobular Ito cells becomes significant.

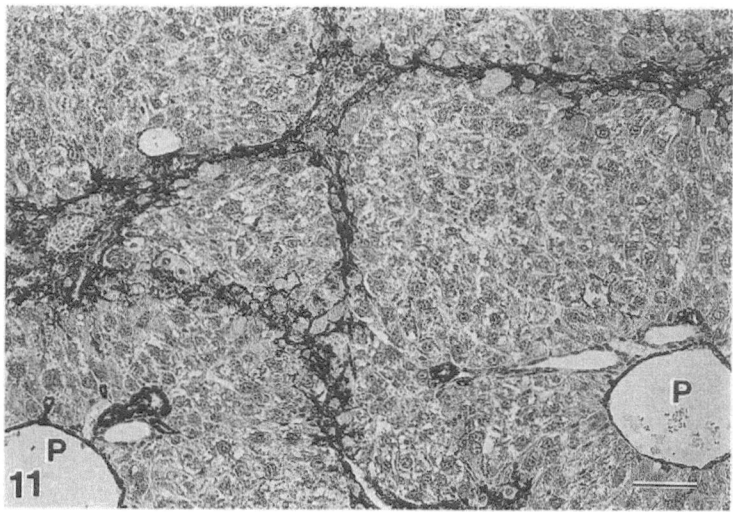

FIG. 11. ASMA expression in CCl₄-induced liver fibrosis in a mouse. The fibrotic areas are mainly composed of ASMA-positive stromal cells and collagen fibers. *P*, portal tract. Bar = 50 μm, ×150

## Relationship Between Myofibroblastic Transformation of Ito Cells in Fibrosis and that in Fetal Livers

In human fetal livers at the 9th to 10th month of gestation, the sinusoidal reticular fibers are more abundantly formed than in adult human livers (Fig. 12a). At that time, almost all Ito cells show myofibroblastic transformation (Fig. 12b), which always occurs in the late stage of fetal liver development. Therefore, the myofibroblastic transformation of Ito cells in liver fibrosis may be a recapitulation of the normal liver development process [10]. The same situation of increased ASMA-expression of stromal cells in both normal development and some diseases with fibrosis has also been identified in mesangial cells in the kidney [11].

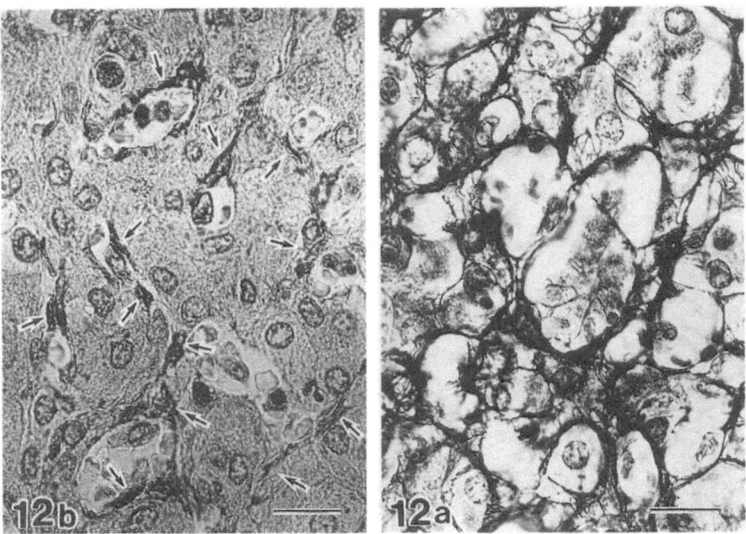

FIG. 12. A human fetal liver at 9 months gestation. **a** A dense network of reticular fibers has formed along the sinusoidal wall. Silver staining. **b** ASMA-positive Ito cells (*arrows*) appear to be swollen and form a loose cellular network. Bar = 20 μm, ×500

## Conclusion

The myofibroblastic transformation of Ito cells is an initial key event in fibrosis and may be a recapitulation of fetal liver development. Future research needs to clarify the mechanism of myofibroblastic transformation of Ito cells in fibrosis on the basis of molecular pathology. In in vivo studies, the significance of a close topographical relationship between Ito cells and various types of infiltrated inflammatory cells in necrotic areas remains to be resolved.

## References

1. Hautekeete ML, Geerts A (1997) The hepatic stellate cell: its role in human liver disease. Virchows Arch 430:195–207
2. Schürch W, Seemayer TA, Gabbiani G (1992) Myofibroblast. In: Sternberg SS (ed) Raven Press, New York, pp 109–144
3. Schürch W, Seemayer TA, Gabbiani G (1998) The myofibroblast. A quarter century after its discovery. Am J Surg Pathol 22:141–147
4. Enzan H, Himeno H, Iwamura S, et al. (1994) Immunohistochemical identification of Ito cells and their myofibroblastic transformation in adult human liver. Virchows Arch 424:249–256
5. Enzan H, Himeno H, Iwamura S, et al. (1995) Sequential changes in human Ito cells and their relation to postnecrotic liver fibrosis in massive and submassive hepatic necrosis. Virchows Arch 426:95–101
6. Enzan H (1985) Proliferation of Ito cells (fat-storing cells) in acute carbon tetrachloride liver injury. A light and electron microscopic autoradiographic study. Acta Pathol Jpn 35:1301–1308

7. Enzan H (1987) Protein synthesis in Ito cells (fat-storing cells) of cultured liver tissue from CCl₄-treated mice. A light and electron microscopic autoradiographic study. Acta Pathol Jpn 37:225–230
8. Enzan H, Hara H (1986) Ito cells (fat-storing cells) and collagen formation in carbon tetrachloride-induced fibrosis. A light and electron microscopic autoradiographic study using ³H-proline as a tracer. In: Kirn A, Knook DL, Wisse E (eds) Cells of the Hepatic Sinusoid, vol 1. Kupffer Cell Foundation, pp 233–238
9. Tuchweber B, Desmoulière A, Bochaton-Piallat M-L, et al. (1996) Proliferation and phenotypic modulation of portal fibroblasts in the early stages of cholestatic fibrosis in the rat. Lab Invest 74:265–278
10. Enzan H, Himeno H, Hiroi M, et al. (1997) Development of hepatic sinusoidal structure with special reference to the Ito cells. Microsc Res Tech 39:336–349
11. Alpers CE, Seifert RA, Hudkins KL, et al. (1992) Developmental patterns of PDGF B-chain, PDGF-receptor, and $\alpha$-actin expression in human glomerulogenesis. Kidney Int 42:390–399

# Retinoids and Liver Fibrosis

MASATAKA OKUNO[1], SEISUKE NAGASE[1], YOSHIMUNE SHIRATORI[1],
HISATAKA MORIWAKI[1], YASUTOSHI MUTO[1], NORIFUMI KAWADA[2],
and SOICHI KOJIMA[3]

*Summary.* The conflicting effects of retinoic acid (an active metabolite of vitamin A) on liver fibrosis were observed between two different animal models either with or without hepatic parenchymal necrosis. In $CCl_4$-treated rats, in which liver fibrosis was accompanied by parenchymal damage, a stable analog of retinoic acid suppressed the progression of fibrosis indirectly by reducing hepatic necrosis. This effect appeared in part to be due to interference with the secretion of tumor necrosis factor-$\alpha$ (TNF-$\alpha$) from Kupffer cells. On the other hand, the same retinoid exacerbated liver fibrosis in porcine serum-treated rats, in which hepatic fibrosis was induced without parenchymal necrosis. In this model, retinoid seemed to act directly on stellate cells; it enhanced plasminogen activator/plasmin levels in stellate cells and thereby activated latent transforming growth factor-$\beta$ (TGF-$\beta$) on the cell surface. The resultant TGF-$\beta$, in turn, auto-stimulated the production of collagen by the cells. Thus, the apparently conflicting effects of retinoic acid on liver fibrosis may partly be explained by the difference in target genes and target cells on which retinoic acid acts under different conditions.

*Key words.* Liver fibrosis, Retinoic acid, Stellate cells, Plasmin, Transforming growth factor-$\beta$

## Introduction

Hepatic stellate cells (SCs) play central roles both in the storage of retinoids (vitamin A and its analogs) and in fibrogenesis of the liver [1, 2]. During the progression of liver fibrosis, SCs lose retinoids from the cytoplasm, transform into myofibroblast-like cells, and start to produce significant amounts of extracellular matrices [1, 2]. There-

---

[1] First Department of the Internal Medicine, Gifu University School of Medicine, 40 Tsukasa-machi, Gifu 500-8076, Japan
[2] Third Department of Internal Medicine, Osaka City University Medical School, 1-4-54 Asahi-machi, Abeno-ku, Osaka 545, Japan
[3] Laboratory of Molecular Cell Science, Tsukuba Life Science Center, The Institute of Physical and Chemical Research (RIKEN), 3-1-1 Koyadai, Tsukuba, Ibaraki 305-0074, Japan

fore, interest has been focused on the relation between the loss of retinoids and the production of extracellular matrices in SCs. So far, contradictory results have been obtained regarding the effects of exogenously added retinoids on liver fibrosis. Senoo and Wake [3] reported that the administration of retinylpalmitate (a storage form of vitamin A) suppressed experimental hepatic fibrosis in rats produced both by carbon tetrachloride ($CCl_4$) and by porcine serum. In support of this, vitamin A deficiency was shown to promote $CCl_4$-induced liver fibrosis [4]. On the other hand, Leo and Lieber [5] reported that vitamin A supplemented with ethanol induces liver fibrosis and cirrhosis in rats. Furthermore, it has been documented that the incidence of human hepatic fibrosis is correlated with the amount of vitamin A intake by patients with vitamin A hepatotoxicity [6]. The suppression of stromelysin and collagenase gene promoters by retinoic acid (RA), an active metabolite of vitamin A [7, 8], may partly account for this fibrosis-enhancing effect. Thus, conflicting effects have been observed in the effect of retinoids on liver fibrosis. The reason for these differences is unclear; however, we address the following two possibilities: (1) the overloading of fat droplets into SCs by the administration of retinylpalmitate would interfere with normal protein synthesis and metabolism in the cells, whereas the administration of RA would directly modulate a certain gene expression by interaction with retinoic acid receptors; (2) the apparent discrepancy might be ascribed to the presence and absence of inflammation in the liver.

Here, we review the opposite effects of RA on liver fibrosis between the $CCl_4$ and porcine serum models to clarify the different mechanisms underlying RA action during the development of liver fibrosis with or without hepatic inflammation.

# Conflicting Effects of RA on Two Liver Fibrosis Models

In the $CCl_4$ model, liver fibrosis was generated and was accompanied by hepatic parenchymal necrosis. A stable analog of RA suppressed liver fibrosis in this model (Fig. 1A) [9]. This suppression seemed to be an indirect result of a reduction in the inflammation in the liver [9]. RA has been shown to down-regulate the action of tumor necrosis factor-$\alpha$ (TNF-$\alpha$) [10], a key cytokine produced by Kupffer cells which induces hepatic necrosis and inflammation [11]. Consistent with this, the retinoid reduced the hepatic necrosis, as indicated by a reduction in serum alanine aminotransferase (ALT) activities (Fig. 1B) as well as by histologic observations. Several previous studies have shown that both RA and retinol (a transport form of vitamin A in plasma) may reduce SC proliferation both in basal conditions [12–14] and following stimulation with growth factors involved in liver inflammation [15]. This RA effect on SC proliferation may also help to explain the suppression of liver fibrosis, because the inflammatory-driven hepatic SC proliferation is likely the most relevant event in the $CCl_4$ model.

On the other hand, porcine serum-induced liver fibrosis was generated without causing hepatic parenchymal necrosis. No elevation of serum ALT activities was found in this model during the entire experimental period (Fig. 2B). The same retinoid as used in the $CCl_4$ model clearly exacerbated liver fibrosis in this model [16], and the tissue hydroxyproline level in the liver increased (Fig. 2A). Davis and co-workers [12, 13, 17] have reported that interstitial collagen and/or TGF-$\beta$ production

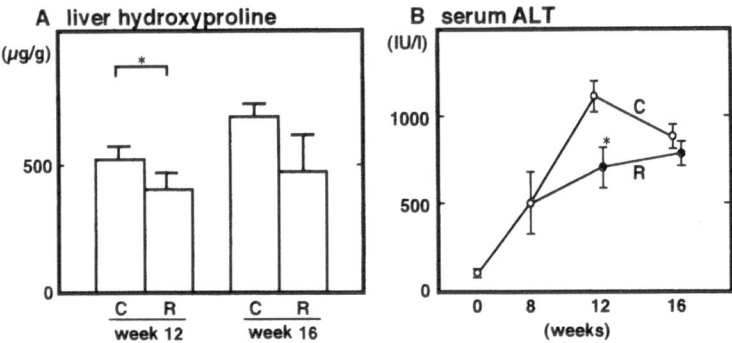

FIG. 1A,B. Suppression of liver fibrosis by a retinoid analog in CCl₄-treated rats. Male Wistar rats received subcutanous injections of CCl₄ mixed with an equal volume of liquid paraffin twice a week at a dose of 0.5 ml/kg body weight. Rats simultaneously received oral administration of either peanut oil or retinoid (80 mg/kg body weight/day) in the control (C) ($n = 15$) and retinoid (R) ($n = 15$) group, respectively, starting at the 8th week. Rats were killed at the 12th ($n = 5$ in each group) and 16th ($n = 10$ in each group) week. Tissue levels of hydroxyproline in the liver, A, and serum activities of alanine aminotransferase (ALT), B, were measured. Each value represents the average ± SD. Asterisks show a significant difference ($P < 0.05$)

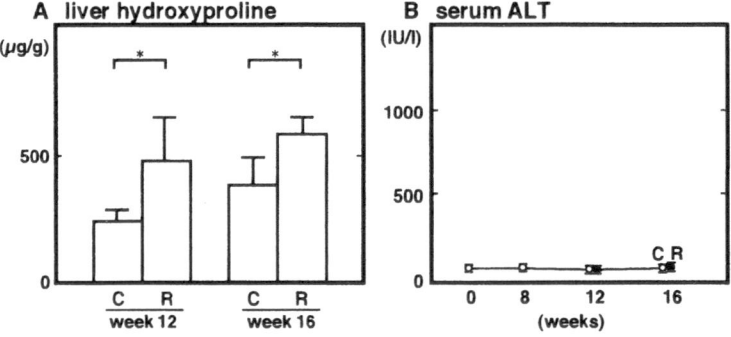

FIG. 2A,B. Exacerbation of liver fibrosis by a retinoid analog in porcine serum-treated rats. Male Wistar rats received intraperitoneal injections of porcine serum twice a week at a dose of 0.5 ml/rat. Rats simultaneously received either peanut oil (control: C) or retinoid (R) as described in Fig. 1. Liver hydroxyproline contents, A, and serum ALT activities, B, were measured. Each value represents the average ± SD. *Asterisks* show a significant difference ($P < 0.05$)

is either increased, unchanged, or reduced by the exposure of rat SCs to all-*trans*-RA or TGF-$\beta$, implying that the difference(s) in the experimental conditions, especially the different stages in the transformation of SCs used for the experiments, caused the opposing effects of RA on liver fibrosis. However, the detailed mechanism remains unclear.

# TGF-$\beta$ and Retinoids

TGF-$\beta$ is the major cytokine implicated in the pathogenesis of liver fibrosis and cirrhosis [1, 2, 18, 19]. TGF-$\beta$ stimulates SCs to transform into myofibroblast-like cells, enhances their production of extracellular matrix proteins [1, 2], and alters the degradation of the extracellular matrix [1, 20]. TGF-$\beta$ suppresses the growth and function of hepatocytes, at least in part, by down-regulating the production of hepatocyte growth factor in SCs [21].

Three subtypes of TGF-$\beta$ (TGF-$\beta$1, -$\beta$2, and -$\beta$3), whose biological properties are almost identical, are found in mammals [22]. TGF-$\beta$s are synthesized and secreted in a biologically latent form (latent TGF-$\beta$, 235–280 kd) which must be activated before it can bind to the receptors and perform biological activities [22, 23]. Activation releases the 25-kd TGF-$\beta$ molecule from the large complex. Plasmin-mediated activation occurs under physiological conditions such as in the co-cultures of endothelial and smooth muscle cells [23–25]. In this system, activation occurs at the cell surface by plasmin generated from serum plasminogen by the action of a plasminogen activator (PA) [25, 26].

The diverse activities of retinoids are primarily mediated by two families of nuclear receptors, retinoic acid receptors and retinoid X receptors [27]. These are ligand-dependent transcription factors that bind to *cis*-acting DNA sequences, called RA responsive elements or retinoid X responsive elements, in the promoter region of the target genes [27]. Retinoic acid receptors bind to RA responsive elements in response to both all-*trans*-RA and 9-*cis*-RA, whereas retinoid X receptors bind to retinoid X responsive elements in response only to 9-*cis*-RA. The effect of certain synthetic retinoids, including an acyclic retinoid used in this study, is also mediated by binding to and transactivating retinoic acid receptors [28]. It has been reported that retinoids enhance the production of PA in many cell types [29]. In bovine endothelial cells, the elevation of surface PA/plasmin [30] levels by retinoids causes the formation of active TGF-$\beta$; this TGF-$\beta$ subsequently mediates some of the retinoid effects on endothelial cells [31, 32].

# Induction of TGF-$\beta$ by RA in SCs [16]

We demonstrated that RA also stimulates the formation of active TGF-$\beta$ in rat SC cultures via plasmin-mediated proteolytic cleavage of latent TGF-$\beta$ on the cell surface (Fig. 3). The resultant active TGF-$\beta$ stimulates its own synthesis by SCs, and consequently a considerable amount of TGF-$\beta$ is produced. TGF-$\beta$ facilitated the production of fibrotic components and suppressed collagenase activities in SC cultures (Fig. 4). In fact, in an in vivo liver fibrosis model induced by porcine serum, the concentration of TGF-$\beta$ in liver tissue increased approximately two-fold in retinoid plus porcine serum-treated rats compared with porcine serum alone-treated rats. We summarize these sequential changes in Fig. 5. However, retinoid treatment alone (without porcine serum) did not cause an increase in TGF-$\beta$ in liver tissue or liver fibrosis. Thus, the retinoid did not directly cause liver fibrosis by itself, but it exacerbated the fibrosis induced by porcine serum. This means that SCs may need to be activated by some stimuli, such as porcine serum, before they become sensitive to RA-treatment.

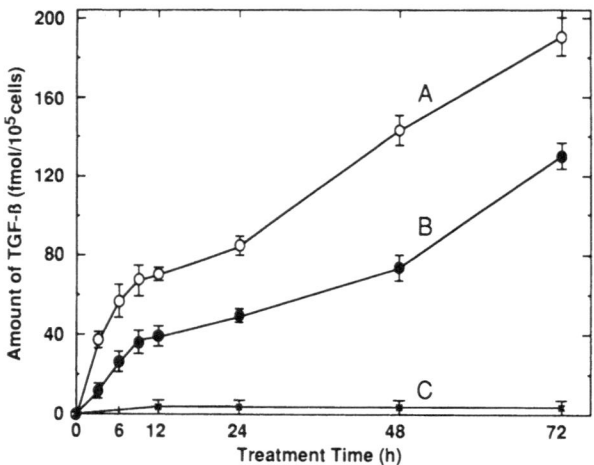

FIG. 3. Time-course of TGF-$\beta$ induction in rat stellate cells (SCs) by 9-*cis*-retinoic acid (RA). Confluent rat SC cultures were incubated either with vehicle (control) or with 1 µM 9-*cis*-RA for varying lengths of time. The culture medium was collected at the times indicated, and both the total and active TGF-$\beta$ concentrations in each culture medium were measured. *Curve A*, the total TGF-$\beta$ concentration in 9-*cis*-RA-treated cultures; *curve B*, the active TGF-$\beta$ concentration in 9-*cis*-RA-treated cultures; *curve C*, the total TGF-$\beta$ concentration in the control cultures. Each value represents the average ± SD ($n = 6$). (From [16], with permission)

A

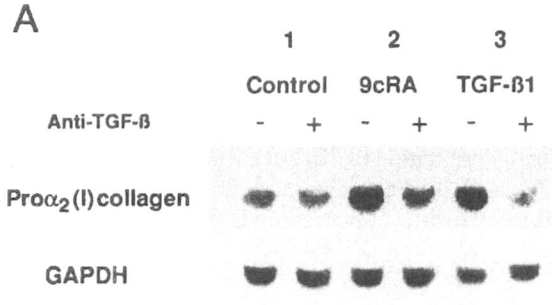

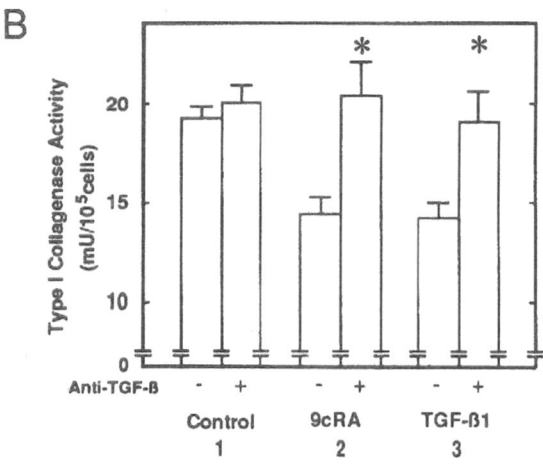

FIG. 4A,B. TGF-$\beta$-dependent stimulation of fibrogenesis by 9-*cis*-retinoic acid (RA) in rat stellate cell (SC) cultures. Confluent rat SC cultures were incubated for 24 h with either vehicle (control, sample 1), 1 µM 9-*cis*-RA (9cRA, sample 2), or 40 pM rTGF-$\beta$1 (sample 3) in the absence (*left side* of each sample) or presence (*right side* of each sample) of 25 µg/ml anti-TGF-$\beta$ antibody (anti-TGF-$\beta$). After the culture medium was collected, cell lysates were prepared. A Proα$_2$ (I) collagen mRNA levels in the lysates were assessed by northern blotting; B the amount of type I collagenase activity in the culture medium measured by monitoring the degradation of fluorescein isothyocyanate-labeled type I collagen. Each value in B represents the average ± SD ($n = 6$). Points marked by an *asterisk* differ significantly ($P < 0.05$) from the control and the samples with the antibody. (From [16], with permission)

236

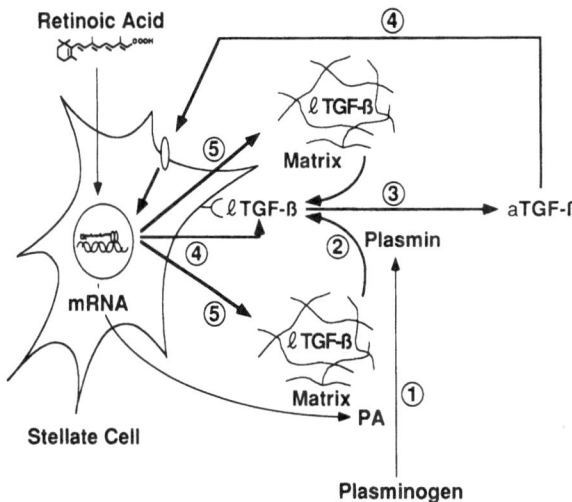

Fig. 5. Illustration of the mechanism of retinoic acid (RA) promotion of liver fibrosis via TGF-$\beta$. RA up-regulates plasminogen activator (*PA*)/plasmin levels in hepatic stellate cells (SCs) (1). This increase elaborates the release (2) and activation (3) of latent TGF-$\beta$ (lTGF-$\beta$) on the cell surface. The active TGF-$\beta$ (aTGF-$\beta$) generated then stimulates its own synthesis (4) and increases the amount of extracellular matrix (5), resulting in a cycle of TGF-$\beta$-extracellular matrix overexpressions and an exacerbation of liver fibrosis

# 9,13-di-*cis*-RA–an Endogenous RA in Fibrotic Liver

The linkage between RA and TGF-$\beta$ has been shown both in vitro and in vivo [16]. However, all these observations were conducted by examining the effect of exogenous RA added to each system, and the effect of endogenously produced RA remained a matter of speculation. This issue is especially critical with regard to the liver fibrosis model. It is well known that the retinylpalmitate contents in SCs decrease with the development of fibrosis [33]. This implies that the loss of retinol observed in the fibrotic liver might be, in part, the result of conversion of retinylpalmitate to all-*trans*-RA and/or to further metabolites including 9-*cis*-RA, 13-*cis*-RA, and several nongeometric isomers. In support of this hypothesis, we discovered a two-fold increase in 9,13-di-*cis*-RA generation in rat fibrotic livers (M. Okuno et al., submitted for publication). Because 9,13-di-*cis*-RA is a major product arising from the in vivo isomerization of 9-*cis*-RA [34, 35] and has been suggested to be an indicator of pre-existing 9-*cis*-RA [34, 36], the elevation in hepatic 9,13-di-*cis*-RA concentration implied that 9-*cis*-RA might be generated during the development of fibrosis. In addition, we found that 9,13-di-*cis*-RA itself can induce the activation of latent TGF-$\beta$ in a plasmin-dependent manner and enhance TGF-$\beta$ biosynthesis (Fig. 6) [37]. This biological action of 9,13-di-*cis*-RA seems to be mediated by RAR$\alpha$.

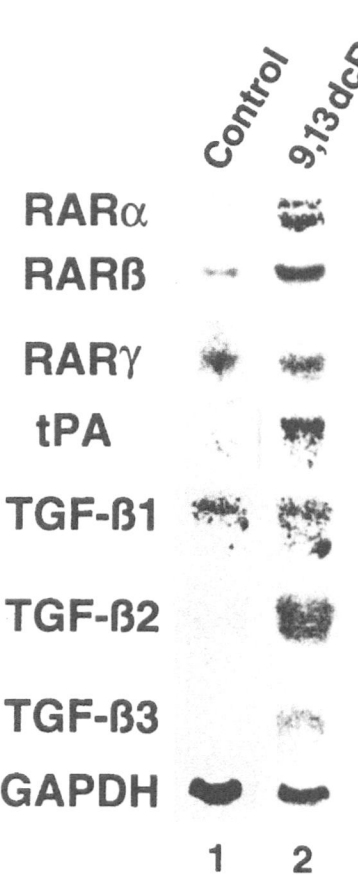

FIG. 6. Changes in the mRNA levels of retinoic acid receptor (*RAR*) $\alpha$, $\beta$, $\gamma$, tissue plasminogen activator (*tPA*), and TGF-$\beta$1, -$\beta$2, -$\beta$3 following the exposure of a human hepatic stellate cell line, LI90, to 9,13-di-*cis*-retinoic acid (9,13dcRA). Confluent LI90 cell cultures were incubated either with vehicle (*control; lane 1*) or with 1 µM 9,13dcRA (*lane 2*) for 12 h. Total RNA was isolated from each cell sample, fractionated through 1% agarose-formaldehyde gels, transferred to nylon membranes and hybridized with $^{32}$P-labeled probe for RAR$\alpha$, $\beta$, $\gamma$, tPA, TGF-$\beta$1, -$\beta$2, -$\beta$3, or GAPDH. The radioactivity of each band was detected on an imaging analyzer. (From [37], with permission)

## Future Directions

Our results suggest two aspects of retinoid action in liver fibrosis. One is the anti-inflammatory effect. In the CCl$_4$ model, RA suppressed liver fibrosis indirectly by reducing parenchymal necrosis. RA would probably act on Kupffer cells to inhibit TNF-$\alpha$ secretion. The other aspect is the profibrogenic effect via TGF-$\beta$. In the porcine serum model, RA appeared to act directly on SCs and stimulate liver fibrosis.

No definitive therapy exists for the treatment of liver fibrosis and cirrhosis. Recently, the use of anti-TGF-$\beta$ antibody against the fibrosis has started to draw attention. However, experimental data are only just beginning to accumulate [38]. The present study may provide an indication of a possible novel therapy against liver fibrosis. Because the induction of TGF-$\beta$ by RA in the SCs was initiated by the proteolytic activation of latent TGF-$\beta$ on the cell surface, the activation of latent TGF-

$\beta$ can be a primary target for therapeutic development, and inhibitors of PA/plasmin could be effective antifibrogenic agents. In fact, very recently, the plasmin-TGF-$\beta$ activation cascade has been shown to take place in human hepatic fibrosis [39]. Interestingly, in previous studies, protease inhibitors and an inhibitor of surface plasmin have been used episodically as cytoprotective agents to reduce liver cell necrosis [1]. The idea is now being successfully tested using animal models (M. Okuno et al., unpublished observation).

*Acknowledgments.* This study was supported partly by Grants-in-Aid from the Ministry of Education, Science, Sports, and Culture (09670533, MO; 08780689, SK), a grant from the Mochida Memorial Foundation for Medical and Pharmaceutical Research (MO), grants for the Biodesign Research Program and Multi-bioprobe Research Program from RIKEN (SK), and grants from The Naito Foundation (SK).

## References

1. Gressner AM, Bachem MG (1995) Molecular mechanisms of liver fibrogenesis—a homage to the role of activated fat-storing cells. Digestion 56:335–346
2. Friedman SL (1993) The cellular basis of hepatic fibrosis. N Engl J Med 328:1828–1835
3. Senoo H, Wake K (1985) Suppression of experimental hepatic fibrosis by administration of vitamin A. Lab Invest 52:182–194
4. Seifert WF, Bosma A, Brouwer A, et al. (1994) Vitamin A deficiency promotes $CCl_4$ liver fibrosis. Hepatology 19:193–201
5. Leo MA, Lieber CS (1983) Hepatic fibrosis after long-term administration of ethanol and moderate vitamin A supplementation in the rat. Hepatology 3:1–11
6. Geubel AP, De Galocsy C, Alves N, et al. (1991) Liver damage caused by therapeutic vitamin A administration: Estimate of dose-related toxicity in 41 cases. Gastroenterology 100:1701–1709
7. Nicholson RC, Mader S, Nagpal S, et al. (1991) Negative regulation of the rat stromelysin gene promoter by retinoic acid is mediated by an AP1 binding site. EMBO J 9:4443–4454
8. Pan L, Eckhoff C, Brinckerhoff CE (1995) Suppression of collagenase gene expression by all-*trans* and 9-*cis* retinoic acid is ligand dependent and requires both RARs and RXRs. J Cell Biochem 57:575–589
9. Okuno M, Muto Y, Moriwaki H, et al. (1990) Inhibitory effect of acyclic retinoid (polyprenoic acid) on hepatic fibrosis in $CCl_4$-treated rats. J Gastroenterol 25:223–229
10. Hanazawa S, Takeshita A, Kitano S (1994) Retinoic acid suppression of c-*fos* gene inhibits expression of tumor necrosis factor-$\alpha$-induced monocyte chemoattractant JE/MCP-1 in clonal osteoblastic MC3T3-E1 cells. J Biol Chem 269:21379–21384
11. Muto Y, Nouri-Aria KT, Meager A, et al. (1988) Enhanced tumor necrosis factor and interleukin-1 in fluminant hepatic failure. Lancet 2:72–74
12. Davis BH, Pratt BM, Madri JA (1987) Retinol and extracellular collagen matrices modulate hepatic Ito cell collagen phenotype and cellular retinol binding protein levels. J Biol Chem 262:10280–10286
13. Davis BH, Kramer RT, Davidson NO (1990) Retinoic acid modulates rat Ito cell proliferation, collagen and transforming growth factor $\beta$ production. J Clin Invest 86:2062–2070
14. Davis BH, Vucic A (1988) The effect of retinol on Ito cell proliferation in vitro. Hepatology 8:788–793

15. Pinzani M, Gentilini P, Abboud HE (1992) Phenotypical modulation of liver fat-storing cells by retinoids. Influence on unstimulated and growth factor-induced cell proliferation. J Hepatol 14:211–220
16. Okuno M, Moriwaki H, Imai S, et al. (1997) Retinoids exacerbate rat liver fibrosis by inducing the activation of latent TGF-$\beta$ in liver stellate cells. Hepatology 26:913–921
17. Davis BH (1988) Transforming growth factor $\beta$ responsiveness is modulated by the extracellular collagen matrix during hepatic Ito cell culture. J Cell Physiol 136:547–553
18. Border WA, Noble NA (1994) Transforming growth factor $\beta$ in tissue fibrosis. N Engl J Med 331:1286–1292
19. Sanderson N, Factor V, Nagy P, et al. (1995) Hepatic expression of mature transforming growth factor $\beta 1$ in transgenic mice results in multiple tissue lesions. Proc Natl Acad Sci USA 92:2572–2576
20. Milani S, Herbst H, Schuppan D, et al. (1994) Differential expression of matrix metalloproteinase-1 and -2 genes in normal and fibrotic human liver. Am J Pathol 144:528–537
21. Ramadori G, Neubauer K, Odenthal M, et al. (1992) The gene of hepatocyte growth factor is expressed in fat-storing cells of rat liver and is down-regulated during cell growth and by transforming growth factor-$\beta$. Biochem Biophys Res Commun 183:739–742
22. Roberts AB, Sporn MB (1990) The transforming growth factor-$\beta$s. In: Sporn MB, Roberts AB (eds) Peptide growth factors and their receptors. I. Handbook of experimental pharmacology. vol 95/I. Springer-Verlag, Berlin, pp 419–472
23. Flaumenhaft R, Kojima S, Abe M, et al. (1993) Activation of latent transforming growth factor $\beta$. In: August JT, Anders MW, Murad F (eds) Advances in pharmacology. vol 24. Academic Press, San Diego, pp 51–76
24. Sato Y, Rifkin DB (1989) Inhibition of endothelial cell movement by pericytes and smooth muscle cells: Activation of a latent transforming growth factor-$\beta 1$-like molecule by plasmin during co-culture. J Cell Biol 109:309–315
25. Sato Y, Tsuboi R, Lyons R, et al. (1990) Characterization of the activation of latent TGF-$\beta$ by co-cultures of endothelial cells and pericytes or smooth muscle cells: A self-regulating system. J Cell Biol 111:757–763
26. Kojima S, Harpel PC, Rifkin DB (1991) Lipoprotein (a) inhibits the generation of transforming growth factor $\beta$: An endogenous inhibitor of smooth muscle cell migration. J Cell Biol 113:1439–1445
27. Mangelsdorf DJ, Umesono K, Evans RM (1994) The retinoid receptors. In: Sporn MB, Roberts AB, Goodman DS (eds) The reitnoids. biology, chemistry, and medicine. 2nd edn. Raven, New York, pp 319–349
28. Yamada Y, Shidoji Y, Fukutomi Y, et al. (1994) Positive and negative regulations of albumin gene expression by retinoids in human hepatoma cell lines. Mol Carcinogenesis 10:151–158
29. Gudas LJ, Sporn MB, Roberts AB (1994) Cellular biology and biochemistry of the retinoids. In: Sporn MB, Roberts AB, Goodman DS (eds) The retinoids. Biology, chemistry, and medicine. 2nd edn. Raven, New York, pp 443–520
30. Krätzschmar J, Haendler B, Kojima S, et al. (1993) Bovine urokinase-type plasminogen activator and its receptor: Cloning and induction by retinoic acid. Gene 125:177–183
31. Kojima S, Nara K, Rifkin DB (1993) Requirement for transglutaminase in the activation of latent transforming growth factor-$\beta$ in bovine endothelial cells. J Cell Biol 121:439–448
32. Kojima S, Rifkin DB (1993) Mechanism of retinoid-induced activation of latent transforming growth factor-$\beta$ in bovine endothelial cells. J Cell Physiol 155:323–332
33. Blomhoff R, Wake K (1991) Perisinusoidal stellate cells of the liver: important roles in retinol metabolism and fibrosis. FASEB J 5:271–277

34. Horst RL, Reinhardt TA, Goff JP, et al. (1995) Identification of 9-*cis*, 13-*cis*-retinoic acid as a major circulating retinoid in plasma. Biochemistry 34:1203–1209
35. Kojima R, Fujimori T, Kiyota N, et al. (1994) In vivo isomerization of retinoic acids. Rapid isomer exchange and gene expression. J Biol Chem 269:32700–32707
36. Arnhold T, Tzimas G, Wittfoht W, et al. (1996) Identification of 9-*cis*-retinoic acid, 9,13-di-*cis*-retinoic acid, and 14-hydroxy-4,14-retro-retinol in human plasma after liver consumption. Life Sci 59:PL169–177
37. Imai S, Okuno M, Moriwaki H, et al. (1997) 9,13-di-*cis*-Retinoic acid induces the production of tPA and activation of latent TGF-$\beta$ via RAR$\alpha$ in a human liver stellate cell line, LI90. FEBS Lett 411:102–106
38. Mavier P, Mallat A (1995) Perspectives in the treatment of liver fibrosis. J Hepatol 22 (suppl 2):111–115
39. Inuzuka S, Ueno T, Torimura T, et al. (1997) The significance of colocalization of plasminogen activator inhibitor-1 and vitronectin in hepatic fibrosis. Scand J Gastroenterol 32:1052–1060

# Hepatic Fibrolysis and Hepatic Sinusoidal Cells

Isao Okazaki[1], Tetsu Watanabe[1], Sigenari Hozawa[1],
Maki Niioka[1], Masao Arai[2], and Katsuya Maruyama[3]

*Summary.* The authors succeeded in inducing MMP-1 production by coculture of fibroblasts and hepatocytes. This abundant MMP-1 production by fibroblasts contributes to massive necrosis or tissue breakdown in vivo. Bhatnagar et al. [26] revealed that rat Kupffer cell stimulation by lipopolysaccharide releases collagenase. Bacterial antigen and endotoxins stimulate Kupffer cells to secrete collagenase. This finding leads to the possibility that the sinusoidal environment may prevent pericellular collagen deposition. The authors also observed the gene expression of interstitial collagense in $CCl_4$-treated rat liver by reverse transcription-polymerase chain reaction (RT-PCR) and in situ hybridization (unpublished data). In normal rats, no signals for interstitial collagenase mRNA were observed in the liver by in situ hybridization. In rats with fatty change induced by treatment with $CCl_4$ for 4 weeks, positive signals for interstitial collagenase mRNA were observed in scattered Ito cells which were identified as $\alpha$-smooth muscle actin-positive cells. In rats treated for 8 weeks, an intense signal for interstitial collagenase mRNA was observed in several kinds of cells within lobules. In contrast, cirrhotic liver in rats treated for 12 weeks revealed weak expression of interstitial collagenase mRNA in Ito cells. RT-PCR analysis also revealed gene expression of interstitial collagenase in rats treated for 8 weeks. No hepatocytes in the liver displayed interstitial collagenase mRNA transcripts, despite $CCl_4$ treatment. Moreover the authors demonstrated evidence of participation of interstitial collagenase in the destruction of matrix in the recovery stage of hepatic fibrosis.

*Key words.* Liver fibrosis, Interstitial collagenase, Ito cells, Kupffer cells

[1] Department of Community Health, Tokai University School of Medicine, Bohseidai, Isehara, Kanagawa 259-1193, Japan
[2] Department of Internal Medicine, Hiratsuka City Hospital, Hiratsuka, Kanagawa 254-0065, Japan
[3] Clinical Research Unit, Kurihama National Hospital, 5-3-1 Nobi, Yokosuka, Kanagawa 239-0841, Japan

# Introduction

Once collagen has formed fibrils followed by linkages with extracellular matrix components, these fibrous tissues had been thought to be stable and resistant to proteolytic enzymes. In 1936, Cameron and Karunaratne [1] published a key paper about hepatic fibrolysis after the removal of the toxic agent in a carbon-tetrachloride-induced cirrhosis model. Since then, hepatic fibrosis induced by thioacetamide [2], $\alpha$-naphthylisothiocyanate [3], ethionine [4], and a choline-deficient diet [5], as well as by ligation of the bile duct [6], and fibrolysis after the removal of causative agents have all been observed.

In 1965, Perez-Tamayo [7] published a stimulating review entitled "Connective Tissue Metabolism in the Liver". In that paper, the following very interesting case was introduced:

Regression of human cirrhosis is not adequately documented although it can occur. Through the courtesy of Dr. Ivan L. Bennett, Jr., I have examined a surgical biopsy specimen from a patient with hemochromatosis and advanced cirrhosis who was treated with repeated bleeding and P32. A new surgical biopsy 10 years later revealed completely normal hepatic structure. The patient died later, however, with primary carcinoma of the liver, and at autopsy there was no cirrhosis.

Excellent reviews [8–12] later discussed the reversibility of hepatic fibrosis. However, it had long been obscure which enzyme participates in recovery from liver cirrhosis until the authors demonstrated the presence of mammalian collagenase in experimental liver fibrosis in rats induced by chronic carbon tetrachloride [13]. The activity of mammalian collagenase, which increased in the early stage of hepatic fibrosis and decreased in cirrhosis [14–16], was confirmed by others both in vivo and in vitro [17–20].

In this chapter, we describe the role of hepatic sinusoidal cells, particularly Ito cells, in the context of matrix metalloproteinase production. Finally, we propose a hypothesis for the mechanism of fibrolysis in the liver.

# Which Matrix Metalloproteinases are Responsible in Hepatic Fibrolysis?

Mammalian collagenase, described in 1974 [13], is now referred to as interstitial collagenase or matrix metalloproteinase-1 (MMP-1). Among 17 MMPs reported until today, representative 12 MMPs are shown in Table 1 [21]. Their activity is regulated by several mechanisms, which include regulation of gene expression by cytokines or hormones, extracellular cleavage of a proenzyme to an active enzyme, and specific inhibition of an active enzyme by endogenous proteins known as tissue inhibitors of metalloproteinases (TIMPs). Interstitial collagenase can degrade type I, type III, and type X collagens, but cannot degrade other types of collagen such as type IV, type V, and type IV, or other components of the extracellular matrix such as proteoglycans and glycoproteins. However, other MMPs, except MMP-1, MMP-8, and MMP-13, cannot degrade type I collagen, which is very stable, and there is net deposition of type I collagen in progressive hepatic fibrosis [8, 10–12]. Therefore, gene expression

TABLE 1. Matrix metalloproteinase family

| Enzyme | Abbreviation | MMP# | MW | Extracellular matrix substrate |
|---|---|---|---|---|
| Fibroblast-type collagenase | FIB-CL | MMP-1 | 57000/52000 | Collagen I, II, III (III >> II), VII, VIII, X, gelatin, proteoglycan (PG) core protein |
| PMN-type collagenase | PMN-CL | MMP-8 | 75000 | Same as FIB-CL (I >> III) |
| Collagenase-3 | CL-3 | MMP-13 | 54000 | Collagen I, II, III |
| Mr 72K gelatinase/ type IV collagenase | Mr 72K GL/ GL-A | MMP-2 | 72000 | Gelatin, collagen IV, V, VII, X, XI, elastin, fibronectin, PG core protein |
| Mr 92K gelatinase/ type IV collagenase | Mr 92K GL/ GL-B | MMP-9 | 92000 | Gelatin, collagen IV, V, elastin, PG core protein |
| Stromelysin-1 | SL-1 | MMP-3 | 60000/55000 | PG core protein, fibronectin, laminin, collagen IV, V, IX, X, elastin, proCL |
| Stromelysin-2 | SL-2 | MMP-10 | 50000/55000 | Same as SL-1 |
| Membrane type-matrix metalloproteinase-1 | MT1-MMP | MMP-14 | 63000 | n.d., potent activator for proMMP-2 |
| Membrane type-matrix metalloproteinase-2 | MT2-MMP | MMP-15 | 72000 | n.d., potent activator for proMMP-2 |
| Stromelysin-3 | SL-3 | MMP-11 | n.d. | n.d. |
| Macrophage metalloelastase | MME | MMP-12 | 53000 | Elastin |
| Putative metalloproteinase-1 | PUMP-1 | MMP-7 | 28000 | Fibronectin, laminin, collagen IV, gelatin, proCL, PG core potein |

of interstitial collagenase in fibrous liver should be important from the standpoint of the amelioration of liver fibrosis.

The rat interstitial collagenase cDNA shares a high degree of homology with human collagenase-3 (MMP-13) [22] and is distinct from human MMP-1 [23]. It is now proposed that this rat collagenase cDNA should be considered the rat homolog of human MMP-13. To date, cDNA of rat MMP-1 has not yet been cloned, and this rat collagenase cDNA is the only known gene coding for interstitial collagenase. We used this rat collagenase cDNA for a recent in situ hybridization study (in preparation).

# Matrix Metalloproteinase Production by Hepatic Sinusoidal Cells

## Interstitial Collagenase (MMP-1 and MMP-13)

We prepared a monolayer culture of fibroblasts derived from rabbit liver in order to clarify the mechanism of interstitial collagenase production by cells obtained from liver [24, 25]. Elucidation of the mechanism for MMP-1 gene expression in liver cirrhosis enabled us to develop a new strategy for the treatment of liver cirrhosis. Figure 1 shows the differences in the mechanism of MMP-1 production between fibroblasts derived from synovium, gastric mucosa, and liver in the same rabbit. All fibroblasts used in this experiment were fourth-passaged cells in order to exclude macrophages and to get uniform cell lines. Synovial fibroblasts secreted a low level of MMP-1 without any treatment, and cells treated with PMA (phorbol myristate acetate) produced high level of MMP-1. Gastric mucosal fibroblasts produced a high level of MMP-1 without any treatment, and after treatment of the cells with PMA, MMP-1 production was further dramatically increased. Liver fibroblasts did not produce MMP-1 even with PMA treatment [24].

The authors succeeded in inducing MMP-1 production by co-culture of fibroblasts and hepatocytes at a cell number ratio of 3:1, as shown in Fig. 2. After a long lately period, a remarkably high level of MMP-1 production was observed [25]. This

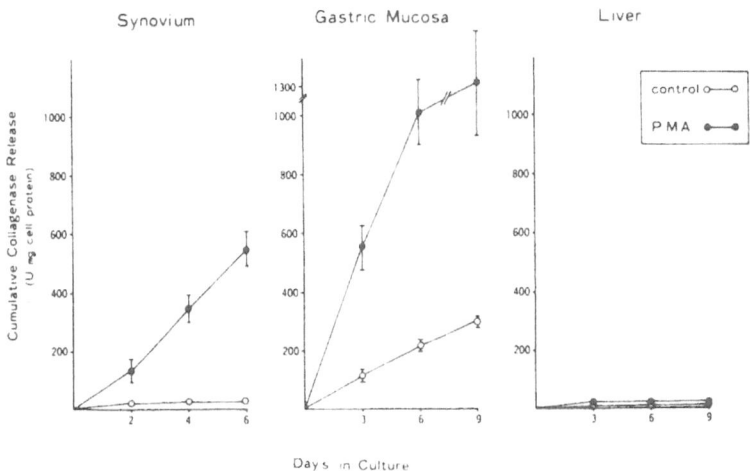

FIG. 1. Collagenase production by fibroblasts obtained from different organs. Fibroblasts derived from synovium, gastric mucosa, and liver from the same rabbit were prepared, and all fibroblasts used in the experiments were the fourth-passaged cells in order to exclude macrophages and to get uniform cell lines. Note the difference in the production mechanism of MMP-1 by fibroblasts of different origin. Liver fibroblasts do not produce MMP-1 even with PMA treatment [24]

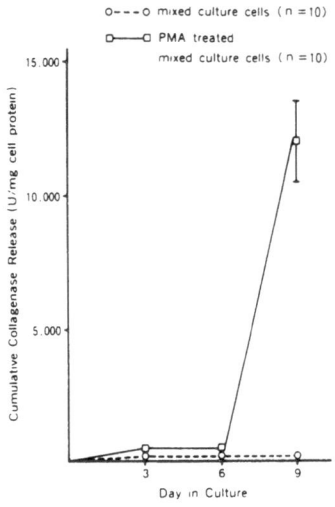

FIG. 2. Collagenase production in co-culture of rabbit liver fibroblasts and hepatocytes. Fibroblasts and hepatocytes were co-cultured at a cell number ratio of 1 : 3 and collagenase activity was measured as described in [25]

abundant of MMP-1 production by fibroblasts contributes to massive necrosis or tissue breakdown in vivo.

Bhatnagar et al. [26] reported that rat Kupffer cells stimulated by lipopolysaccharide (LPS) release collagenase. Bacterial antigen and endotoxins also stimulate Kupffer cells to secrete collagenase. This finding led to the new concept that the sinusoidal environment may prevent pericellular collagen deposition. Otherwise sinusoidal capillarization may occur [27]. Kashiwazaki et al. [28] reported that perisinusoidal cells cultured in conditioned media can secrete some MMP-1, as shown in Fig. 3. They cultured isolated rat hepatocytes in culture media containing LPS, and spent media were used as conditioned media. This mechanism may also be necessary for cleaning around hepatocytes and sinusoids to prevent perihepatocellular fibrosis.

Recently the authors observed the gene expression of interstitial collagense in CCl$_4$-treated rat liver by reverse transcription-polymerase chain reaction (RT-PCR) and in situ hybridization (submitted). In normal rats, no signals for interstitial collagenase mRNA were observed in the liver by in situ hybridization. In rats with fatty change induced by treatment with CCl$_4$ for 4 weeks positive signals for interstitial collagenase mRNA were observed in scattered Ito cells, and these were identified as $\alpha$-smooth muscle actin positive cells. In rats treated for 8 weeks, an intensive signal for interstitial collagenase mRNA was observed in several kinds of cells within lobules. On the other hand, cirrhotic liver in rats treated for 12 weeks revealed weak expression of interstitial collagenase mRNA in Ito cells. RT-PCR analysis also revealed gene expression of interstitial collagenase in rats treated for 8 weeks. No hepatocytes in the liver displayed interstitial collagenase mRNA transcripts regardless of CCl$_4$ treatment.

The authors observed positive signals in activated Ito cells. Activated Ito cells can produce matrix components as well as MMP-1, as reported by Iredale et al. [29] in autoimmune chronic active hepatitis. Their results suggested that Ito cells produce MMP-1 to accumulate fibrosis. There are no published reports of MMP-1 production by Ito cells in the process of hepatic fibrolysis.

FIG. 3. Cumulative collagenase activity by hepatic perisinusoidal cells and hepatic fibroblasts. Perisinusoidal cells cultured in conditioned media can secrete some MMP-1. Conditioned media were prepared as described in [28]

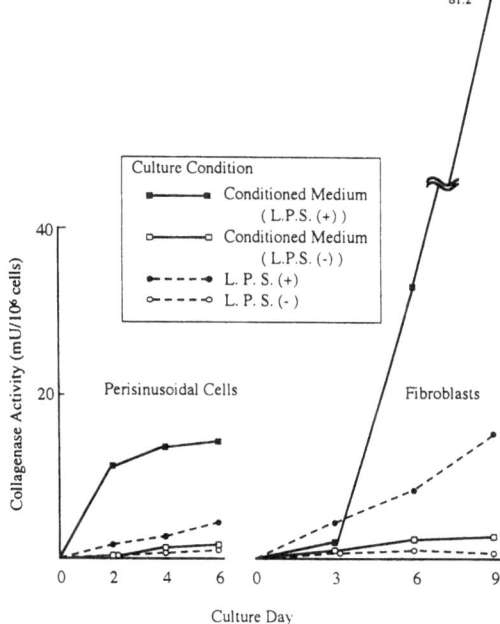

The authors demonstrated their recent data at this Memorial Symposium. The evidence for the participation of interstitial collagenase to destroy matrix in the recovery stage of hepatic fibrosis has not been reported. The aim of present study is to elucidate the gene expression of interstitial collagenase in the recovery stage of experimental rat liver fibrosis.

Generally speaking, as mentioned above, gene expression of interstitial collagenase is weak in the process of rat hepatic fibrosis from chronic CCl₄ intoxication. Conversely, in the recovery stage of hepatic fibrosis, that is 5 days after the last injection of the 8-week-long CCl₄ treatment, a very strong expression of interstitial collagenase mRNA was observed in Ito cells as well as in hepatocytes. Intense signals were seen in Ito cells within or close to disappearing fibrous bands and neighboring hepatocytes, especially at the front edge of resorption. These results indicate the participation of interstitial collagenase expressed in hepatocytes and Ito cells in matrix degradation in the recovery stage of experimental rat liver fibrosis (in preparation).

## MMP-2, MMP-3, MT1-MMP, and Other MMPs

Arthur and co-workers [30, 31] reported that Ito cells secreted neutral metalloproteinase which can degrade type IV collagen (a component of basement membrane). This was 72 kDa type IV collagenase/gelatinase (MMP-2). MMP-2 gene expression is up-regulated by TGFβ 1 while MMP-1 gene expression is down-regulated by TGFβ 1. Takahara et al. [32] reported the MMP-2 gene expression is increased in the process of experimental hepatic fibrosis and is decreased in cirrhosis. In the recovery stage from experimental hepatic fibrosis they showed increased gene expression of MMP-2 on the 3rd and 7th day after the discontinuation of treatment and decreased expression on the 14th day. The destruction of pericellular fibrosis may occur at a very early stage of recovery.

In situ hybridization of MMP-2 [33] revealed that vimentin-positive, CD-68 negative mesenchymal cells which should be Ito cells showed high transcript levels of TGF$\beta$ as well as MMP-2. They observed this gene expression in the process of hepatic fibrosis in chronic hepatitis. Very recently, Takahara et al. [34] demonstrated that dual expression of MMP-2 and MT1-MMP in chronic hepatitis and cirrhosis, and cytoplasmic and membranous immunodeposits of both MMPs, were found in endothelial cells, Kupffer cells, capillary endothelial cells, and lymphocytes. In particular they observed over-expression of MMPs in Ito cells and fibroblasts, and suggested that MT1-MMP activates Pro-MMP-2, and then activated MMP-2 may remodel liver parenchyma during the process of liver fibrosis. However, MMP-2 gene expression has not been observed during the process of fibrolysis in the liver by in situ hybridization.

Vyas et al. [35] reported that cultured rat Ito cells synthesize and secrete transin (stromelysin). Herbst et al. [36] reported that gene expression of MMP-3 in hepatocytes was observed during the early phase of rat liver regeneration after a single injection of $CCl_4$. At the site of this gene expression both c-fos and c-jun transcripts were also observed by in situ hybridization. Winwood et al. [37] reported that Kupffer cells secreted 95-kd type IV collagenase/gelatinase B. MMP-3 and MMP-9 should be investigated by a more specific technique in relation to perihepatocellular fibrosis. MMP-3 gene expression has not been observed during the process of fibrolysis in hepatic fibrosis. There have been no studies on gene expression of MT1-MMP and other MMPs in the context of fibrolysis in the liver.

## Production of TIMPs by Hepatic Sinusoidal Cells

Recent studies have emphasized the importance of TIMPs in liver fibrosis [38–41]. Iredale et al. [38] and Roeb et al. [40] demonstrated that TIMP-1 mRNA increased during the early phase of $CCl_4$ treatment; it then decreased and stayed at a low level during the remainder of the experiment. The net activity of MMPs is determined by the balance between the activities of MMPs and their inhibitors. Herbst et al. [41] reported that TIMP-1 and TIMP-2 transcripts were present at high levels in all fibrotic rat and human livers, predominantly in Ito cells. However, TIMPs have not been examined during the recovery phase of experimental hepatic fibrosis.

## Conclusion

Not all of the mechanisms involved in the fibrolysis of hepatic fibrosis have been classified. However, we now have some very useful tools to help us to analyze this process. Advances in understanding the mechanisms of fibrolysis will make it possible to develop a new strategy for the treatment of liver cirrhosis. This paper investigated gene expression of rat interstitial collagenase in hepatocytes as well as Ito cells in the process of fibrolysis in experimental hepatic fibrosis. A summary of a possible mechanism of fibrolysis in the liver is shown schematically in Fig. 4. In this figure the gene

FIG. 4. Scheme of fibrolysis in the liver

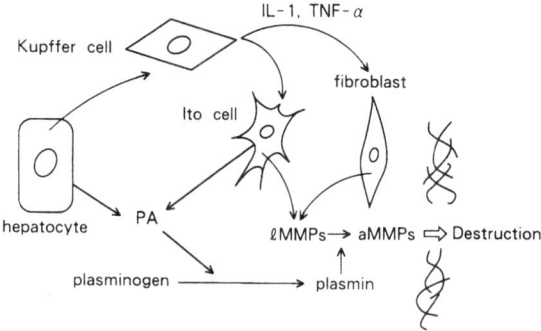

expression in hepatocytes is not described. The precise mechanism of fibrolysis in hepatic fibrosis remains to be clarified.

## References

1. Cameron GR, Karunaratne WAE (1936) Carbon tetrachloride cirrhosis in relation to liver regeneration. J Pathol Bacteriol 42:1–21
2. Quinn PS, Higginson J (1965) Reversible and irreversible changes in experimental cirrhosis. Am J Pathol 47:353–369
3. Morrione TG, Levine J (1967) Collagenolytic activity and collagen resorption in experimental cirrhosis. Arch Pathol 84:59–63
4. Hutterer F, Rubin E, Popper H (1964) Mechanism of collagen resorption in reversible hepatic fibrosis. Exp Mol Pathol 3:215–223
5. Takada A, Porta EA, Hartroft WS (1967) The recovery of experimental dietary cirrhosis. Am J Pathol 51:929–957, 959–976
6. Jacques WE, McAdams AI (1957) Reversible biliary cirrhosis in rat after partial ligation of common bile duct. AMA Arch Pathol 63:149–153
7. Perez-Tamayo R (1965) Some aspects of connective tissue of the liver. In: Popper H, Schaffner F (eds) Progress in liver diseases. vol 2. Grune & Stratton, New York/London, pp 204–210
8. Rojkind M, Dunn M (1979) Hepatic fibrosis. Gastroenterology 76:849–863
9. Okazaki I, Maruyama K (1980) Mammalian collagenase in the process of hepatic fibrosis. J Univ Occupat Environ Health 2:401–424
10. Bissell DM, Friedman SL, Maher JJ, et al. (1990) Connective tissue biology and hepatic fibrosis: Report of a conference. Hepatology 11:488–498
11. Friedman S (1993) The cellular basis of hepatic fibrosis: Mechanisms and treatment strategies. N Engl J Med 328:1828–1835
12. Arthur MJP (1995) Role of Ito cells in the degradation of matrix in liver. J Gastroenterol Hepatol 10:S57–S62
13. Okazaki I, Maruyama K (1974) Collagenase activity in experimental hepatic fibrosis. Nature 252:49–50
14. Maruyama K, Feinman L, Okazaki I, et al. (1981) Direct measurement of neutral collagenase activity in homogenates from baboon and human liver. Biochim Biophys Acta 658:124–131
15. Maruyama K, Feinman L, Fainsilber Z, et al. (1982) Mammalian collagenase increases in early alcoholic liver disease and decreases with cirrhosis. Life Sci 30:1379–1384
16. Okazaki I, Feinman L, Lieber C (1977) Hepatic mammalian collagenase: Development of an assay and demonstration of increased activity after ethanol consumption. Gastroenterology 73:1236

17. Montfort I, Perez-Tamayo R (1978) Collagenase in experimental carbon tetrachloride cirrhosis of the liver. Am J Pathol 92:411–420
18. Carter E, Mccarron M, Alpert E, et al. (1982) Lysyl oxidase and collagenase in experimental acute and chronic liver injury. Gastroenterology 82:526–534
19. Montfort I, Perez-Tamayo R, Alvizouri A, et al. (1990) Collagenase of hepatocytes and sinusoidal liver cells in the reversibility of experimental cirrhosis of the liver. Virchows Archiv B Cell Pathol 59:281–289
20. Lindblad W, Fuller G (1983) Hepatic collagenase activity during carbon tetrachloride-induced fibrosis. Fundam Appl Toxicol 3:34–40
21. Nagase H, Barret A, Woessner J (1992) Nomenclature and glossary of the matrix metalloproteinases. Matrix (Suppl) 1:421–424
22. Freije JMP, Diez-Itza I, Balbin M, et al. (1994) Molecular cloning and expression of collagenase-3, a novel human matrix metalloproteinase produced by breast carcinomas. J Biol Chem 269:16766–16773
23. Knauper V, Lopez-Otin C, Smith B, et al. (1996) Biochemical characterization of human collagenase-3. J Biol Chem 271:1544–1550
24. Okazaki I, Maruyama K, Kashiwazaki K, et al. (1985) Mechanism of collagenase production by liver cells. In: Hirayama C, Kivirikko K (eds) Pathobiology of hepatic fibrosis. Elsevier Amsterdam, pp 141–149
25. Maruyama K, Okazaki I, Kobayashi T, et al. (1983) Collagenase production by rabbit liver cells in monolayer culture. J Lab Clin Med 102:543–550
26. Bhatnagar R, Schade U, Rietschel E, et al. (1982) Involvement of prostaglandin E and adenosine 3'5'-monophosphate in lipopolysaccharide-stimulated collagenase release by rat Kupffer cells. Eur J Biochem 124:2405–2409
27. Okazaki I, Tsuchiya M, Kamegaya K, et al. (1973) Capillarization of hepatic sinusoids in carbon-tetrachloride-induced hepatic fibrosis. Bibl Anat 12:476–483
28. Kashiwazaki K, Hibbs M, Seyer J, et al. (1986) Stimulation of interstitial collagenase in co-cultures of rat hepatocytes and sinusoidal cells. Gastroenterology 90:829–836
29. Iredale J, Goddard S, Murphy G, et al. (1995) Tissue inhibitor of metalloproteinase-1 and interstitial collagenase expression in autoimmune chronic active hepatitis and activated human hepatic lipocytes. Clin Sci 89:75–81
30. Arthur M, Friedman S, Roll F, et al. (1989) Lipocytes from normal rat liver release a neutral metalloproteinase that degrades basement membrane (type IV) collagen. J Clin Invest 84:1076–1085
31. Arthur M, Stanley A, Iredale J, et al. (1992) Secretion of 72 kDa type IV collagenase/gelatinase by cultured human lipocytes. Biochem J 287:701–707
32. Takahara T, Furui K, Funaki J, et al. (1995) Increased expression of matrix metalloproteinase-II in experimental liver fibrosis in rats. Hepatology 21:787–795
33. Milani S, Herbst H, Schuppan D, et al. (1994) Differential expression of matrix-metalloproteinase-1 and -2 genes in normal and fibrotic human liver. Am J Pathol 144:528–537
34. Takahara T, Furui K, Yata Y, et al. (1997) Dual expression of matrix metalloproteinase-2 and membrane-type 1-matrix metalloproteinase in fibrotic human livers. Hepatology 26:1521–1529
35. Vyas SK, Leyland H, Gentry J, et al. (1995) Rat hepatic lipocytes synthesize and secrete transin (stromelysin) in early primary culture. Gastroenterol 109:889–898
36. Herbst H, Heinrichs O, Schuppan D, et al. (1991) Temporal and spatial patterns of transin/stromelysin RNA expression following toxic injury in rat liver. Virchows Archiv B Cell Pathol 60:295–300
37. Winwood PJ, Schuppan D, Iredale JP, et al. (1995) Kupffer cell-derived 95-kd type IV collagenase/gelatinase B: Characterization and expression in cultured cells. Hepatology 22:304–315

38. Iredale JP, Murphy G, Hembry RM, et al. (1992) Human hepatic lipocytes synthesize tissue inhibitor of metalloproteinases-1. J Clin Invest 90:282–287
39. Iredale J, Benyon R, Arthur M, et al. (1996) Tissue inhibitor of metalloproteinase-1 messenger RNA expression is enhanced relative to interstitial collagenase messenger RNA in experimental liver injury and fibrosis. Hepatology 24:176–184
40. Roeb E, Purucker E, Breuer B, et al. (1997) TIMP expression in toxic and cholestatic liver injury in rat. J Hepatology 27:535–544
41. Herbst H, Wege T, Milani S, et al. (1997) Tissue inhibitor of metalloproteinase-1 and -2 RNA expression in rat and human liver fibrosis. Am J Pathol 150:1647–1659

# Diagnosis and Treatment of Hepatic Fibrosis and Hepatic Sinusoidal Cells

Takato Ueno[1], Seishu Tamaki[1], Hiroshi Sugawara[2],
Kodo Sujaku[1], Riko Ogata[1], Kichol Kim[1], Takuji Torimura[1],
Michio Sata[1], and Kyuichi Tanikawa[3]

*Summary.* Hepatic fibrosis is a common response to chronic liver injury from many causes, including alcohol, chronic viral infections, metabolic liver disorders, and autoimmune hepatitis. Hepatic fibrosis results from an imbalance in extracellular matrix (ECM) synthesis (fibrogenesis) and ECM degradation (fibrolysis). The dynamic process of hepatic fibrosis and the cells producing ECM or matrix metalloproteinases (MMP) have largely been elucidated; it is mainly hepatic stellate cells (HSCs) and Kupffer cells which are involved in fibrogenesis and fibrolysis, respectively. Based on an understanding of connective tissue metabolism, new perspectives for specific antifibrotic therapy in hepatic fibrosis are been developed. The new potential strategies for this therapy are the inhibition of ECM synthesis, augmentation of ECM degradation, inhibition of HSC activation, neutralization of proliferative or fibrogenic mediators, and gene therapy. These approaches are expected to prevent progressive hepatic fibrosis and cirrhosis in the future.

*Key words.* Hepatic fibrosis, Hepatic fibrolysis, Hepatic sinusoidal cells, Cytokines, Antifibrotic therapy

## Introduction

Hepatic fibrosis is characterized by an increase in extracellular matrix (ECM) constituents. Fibrosis is defined as a dynamic process resulting from an imbalance between ECM synthesis (fibrogenesis) and ECM degradation (fibrolysis). Advances in the isolation and usefulness of liver cells, and progress in ECM and cytokine biology have led to important new information about hepatic fibrosis. In particular, hepatic stellate cells (HSCs) (also known as fat-storing cells, Ito cells, or lipocytes) have been clearly identified as the primary cellular source of ECM in hepatic fibrosis. It was

[1] The Second Department of Internal Medicine, Research Center for Innovative Cancer Therapy, Kurume University School of Medicine, 67 Asahi-machi, Kurume, Fukuoka 830-0011, Japan
[2] National Kyushu Medical Center Hospital, Clinical Research Insitute, 1-8-1 Jigyohama, Chuo-ku, Fukuoka 810-8563, Japan
[3] International Institute for Liver Research, Kurume Research Center, 2432-2 Aikawa-machi, Kurume, Fukuoka 830-0861, Japan

recently demonstrated that proliferative cytokines such as platelet-derived growth factor (PDGF) [1, 2], and fibrogenic cytokines including transforming growth factor-$\beta_1$ (TGF-$\beta_1$) [3], are major cytokines in the activation process causing the HSC proliferation and in ECM synthesis by HSCs in hepatic fibrosis. In this review, we emphasize the relationship between hepatic fibrosis and hepatic sinusoidal cells, especially HSCs, and the relationship between the diagnosis and treatment of hepatic fibrosis and hepatic sinusoidal cells.

## Hepatic Fibrosis and Hepatic Sinusoidal Cells

In the normal liver, ECM is localized around portal veins, hepatic arteries, and bile ducts in the portal area, the space of Disse, and central veins. In a cirrhotic liver, the volume of ECM increases markedly to scores of ten compared with those of normal liver. In the normal liver, the subendothelial space contains ECM of basement-membrane constituents that are not electron-dense. In liver cirrhosis, this may be replaced by abundant ECM. This morphometric feature is termed "hepatic sinusoidal capillarization" (Fig. 1) [4, 5]. In this stage, on a cellular level, increased ECM deposi-

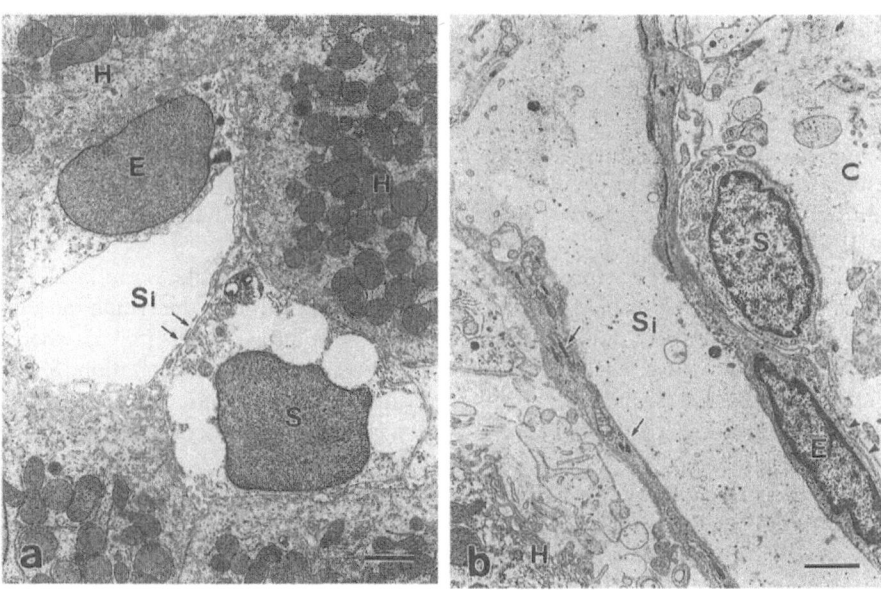

FIG. 1a,b. Electron micrographs showing hepatic sinusoidal areas of normal and cirrhotic livers. **a** Human normal liver. A sinusoidal endothelial cell (SEC) (*E*) shows many fenestrae (*arrows*), but there are no basement membranes on the basal side of the cell. A hepatic stellate cell (HSC) (*S*) containing a few fat droplets in the cytoplasm is visible in the space of Disse. *Si*, sinusoid; H, hepatocyte. (From [5]). **b** Human cirrhotic liver. SECs (*E*) show no fenestrae, but contain many Weibel–Palade bodies containing factor VIII-related antigen (*arrows*) in the cytoplasm. The cells also have visible continuous basal membranes (*arrowheads*) on the basal side of the cells. The spaces of Disse are filled with extracellular matrix (ECM) (*C*). Fat droplets are not visible in the HSC (*S*) in the space of Disse. Typical hepatic sinusoidal capillarization is shown. *Si*, sinusoid; *H*, hepatocyte. (From [5])

tion may underlie the impaired functioning of hepatocytes and the loss of endothelial-cell fenestrae. Fibrosis may also impede the rapid exchange of solutes between the sinusoidal spaces and hepatocytes.

Although HSCs in the normal liver contain prominent intracellular fat droplets containing vitamin A, these vitamin-A-rich cells are replaced by myofibroblast-like cells (MFLCs) (also called transitional cells) which have only a few vitamin A droplets (Fig. 1). Such transitional cells are identified in close association with ECM.

The MFLCs express messenger RNA-encoding ECM components, and produce the various ECM components [6]. However, little or no ECM messenger RNA is expressed in parenchymal cells. The possibility of an early contribution to ECM production by HSCs has not been excluded.

## Diagnosis of Hepatic Fibrosis Using Serum Fibrosis Markers and Hepatic Sinusoidal Cells

Generally, serum fibrosis marker levels are elevated in patients with hepatic fibrosis [7]. The measurement of serum type III procollagen N-terminal peptide (PIII P), type IV collagen, laminin, and hyaluronan (HA) concentrations is used to estimate the degree of hepatic fibrosis. Commonly, these serum markers are elevated with the progression of hepatic fibrosis, and are significantly higher in cirrhotic than in noncirrhotic patients (Fig. 2) [5, 7]. The serum P III P level in particular is involved in histological activity and fibrogenesis. Serum levels of laminin and type IV collagen are usually correlated with the fibrosis score rather than with the histological activity. In addition, these serum markers are usually higher in alcoholic than in nonalcoholic patients [7].

HA (hyaluronic acid, hyaluronate), a glycosaminoglycan molecule, is produced by HSCs in the liver. HA in tissue enters the blood stream through the lymph, and is rapidly taken up via receptors into hepatic sinusoidal endothelial cells (SECs), where degradation then takes place. However, in hepatic sinusoidal capillarization, SECs show morphological changes resembling the characteristics of vascular endothelial cells, and decrease HA uptake via HA receptors, resulting in an increase in the blood HA level (Figs. 3 and 4) [5].

Several investigators have reported that measurement of the serum HA concentration is useful in the diagnosis of liver cirrhosis [5, 8, 9]. To test the differential diagnosis between liver cirrhosis and noncirrhosis, we searched for the cut-off levels of HA, type IV collagen, laminin, P III P, indocyanine green 15 min retention rate (ICGR15), and the platelet count in blood using receiver operating characteristic curves according to various liver pathological diagnoses [8]. The cut-off levels for HA, type IV collagen, laminin, P III P, ICGR15, and platelet count were 130 ng/ml, 250 ng/ml, 2.5 U/ml, 18 ng/ml, 18%, and $14 \times 10^4/mm^3$, respectively. The diagnostic efficiencies at these levels were 91% for laminin, 90% for HA, 83% for type IV collagen, 74% for platelet count, 64% for ICGR15, and 58% for P III P. Moreover, the diagnostic efficiency for liver cirrhosis was 96% in patients showing an HA level over 130 ng/ml and a type IV collagen level exceeding 250 ng/ml. The measurement of serum HA or the serum HA and type IV collagen concentrations is therefore useful in the diagnosis of liver cirrhosis (Table 1) [9].

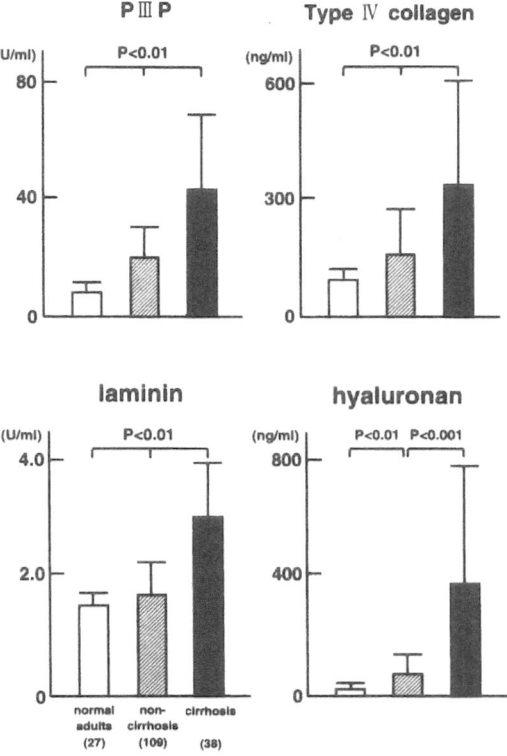

FIG. 2. Serum fibrosis marker levels in patients with or without cirrhosis. Each fibrosis marker level is significantly higher in the cirrhosis group than in the non-cirrhosis group

TABLE 1. Diagnosis of liver cirrhosis by fibrosis markers, ICG 15', and platelets in blood (cut-off value)

| | Laminin (2.5 U/ml) | Hyaluronan (130 ng/ml) | Type IV collagen (250 ng/ml) | Hyaluronan type IV collagen | Platelets $(14 \times 10^4/mm^3)$ | ICG 15' (18%) | P III P (18 ng/ml) |
|---|---|---|---|---|---|---|---|
| Sensitivity (%) | 56 | 87 | 77 | 68 | 67 | 64 | 60 |
| Specificity (%) | 96 | 90 | 86 | 95 | 72 | 63 | 57 |
| Accuracy (%) | 91 | 90 | 83 | 96 | 74 | 64 | 58 |

ICG 15, indocyanine green 15 min retention rate; P III P, type III procollagen N-terminal peptide. Data are from [9].

## NORMAL LIVER

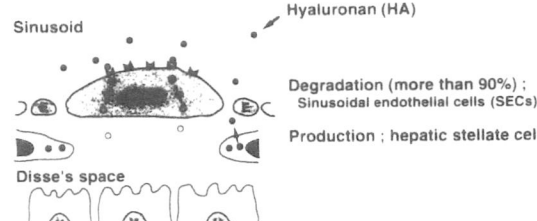

Sinusoid

Hyaluronan (HA)

Degradation (more than 90%) ;
Sinusoidal endothelial cells (SECs)

Production ; hepatic stellate cells

Disse's space

FIG. 3. The relationship between SECs and hyaluronan (HA) in blood in a normal liver and a cirrhotic liver. More than 90% of the circulating HA is degraded in SECs via HA receptors. However, in liver cirrhosis, HA receptors on SECs and the amount of HA binding to the cells are decreased, and the serum HA level is increased

## LIVER CIRRHOSIS

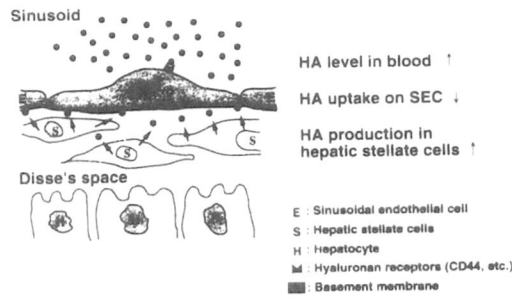

Sinusoid

HA level in blood ↑

HA uptake on SEC ↓

HA production in
hepatic stellate cells ↑

Disse's space

E : Sinusoidal endothelial cell
S : Hepatic stellate cells
H : Hepatocyte
M : Hyaluronan receptors (CD44, etc.)
▓ : Basement membrane

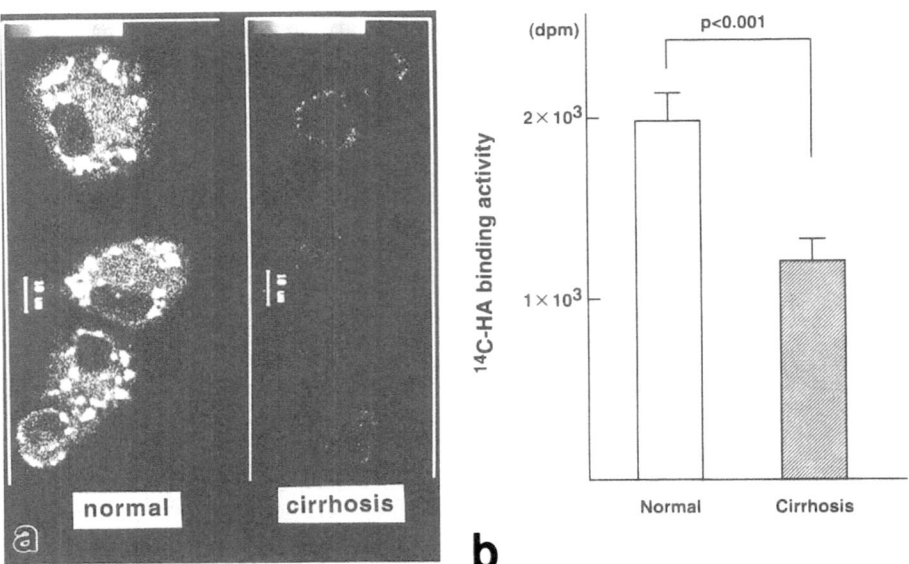

FIG. 4a,b. HA receptor (CD 44) immunolocalization and HA uptake in SECs of normal and cirrhotic rat livers. a Confocal laser-scanning micrographs showing the immunolocalization of anti-CD44 in cultured rat SECs. The intensity of fluorescence is clearly reduced in the cirrhosis group compared with the normal group. (From [8]). b The amount of [$^{14}$C] HA binding to cultured SECs is significantly reduced in the cirrhosis group compared with the normal group. (From [8])

# Treatment of Hepatic Fibrosis and Hepatic Sinusoidal Cells

For the treatment of hepatic fibrosis, removal of the inciting stimulus is clearly the best way to prevent its progression: antihelminthic agents for helminthiasis, abstinence from alcohol for alcoholic fibrosis, discontinuation of hepatotoxic drugs such as methotrexate, and antiviral therapy in patients with chronic viral hepatitis [10].

Anti-inflammatory medications such as corticosteroids are currently used for the suppression of the release of proliferative or fibrogenic cytokines in some liver diseases. Nevertheless, recovery from fibrosis is rarely complete [6].

Based on the growing understanding of connective tissue metabolism, the involvement of cytokines in fibrogenesis or fibrolysis, and the intracellular signaling of ECM-producing cells or matrix metalloproteinase (MMP)-producing cells by cytokines, new perspectives for specific antifibrotic therapy in liver fibrosis have recently been developed. These include the inhibition of ECM synthesis, augmentation of matrix degradation, inhibition of HSC activation, neutralization of proliferative or fibrogenic mediators, and gene therapy, among others [11].

Regarding the inhibition of ECM synthesis, an inhibitor of prolyl-4-hydroxylase, HOE 077, suppressed the production of collagen in HSCs and the progression of hepatic fibrosis in a rat hepatic fibrosis model [12, 13]. Tumor necrosis factor-$\alpha$ (TNF-$\alpha$) inhibits collagen $\alpha$ 1 (1) gene expression in rat HSCs through a G protein [14]. The enhancement of matrix degradation may prove particularly valuable when ECM deposition in response to injury is already extensive. In recent years, in vitro studies have detected MMP-producing cells in the hepatic sinusoidal walls [15–18]. It has been shown that MMPs-1, -2, and -3 are produced by HSCs [15–17], and that MMP-9 is produced by Kupffer cells [18]. We also showed that cultured rat Kupffer cells secreted MMP-9 following treatment with OK-432 (a biological response modifier) (Fig. 5) [19]. In in vivo studies, MMP-2 expression increased in liver tissue once hepatic fibrosis occurred. The expression of active MMP-2 was maximal during the process of hepatic fibrosis, but decreased in liver cirrhosis [20]. In patients with liver cirrhosis, the function of Kupffer cells is reduced compared with that in patients with chronic hepatitis, and the number of Kupffer cells is decreased [21–23]. That is, the changes in the function and number of Kupffer cells closely contribute to the development of hepatic fibrosis. In vivo studies have demonstrated that OK-432 treatment increases the number and activity of Kupffer cells [24].

The control of HSC activation is an especially attractive approach to hepatic fibrogenesis. Interferon gamma inhibits HSC activation in culture [25]. Retinoids may also prove useful for down-regulating HSC proliferation [26]. Hepatocyte growth factor (HGF) by intravenous administration to dimethylnitrosamine or carbon tetrachloride fibrosis model rats suppressed the onset of hepatic fibrosis [27]. A deletion variant of HGF is more mitogenic than HGF for rat hepatocytes or HSCs. This agent reduces messenger RNA levels of procollagens and TGF-$\beta$1 by inhibiting HSC activation and thus suppresses hepatic fibrosis [28]. Gene therapy using the HGF gene is also being explored. Human HGF with SR$\alpha$ promoter was introduced using hemmagglutinating virus of Japan (HVJ)-liposomes into the skeletal muscle of hepatic fibrosis model rats treated with dimethylnitrosamine. The HGF level in the

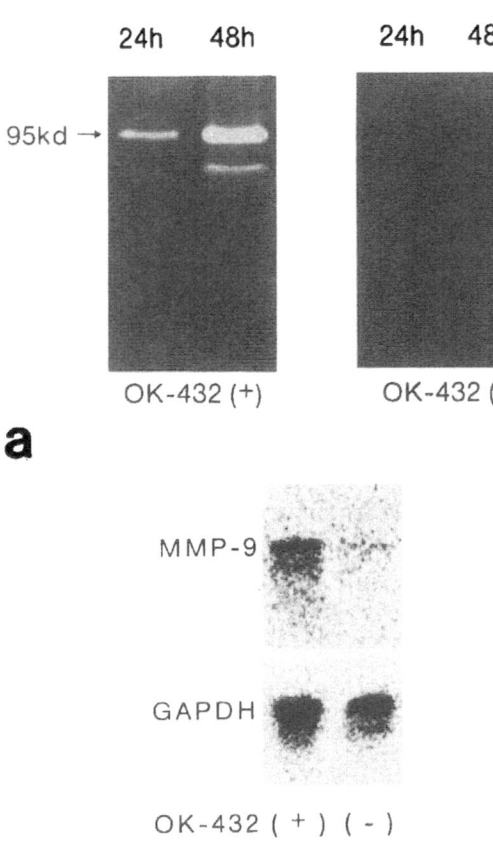

**a**

**b**

FIG. 5a,b. MMP-9 activity shown by gelatin zymography and a Northern blot analysis of MMP-9 messenger RNA. **a** MMP-9 activity by gelatin zymography. In the OK-432-treated group, a 95-kd band and a less than 95-kd band were detected 24 and 48 h after the OK-432 treatment. These bands have clearly increased at 48 h after the OK-432 treatment. In the OK-432 nontreated group, these bands are hardly detectable 24 and 48 h after treatment with OK-432-free medium. (From [19]). **b** Northern blot analysis of MMP-9 messenger RNA. In OK-432-stimulated rat Kupffer cells, single hybridization signals suggesting MMP-messenger RNA are detected. In total RNA from OK-432 unstimulated Kupffer cells, no signals are detected. Lane 1, OK-432 (+); Lane 2, OK-432 (−). (From [19])

blood increased, c-met protein (the receptor for HGF) increased in the liver, and hepatic fibrosis markedly improved [29].

Neutralization of proliferative or fibrogenic mediators by either direct ligand binding or receptor blockade seems achievable with current techniques. In liver diseases, platelet-derived growth factor (PDGF) and TGFβ1 are especially relevant given their roles in HSC proliferation and fibrogenesis. This approach has already shown promise at other sites of experimental tissue injury [6]. The groundwork to neutralize PDGF activity is developing [1, 2]. For PDGF–PDGF receptors there are at least two major pathways of signaling, one involving phosphatidylinositol-3 kinase (PI-3 kinase) and the other involving mitogen-activated protein kinase (MAP kinase). Both pathways begin with the transphosphorylation of tyrosines. The MAP kinase cascade is characterized by a series of phosphorylations involving the accessory factors Src, Grb 2, Ras, Raf, and ERK. PI-3 kinase binds directly to phosphorylated tyrosines of PDGF receptors. The binding of dimeric PDGF to the dimeric PDGF receptor leads to phosphorylation of the intracellular domain, and the interaction of PI-3 kinase with

Fig. 6a,b. Effects of OPC-15161 on inositol triphosphate and $Ca^{2+}$ mobilization in HSCs. **a** Effect of OPC-15161 on inositol triphosphate ($IP_3$) in HSCs. The $IP_3$ level in HSCs treated with interleukin (IL)-1$\beta$ and OPC-15161 is significantly decreased compared with that in HSCs treated with IL-1$\beta$ alone (8.96 $\pm$ 1.70 pmol/tube vs. 1.99 $\pm$ 1.74 pmol/tube; $P < 0.001$). (From [32]). **b** Effect of OPC-15161 on $Ca^{2+}$ mobilization in HSCs. The addition of IL-1$\beta$ rapidly increases the intracellular $Ca^{2+}$ level. After 1 min, OPC-15161 was added. The intracellular-$Ca^{2+}$ level rapidly decreased below the level observed before IL-1$\beta$ treatment. (From [32])

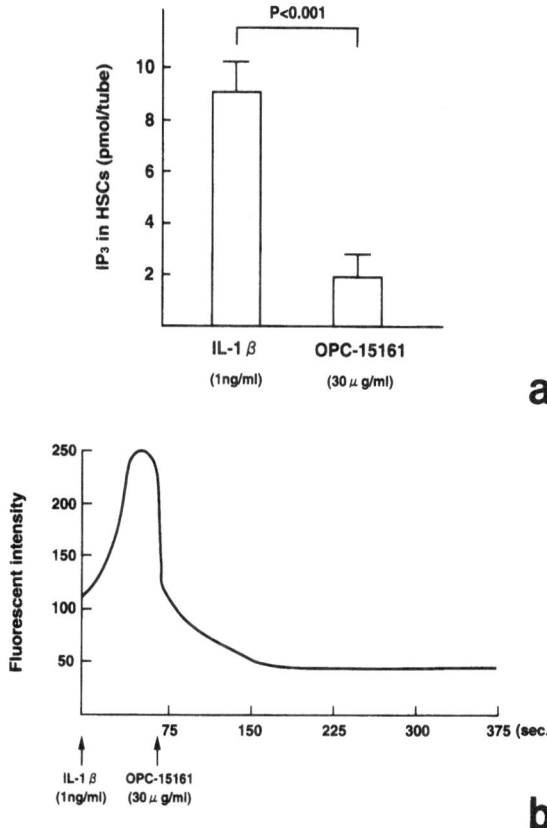

the receptor results in the phosphorylation of phosphoinositol substrates, which are inhibited by wortmannin [2]. Wortmannin is a fungal metabolite that has been used as a PI-3 kinase inhibitor [30]. The proliferation of HSCs is also inhibited by the phosphorylation of the adenosine 3',5'-monophosphate (cAMP) response element-binding protein (CREB) on serine 133 in the nucleus [31]. This finding may be useful for the treatment of hepatic fibrogenesis. We demonstrated that OPC-15161, a fungal metabolite, interferes with the inositol triphosphate-$Ca^{2+}$ pathway (Fig. 6) and inhibits proliferation in cultured rat HSCs treated with interleukin (IL)-1$\beta$ [32] (Fig. 7).

In fibrotic liver, the TGF-$\beta$1 expression is increased in HSCs and SECs [33]. In human liver, TGF-$\beta$1-induced collagen synthesis in myofibroblasts is inhibited by $\alpha$2-macroglobulin [34]. The reduction of TGF-$\beta$1 activity by $\alpha$2-macroglobulin may be explained by the receptor-mediated clearance of TGF-$\beta$1-$\alpha$2-macroglobulin complex. In addition, TGF-$\beta$ receptors exist in rat-cultured HSCs, and the receptors are regulated by TGF-$\beta$ [35]. TGF-$\beta$ signaling from the cell membrane to the nucleus is translocated through the small mother against dpp (SMAD) family [36]. Pathway-restricted SMADs (SMADs 2 and 3) are phosphorylated by specific cell-surface receptors that have serine/threonine kinase activity, and they then oligomerize with SMAD4 and translocate to the nucleus where they direct transcription to affect the

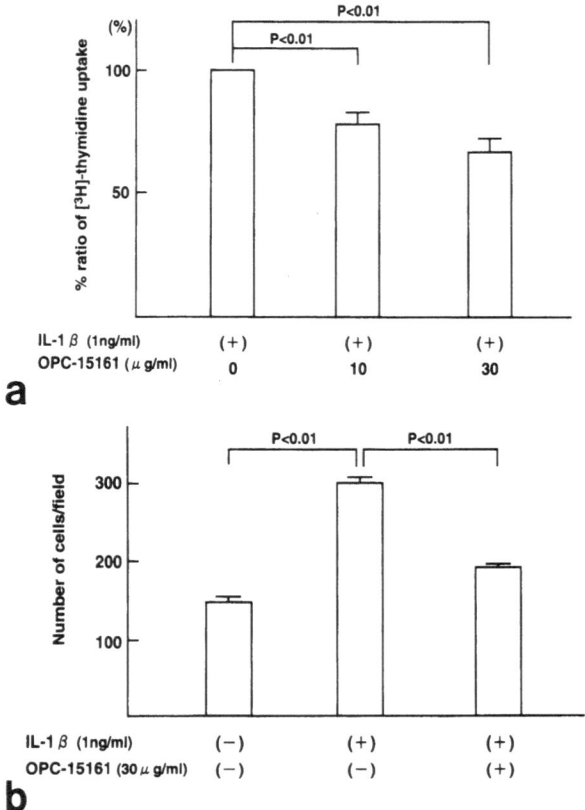

FIG. 7a,b. Effect of OPC-15161 on the proliferation of HSCs. a Inhibitory effect of OPC-15161 on the uptake of [³H]-thymidine in HSCs. The uptake of [³H]-thymidine is significantly inhibited dose-dependently by OPC-15161. (From [32]). b Changes in the cell number of HSCs treated with OPC-15161. The addition of IL-1β significantly increased the number of HSCs compared with that of HSCs in the nontreated group. The addition of OPC-15161 (30 μg/ml) significantly inhibited the number of HSCs. (From [32])

cells response to TGF-β. It has been shown that inhibitory SMADs (SMADs 6 and 7) block the activation of these pathway-restricted SMADs. The antagonistic effect of SMADs 6 or 7 may participate in a negative feedback loop to control TGF-β responses, and has been suggested as a useful treatment for hepatic fibrosis [37, 38].

Various approaches, including the inhibition of ECM synthesis, augmentation of ECM degradation, inhibition of HSC activation, neutralization of proliferative or fibrogenic mediators, and gene therapy, are expected to prevent hepatic fibrosis or cirrhosis in the future.

## References

1. Friedman SL (1997) Closing in on the signals of hepatic fibrosis. Gastroenterology 112:1406–1414
2. Marra F, Gentilini A, Pinzani M, et al. (1997) Phosphatidylinositol 3-kinase is required for platelet-derived growth factor's actions on hepatic stellate cells. Gastroenterology 112:1297–1306
3. Czaja MJ, Weiner FR, Flanders KC, et al. (1989) In vitro and in vivo association of transforming growth factor-β1 with hepatic fibrosis. J Cell Biol 108:2477–2482
4. Schaffner F, Popper H (1963) Capillarization of hepatic sinusoids in man. Gastroenterology 44:239–242

5. Ueno T, Inuzuka S, Torimura T, et al. (1993) Serum hyaluronate reflects hepatic sinusoidal capillarization. Gastroenterology 105:475–481
6. Friedman SL (1993) The cellular basis of hepatic fibrosis: Mechanisms and treatment strategies. N Engl J Med 328:1828–1835
7. Trinchet JC (1995) Clinical use of serum markers of fibrosis in chronic hepatitis. J Hepatol 22(Suppl 2):89–95
8. Tamaki S, Ueno T, Torimura T, et al. (1996) Evaluation of hyaluronic acid binding ability of hepatic sinusoidal endothelial cells in rats with liver cirrhosis. Gastroenterology 110:1049–1057
9. Ueno T, Tanikawa K (1997) Liver injury and serum hyaluronan. In: Rana SVS, Takeda K (eds) Liver and environmental xenobiotics. Narosa Publishing, New Delhi, pp 61–71
10. Oberti F, Valsesia E, Pilette C, et al. (1997) Noninvasive diagnosis of hepatic fibrosis or cirrhosis. Gastroenterology 113:1609–1616
11. Strobel D, Hahn EG (1997) Pathogenesis of liver fibrogenesis. Digestion 58(Suppl 1):37–38
12. Sakaida I, Matsumura Y, Kubota N, et al. (1996) The prolyl 4-hydroxylase inhibitor HOE 077 prevents activation of Ito cells, reducing procollagen gene expression in rat liver fibrosis induced by choline-deficient L-amino acid-defined diet. Hepatology 23:755–763
13. Wang YJ, Wang SS, Bickel M, et al. (1998) Two novel antifibrotics, HOE 077 and safironil, modulate stellate cell activation in rat liver injury. Am J Pathol 152:279–287
14. Hernández-Muñoz I, Torre PDL, Sánchez-Alcázar JA, et al. (1997) Tumor necrosis factor $\alpha$ inhibits collagen $\alpha 1$ (1) gene expression in rats hepatic stellate cells through a G protein. Gastroenterology 113:625–640
15. Milani S, Herbst H, Schuppan D, et al. (1994) Differential expression of matrix-metalloproteinase-1 and -2 genes in normal and fibrotic human liver. Am J Pathol 144:528–537
16. Iredale JP, Benyon RC, Arthur MJP, et al. (1996) Tissue inhibitor of metalloproteinase-1 messenger RNA expression is enhanced relative to interstitial collagenase messenger RNA in experimental liver injury and fibrosis. Hepatology 24:176–184
17. Vyas SK, Leyland H, Gentry J, et al. (1995) Rat hepatic lipocytes synthesize and secrete transin (Stromelysin) in early primary culture. Gastroenterology 109:888–898
18. Winwood PJ, Schuppan D, Iredale JP, et al. (1995) Kupffer cell-derived 95-kd type IV collagenase/gelatinase B: Characterization and expression in cultured cells. Hepatology 22:304–315
19. Sujaku K, Ueno T, Torimura T, et al. (1998) Effects of OK-432 on matrix metalloproteinase-9 expression and activity in rat-cultured Kupffer cells. Hepatol Res 10:91–100
20. Takahara T, Furui K, Funaki J, et al. (1995) Increased expression of matrix metalloproteinase-II in experimental liver fibrosis in rats. Hepatology 21:787–795
21. Petermann H, Heymann S, Vogel S, et al. (1996) Phagocytic function and metabolite production in thioacetamide-induced liver cirrhosis: A comparative study in perfused livers and cultured Kupffer cells. J Hepatol 24:468–477
22. Kamimura S, Tsukamoto H (1995) Cytokine gene expression by Kupffer cells in experimental alcoholic liver disease. Hepatology 21:1304–1309
23. Tomita M, Yamamoto K, Kobayashi H, et al. (1994) Immunohistochemical phenotyping of liver macrophages in normal and diseased human liver. Hepatology 20:317–325
24. Bouwens L, Wisse E (1988) Tissue localization and kinetics of pit cells or large granular lymphocytes in the liver of rats treated with biological response modifiers. Hepatology 8:46–52

25. Rockey DC, Maher JJ, Jarnagin WR, et al. (1992) Inhibition of rat hepatic lipocyte activation in culture by interferon-γ. Hepatology 16:776–784
26. Davis BH, Kramer RT, Davidson NO (1990) Retinoic acid modulates rat Ito cell proliferation, collagen, and transforming growth factor β production. J Clin Invest 86:2062–2070
27. Matsuda Y, Matsumoto K, Yamada A, et al. (1997) Preventive and therapeutic effects in rats of hepatocyte growth factor infusion on liver fibrosis/cirrhosis. Hepatology 26:81–89
28. Yasuda H, Imai E, Shiota A et al. (1996) Antifibrogenic effect of a deletion variant of hepatocyte growth factor on liver fibrosis in rats. Hepatology 24:636–642
29. Ueki T, Hirano T, Okamoto E, et al. (1997) Gene therapy for rat liver cirrhosis by skeletal muscle secretion of hepatocyte growth factor. Hepatology 26:192A
30. Ui M, Okada T, Hazeki K, et al. (1995) Wortmannin as a unique probe for an intracellular signalling protein, phosphoinositide 3-kinase. TIBS 20:303–307
31. Houglum K, Lee KS, Chojkier M (1997) Proliferation of hepatic stellate cells is inhibited by phosphorylation of CREB on serine 133. J Clin Invest 99:1322–1328
32. Sugawara H, Ueno T, Torimura T, et al. (1998) Inhibitory effect of OPC-15161, a component of fugus *Thielavia minor*, on proliferation and extracellular matrix production of rat cultured hepatic stellate cells. J Cell Physiol 174:398–406
33. De Bleser PJ, Niki T, Rogiers V, et al. (1997) Transforming growth factor-β gene expression in normal and fibrotic rat liver. J Hepatol 26:886–893
34. Tiggelman AMBC, Linthorst C, Boers W, et al. (1997) Transforming growth factor-β-induced collagen synthesis by human liver myofibroblasts is inhibited by $\alpha_2$-macroglobulin. J Hepatol 26:1220–1228
35. Knittel T, Janneck T, Müller L, et al. (1996) Transforming growth factor-β1-regulated gene expression of Ito cells. Hepatology 24:352–360
36. Heldin CH, Miyazono K, Dijke PT (1997) TGF-β signalling from cell membrane to nucleus through SMAD proteins. Nature 390:465–471
37. Imamura T, Takase M, Nishihara A, et al. (1997) Smad 6 inhibits signalling by the TGF-β superfamily. Nature 389:622–626
38. Nakao A, Afrakhte M, Morén A, et al. (1997) Identification of smad 7, a TGF β-inducible antagonist of TGF-β signalling. Nature 389:631–635

# Anti-Fibrotic Agent Reduces Enzyme-Altered Lesions and Neoplasms in the Rat Liver

Isao Sakaida and Kiwamu Okita

*Summary.* A choline-deficient L-amino acid-defined (CDAA) diet led to the development of liver cirrhosis in 100% of male Wistar rats after 15 weeks and to liver neoplasms in 90% of rats after 1 year.

Concurrent administration of a prolyl 4-hydroxylase inhibitor (HOE 077), [2,4-pyridine dicarboxylic acid bis (2-methoxyethyl amide)] as an antifibrotic agent to rats fed a CDAA diet reduced the increase in liver hydroxyproline content in a dose-dependent manner for doses up to 200 p.p.m. without reduction of serum alanine aminotransferase (ALT). HOE 077 prevented the histological activation of stellate cells as well as the expression of procollagen type I mRNA, resulting in a reduced hydroxyproline content in the liver and a reduced number of pseudolobuli and thinner fibrous septa. Also, the administration of a CDAA diet for 15 weeks led to a substantial induction of glutathione S-transferase placental form (GSTP)-positive lesions in the liver. The concurrent administration of HOE 077 reduced the percentage area of GSTP-positive lesions in a dose-dependent manner, in parallel with the reduction in hydroxyproline content. Administration of HOE 077 for 1 year reduced the development of liver neoplasms to 50% of those in rats fed a CDAA diet.

These data suggest that inhibition of fibrosis may prevent the development of neoplasms.

*Key words.* Fibrosis, Carcinogenesis, Prolyl 4-hydroxylase inhibitor, Enzyme-altered lesions, Stellate cell

## Introduction

Liver cirrhosis is a very common disease in Japan as well as in other countries. and hepatocellular carcinoma is usually associated with liver cirrhosis, mainly as a consequence of chronic hepatitis or alcohol consumption, although the relationships between carcinogenesis and fibrosis (liver cirrhosis) are unknown. There have been two

First Department of Internal Medicine, School of Medicine, Yamaguchi University, Kogushi 1144 Ube, Yamaguchi 755-8505, Japan

basic approaches to the prevention of liver cancer. The first approach is causation prevention, in which causative agents are eliminated or reduced. Hepatitis, alcohol, and aflatoxins are major causes which have been identified, and the prevention of liver cancer by the elimination of such causes has considerable potential. The second approach is interventional prevention, in which a protective agent, either chemical (chemoprevention) or biological, is administered to prevent or reduce carcinogenesis. In situations where the causes are unknown or cannot be completely eliminated, such as in chronic hepatitis B or C, only interventional prevention is available. There have been many reports about the prevention of liver cancer in rodents by butylated hydroxytoluene (BHT), retinoids, S-adenosyl-L-methionine, and other agents [1–3], but to date there is no effective agent for chemoprevention in clinical practice.

In the present study, we tried the effect of prolyl 4-hydroxylase inhibitor (HOE 077), [2,4-pyridine dicarboxylic acid bis (2-methoxyethyl amide)], on the development of enzyme-altered lesions of glutathione S-transferase placental form (GSTP) as preneoplastic lesions in rat liver cirrhosis induced by the administration of a choline-deficient L-amino acid-defined (CDAA) diet for 15 weeks, as well as on the development of hepatocellular carcinoma for 52 weeks. Our data suggest that inhibition of fibrosis (liver cirrhosis) may prevent the development of liver neoplasms, and this will be a new approach to the prevention of liver neoplasms.

# Materials and Methods

## Animals

Male Wistar rats, 6 weeks of age and weighing 140–150 g (Nippon SLC, Shizuoka, Japan) were obtained, quarantined for 1 week, and housed in a room under controlled temperature (25°C), humidity, and lighting (12h light, 12h dark). Access to food and tap water was ad libitum throughout the study period. After a 1-week acclimation period on a basal diet (Oriental MF Diet, Oriental Yeast, Tokyo, Japan), the rats were divided into experimental groups.

## Diets

The CDAA and choline-supplemented L-amino acid defined (CSAA) diets were obtained in powdered form (Dyets Bethlehem, PA, USA; product numbers 518753, 518754). The detailed compositions of these diets have been described in a previous report [4].

A prolyl 4-hydroxylase inhibitor (HOE 077), 2,4-pyridine dicarboxylic acid bis [(2-methoxyethyl amide)] (Hoechst Pharmaceutical, Frankfurt, Germany) in powdered form (M.W. 281, white powder, melting point 86°C, soluble in water, purity more than 99.9%) was mixed evenly into the CDAA diet at various concentrations as described in the experimental protocol. Whether appropriate concentrations of HOE 077 were present in diets was examined by HPLC. Diets with or without HOE 077 were stored at 4°C immediately after preparation, and were consumed within 1 week.

## Experimental Protocol

The total study periods were 15 or 52 weeks. For the short-term experiment, the groups for assessing the effect of HOE 077 on hydroxyproline content consisted of 20 or 3 rats each. Three groups of 20 rats received a CDAA diet with HOE 077 concentrations of 200, 100, or 0 p.p.m. One group of 3 rats received a CSAA diet as a control. For the long-term experiment, two groups of 10 rats each received a CDAA diet with or without 200 p.p.m. HOE 077 for 52 weeks. Food was replaced every Monday, Wednesday, and Friday to ensure an adequate supply.

At the end of the study, all rats were killed under ether anesthesia. Blood was obtained from the bifurcation of the abdominal aorta and the liver was excised. The livers were weighed, and then immediately frozen for hydroxyproline measurements or fixed in an ice-cold 19:1 mixture of dehydrated ethyl alcohol and glacial acetic acid for 3 h, followed by overnight incubation in 99.5% ethyl alcohol at 4°C and embedded in paraffin, as described previously [5].

## Histology and Immunohistochemical Examination

Sections of 5-μm thickness of the right lobe of all rat livers were processed routinely for hematoxylin and eosin and Azan–Mallory staining and examined immunohistochemically for $\alpha$ smooth muscle actin ($\alpha$SMA) and glutathione-S-transferase placental form (GSTP) by the advidin–biotin–peroxidase complex method, as described previously [6]. Anti-$\alpha$ smooth muscle actin ($\alpha$SMA) monoclonal antibody and rabbit anti-rat GSTP antibody (DAKO, Kyoto, Japan) were employed [6, 7]. Quantitative analyses of $\alpha$SMA-positive cells and GSTP-positive lesions were then carried out with an image analysis system (Personal Image Analysis System LA-555, Pias, Osaka, Japan). The area of $\alpha$SMA-positive cells and GSTP-positive lesions was expressed as a percentage of the total area of the specimen, as described previously [4, 5].

The incidence of hepatocellular carcinomas was assessed by macroscopic findings. The suspected lesions were excised and confirmed by histological examination.

## Hydroxyproline Content

Hydroxyproline content was determined by the modified Kivirikko's method, as described previously [5].

## Probes

The following probes were used in this study. The complementary deoxynucleic acid (cDNA) of type I procollagen alpha 2 and G3PDH (glyceraldehyde-3-phosphate dehydrogenase) were used [8].

## Northern Blot Analysis

Northern blot analysis was performed after isolation of total RNA from the liver tissue by extraction of guanidine isothiocyanate, as described previously [8].

TABLE 1. Effect of HOE 077 on various markers after a 15-week experiment

| Treatment (number of rats) | Hydroxyproline (μg/g wet wt) | GSTP-positive lesions (%) | αSMA-positive cells (%) | ALT (U/L) |
|---|---|---|---|---|
| CDAA (20) | 787 ± 128 | 6.12 ± 2.57 | 4.33 ± 2.03 | 228 ± 88 |
| +HOE 077 /100 p.p.m. (20) | 717 ± 122 | 5.52 ± 2.87 | 3.96 ± 2.33 | 246 ± 92 |
| +HOE 077 /200 p.p.m. (20) | 598 ± 155** | 4.13 ± 2.15* | 3.02 ± 1.71* | 276 ± 75 |
| CSAA (3) | 136 ± 57 | — | — | 58 ± 7 |

Each number represents mean ± SD.
GSTP, glutathione S-transferase placental form; αSMA, α smooth muscle actine; CDAA, choline-deficient L-amino acid-defined; CSAA, choline-supplemented L-amino acid-defined; HOE 077, 2,4-pyridine dicarboxylic acid bis [(2-methoxyethyl amide)].
* $P < 0.05$ versus CDAA group; ** $P < 0.01$ versus CDAA group.

## Statistical Methods

Results are expressed as the mean ± SD, and the data were evaluated by ANOVA as appropriate. The level of significance was set at $P < 0.05$ for each analysis.

## Results

Table 1 indicates that Rats fed a CDAA diet for 15 weeks showed an increased liver hydroxyproline content of 787 ± 128 μg/g wet weight compared with 136 ± 57 μg/g wet weight for rats fed a CSAA diet. Concurrent administration of HOE 077 at 200 p.p.m. significantly reduced this increase in hydroxyproline content to 598 ± 155 μg/g wet weight.

HOE 077 at 200 p.p.m. prevented the formation of pseudolobuli and reduced the thickness of fibrous septa seen by light microscopy (Fig. 1) in parallel with the reduction in the hydroxyproline content of the liver (Table 1). Administration of HOE 077 at doses up to 200 p.p.m. did not notably change the histological findings other than the reduced formation of fibrous septa, e.g., liver cell necrosis or fatty changes, which may have influenced the development of enzyme-altered lesions. The inhibition of fibrosis by HOE 077 cannot be attributed to the reduced cell damage, because HOE 077 did not reduce the increased serum ALT level of rats fed a CDAA diet .

Activated stellate cells which express α smooth muscle actin (αSMA) are called myofibroblast-like cells, and are now considered to be the main collagen-producing cells. These cells markedly proliferated in the liver of rats fed a CDAA diet for 15 weeks (Fig. 2A). HOE 077 at 200 p.p.m. again reduced the number of αSMA-positive cells in the liver (Fig. 2B). Thus, the prevention of fibrogenesis by HOE 077 is somehow related to inhibition of the activation of stellate cells. The results of quantitative analysis of αSMA-positive cells are summarized in Table 1. HOE 077 (200 p.p.m.) significantly reduced the expression of αSMA-positive cells.

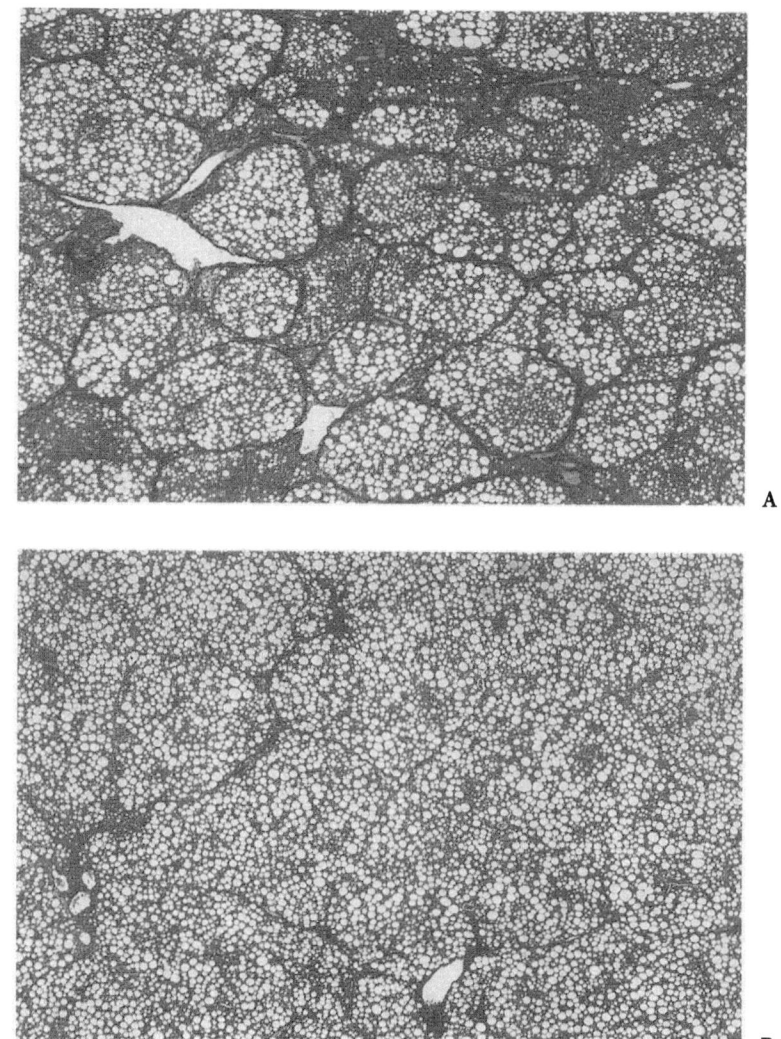

FIG. 1. Photomicrograph of a liver section stained with Azan–Mallory **A** from a male Wistar rat fed a CDAA diet for 15 weeks, and **B** from a rat fed a CDAA diet with concomitant administration of 200 p.p.m. of HOE 077 for 15 weeks. (×40)

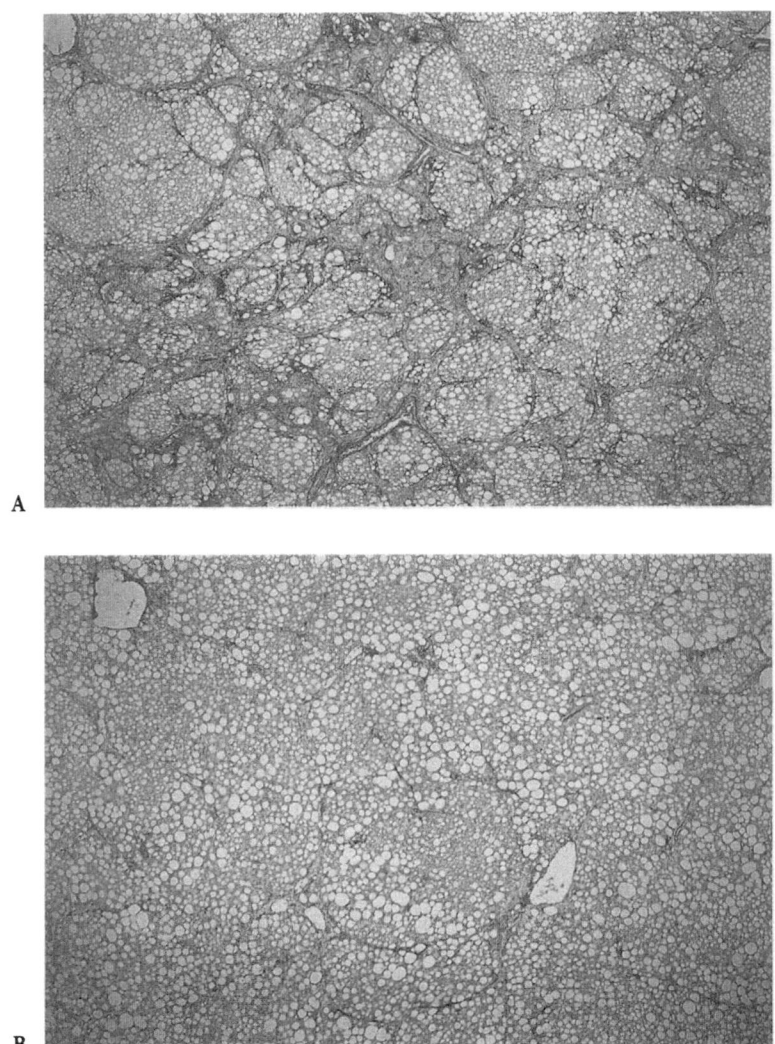

FIG. 2. Photomicrographs of liver sections stained with anti-rat $\alpha$-smooth muscle actin antibody **A** from a male Wistar rat fed a CDAA diet for 15 weeks, and **B** from a rat fed a CDAA diet with concomitant administration of 200 p.p.m. of HOE 077 for 15 weeks. ($\times$40)

FIG. 3. Messenger RNA expression of $\alpha_2$ (I) procollagen and G3PDH in the livers of rats fed a CDAA diet alone (*lane 1*) or a CDAA diet with 200 p.p.m. of HOE 077 for 15 weeks (*lane 2*) or a CSAA diet (*lane 3*). The figure shows a representative sample of six independent Northern blots

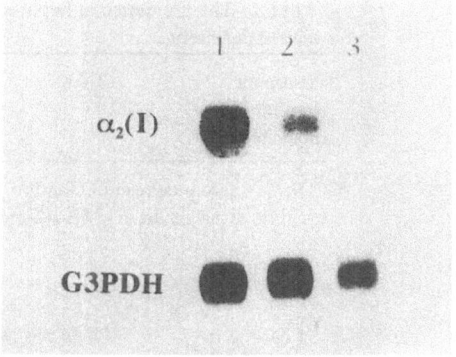

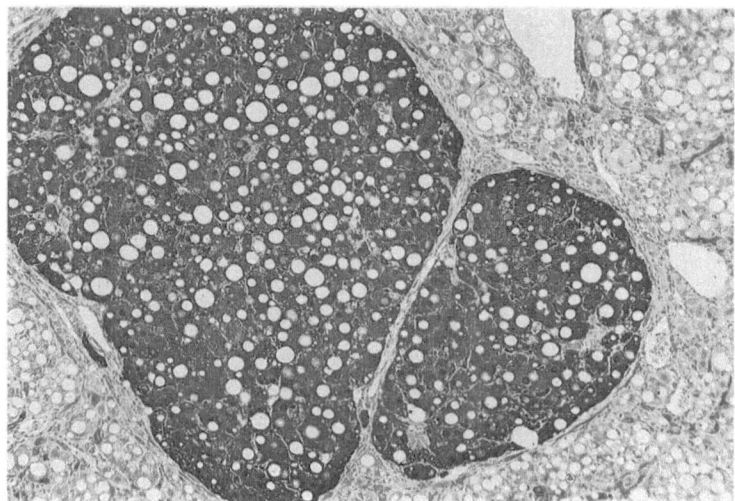

FIG. 4. Typical photomicrograph of GSTP-positive nodules surrounded by fibrous septa in a liver section from a male Wistar rat fed a CDAA diet for 15 weeks. ($\times 40$)

$\alpha_2$(I) procollagen transcript was clearly demonstrated by the Northern-blot analysis of poly (A)$^+$ RNA isolated from the livers of the rats fed the CDAA diet alone or with 200 p.p.m. HOE 077. The levels of $\alpha_2$(I) procollagen mRNA expression were clearly decreased in the livers of rats fed a CDAA diet with 200 p.p.m. HOE 077 for 15 weeks (Fig. 3). Densitometric analysis of $\alpha_2$(I) procollagen after standardization with the expression of G3PDH (Fig. 3) showed significant ($P < 0.05$) suppression by 200 p.p.m. HOE 077 ($1.18 \pm 0.37$ vs. $0.57 \pm 0.33$, $n = 6$). Thus, the prevention of fibrosis by prolyl 4-hydroxylase inhibitor (HOE 077) can be attributed not only to the inhibition of hydroxylation of the proline, but also to the prevention of stellate cell activation resulting in reduced gene expression of procollagen.

Typical GSTP-positive nodules surrounded by fibrous septa are shown in Fig. 4. In this model at 15 weeks, GSTP-positive lesions mainly consist of these nodules.

TABLE 2. The incidence of hepatocellular carcinomas after a 52-week experiment

| Treatment | CDAA | CDAA + 200 p.p.m. HOE 077 |
| --- | --- | --- |
| Number of rats | 10 | 10 |
| Incidence | 90% | 50% |

CDAA, choline-deficient L-amino acid-defined; HOE 077, 2,4-pyridine dicarboxylic acid bis [(2-methoxyethyl amide)].

FIG. 5. Typical histological appearance of a hepatocellular carcinoma stained with hematoxylin and eosin found in a rat fed a CDAA diet for 52 weeks (Magnification: ×40)

The results of quantitative analysis of GSTP-positive lesions of the liver at the end of the study are also summarized in Table 1. A CDAA diet for 15 weeks was associated with the development of a large number of GSTP-positive lesions. The concomitant administration of HOE 077 significantly reduced such lesions in a dose-dependent manner, in parallel with the reduced hydroxyproline content.

The administration of a CDAA diet for 52 weeks resulted in hepatocellular carcinomas in 90% of rats (Table 2; Fig. 5). HOE 077 at 200 p.p.m. reduced the incidence of liver neoplasms to 50% even without a significant difference.

## Discussion

Using the rat liver fibrosis induced by a CDAA diet, the effects of a prolyl 4-hydroxylase inhibitor (HOE 077) on the development of preneoplastic lesions and liver neoplasms were investigated.

HOE 077 is designed as a prodrug. In its original state, it is not an effective inhibitor of prolyl 4-hydroxylase, but it is able to cross biological membranes. It is well absorbed from the gastrointestinal tract and is taken up by the liver, where it is converted to active metabolites which are competitive inhibitors of prolyl 4-hydroxylase within the hepatocytes [9]. In primary human and rat hepatocytes, HOE 077 was also effective in preventing the hydroxylation of proline in a dose-dependent manner [10]. The inhibition of prolyl 4-hydroxylase results in the formation of underhydroxylated collagen species that are not able to form the stable triple helix of procollagen molecules. These are then rapidly degraded.

Stellate cells are now considered to be the main collagen-producing cells under nonphysiological conditions [11] as well as in our experimental model [12]. As already mentioned, this prolyl 4-hydroxylase inhibitor is a hydrophobic prodrug which can be converted to active hydrophilic metabolites only within hepatocytes, and the effect of fibrosuppression was proved to be liver-specific [13].

Our results indicate that HOE 077 reduced the liver hydroxyproline content in rats fed a CDAA diet in a dose-dependent manner up to a dose of 200 p.p.m. A CDAA diet alone dramatically increased the hydroxyproline content of the liver by a factor of more than five compared with a CSAA diet. The administration of 200 p.p.m. HOE 077 was found to result in almost 30% inhibition of this hydroxyproline accumulation without reducing the increased serum ALT level (Table 1). Thus, the inhibition of fibrosis by HOE 077 cannot be attributed to any direct action of preventing liver cell death.

Histologically, a reduced number of pseudolobuli and the incomplete formation of pseudolobuli were found, as well as thinner fibrous septa, in accordance with the reduced hydroxyproline content of the liver. These results indicate that this prolyl 4-hydroxylase inhibitor effectively retarded the development of liver cirrhosis in rats fed a CDAA diet.

However, the mechanism of prevention of liver fibrosis seems to be different from what was expected from the character of this drug as a prolyl 4-hydroxylase inhibitor.

A paper published in 1986 [14] suggested the mechanism of fibrosuppression by HOE 077, and reported that the COOH or $NH_2$ terminal propeptides of collagen inhibit the synthesis of collagen in culture or in a cell-free system. These findings agree with ours in these interpretation of post-transcriptional down-regulation. Our results indicate that prolyl 4-hydroxylase inhibitor can prevent fibrosis by inhibiting not only the hydroxylation of proline, but also expression of the mRNA of procollagen, presumably by inhibiting the activation of stellate cells.

The sequence of cellular changes in the liver proceeds from hepatocytes to enzyme-altered foci and then to hepatocellular neoplasms [15]. Thus, the induction of enzyme-altered foci or nodules can serve as an indicator of preneoplastic change. GSTP-positive lesions, in particular, have been used as a marker for preneoplastic lesions [16], and the extent of GSTP-positive lesions was in parallel with the generation of 8OHdG formation in DNAs, which has been construed to be the major molecular lesion stemming from the same model of choline-deficient L-amino acid-defined diet [17].

At 15 weeks with a CDAA diet alone, GSTP-positive lesions mainly consisted of nodules surrounded by fibrous septa, resulting in the formation of pseudolobuli (Fig.

4). HOE 077 reduced, in a dose-dependent manner, the percent age area of GSTP-positive lesions. The inhibition of the formation of GSTP-positive lesions by this antifibrous agent is in parallel with the reduction in the hydroxyproline content of the liver. The liver hydroxyproline content reflects the amount of collagen fibers making up the fibrous septa [18]. Therefore, the inhibition of GSTP-positive lesions by HOE 077 can be presumed to be attributable to the prevention of pseudolobule formation by fibrous septa.

Our long-term experiment indicates that fibrosuppresion may prevent the development of liver neoplasms. However, as the mechanism of cancer prevention by fibrosuppression is still obscure, further research are necessary.

The inhibition of carcinogenesis by HOE 077 could be attributed, for example, to the prevention of hypomethylated DNA [19]. However, this prevention of hypomethylated DNA could also be attributed to inhibition of fibrosis, because the fibrosis (liver cirrhosis) may interfere with the methyl delivery through the blood flow. Thus, the emphasis in the present study was on finding at least some correlation between fibrosis and preneoplastic lesions or liver neoplasms.

To date, clinically useful chemoprevention has not been found. Therefore, the prevention of fibrosis will be a new approach to the prevention of liver neoplasms.

## References

1. Williams GM, Tanaka, T, Maruyama H, et al. (1982) Modulation by butylated hydroxytoluene of liver and bladder carcinogenesis induced by chronic low level exposure to 2-acetylaminofluorene. Cancer Res 51:6224–6230
2. Williams GM, Tanaka T, Maeura Y (1986) Dose-dependent inhibition of aflatoxin B1 induced hepatocarcinogenesis by the phenolic antioxidants, butylated hydroxyanisole and butylated hydroxytoluene. Carcinogenesis 7:1043–1050
3. Hill DL, Grubbs CJ (1992) Retinoids and cancer prevention. Annu Rev Nutr 12:161–181
4. Sakaida I, Matsumura Y, Kubota M, et al. (1996) The prolyl 4-hydroxylase inhibitor (HOE 077) prevents activation of Ito cells, reducing procollagen gene expression in rat liver fibrosis induced by choline-deficient L-amino acid-defined diet. Hepatology 23:755–763
5. Sakaida I, Kubota M, Kayano K, et al. (1994) Prevention of fibrosis reduces enzyme-altered lesions in the rat liver. Carcinogenesis 15:2201–2206
6. Sakaida I, Matsumura Y, Akiyama S, et al. Herbal medicine Sho-saiko-to (TJ-9) prevents liver fibrosis and enzyme-altered lesions in rat liver cirrhosis induced by a choline-deficient L-amino acid-defined diet. J Hepatol 28:298–306
7. Sakaida I, Uchida K, Matsumura Y, et al. Interferon gamma treatment prevents procollagen gene expression without affecting TGF-$\beta$1 expression in pig serum-induced rat liver fibrosis. J Hepatol 28:471–479
8. Matsumura Y, Sakaida I, Uchida K, et al. (1997) Prolyl 4-hydroxylase inhibitor (HOE 077) inhibits pig serum-induced rat liver fibrosis by preventing stellate cell activation. J Hepatol 27:185–192
9. Hanauske-Abel HM (1991) Prolyl 4-hydroxylase, a target enzyme for drug developement: Design of suppressive agents and the in vitro effects of inhibitors and proinhibitors. J Hepatol 13(Suppl. 3):S8–S16
10. Clement B, Chesne C, Satie AP, et al. (1991) Effects of the prolyl 4-hydroxylase proinhibitor HOE 077 on human and rat hepatocytes in primary culture. J Hepatol 13(Suppl. 3):S41–S47
11. Friedman SL (1993) The cellular basis of hepatic fibrosis. N Engl J Med 328:1828–1835

12. Sakaida I (1996) Hepatic fibrogenesis and carcinogenesis. Bull Yamaguchi Med Sch 43:45–48
13. Bickel M, Baader E, Brocks DG, et al. (1991) Beneficial effects of inhibitors of prolyl 4-hydroxylase in CCl₄-induced fibrosis of the liver in rats. J Hepatol 13:(Suppl. 3) S26–S34
14. Wu CH, Donovan CB, Wu GY (1986) Evidence for pretranslational regulation of collagen synthesis by procollagen propepides. J Biol Chem 261:10482–10484
15. Kitahara A, Satoh K, Nishimura K, et al. (1984) Changes in molecular forms of rat hepatic glutathione S-transferase during chemical hepatocarcinogenesis. Cancer Res 44:2698–2703
16. Satoh K, Kitahara A, Soma Y, et al. (1985) Purification, induction and distribution of placental glutathione transferase: A new marker enzyme for preneoplastic cells in the rat chemical hepatocarcinogenesis. Proc Natl Acad Sci USA 82:3964–3968
17. Yoshiji H, Nakae D, Mizumoto Y, et al. (1992) Inhibitory effect of dietary iron deficiency on inductions of putative preneoplastic lesions as well as 8-hydroxydeoxyguanosine in DNA and lipid peroxidation in the livers of rats caused by exposure to a choline-deficient L-amino acid defined diet. Carcinogenesis 13:1227–1233
18. Nakano M (1986) Morphogenesis of septa in hepatic fibrosis induced by choline deficiency in rats. Acta Pathol Jpn 36:1643–1652
19. Wainfan E, Dizik M, Stender M, et al. (1989) Rapid appearance of hypomethylated DNA in livers of rats fed cancer-promoting, methyl-deficient diets. Cancer Res 49:4094–4097

# VEGF Participates in Neovascularization and Sinusoidal Capillarization in HCC

Takuji Torimura[1], Takato Ueno[1], Motoaki Kin[1], Riko Ogata[1], Michio Sata[1], and Kyuichi Tanikawa[2]

*Summary.* Early in hepatocarcinogenesis, hepatocellular carcinomas do not show hypervascularity, but at later stages they require abundant arterial blood supply. Vascular endothelial growth factor is one of the most direct-acting angiogenic factors. We have clarified the participation of vascular endothelial growth factor in the development of neovascularization and sinusoidal capillarization in hepatocellular carcinoma.

Vascular endothelial growth factor expression was detected in hepatoma cells and hepatic stellate cells by immunoelectron microscopy and in situ hybridization. The major vascular endothelial growth factor isoforms expressed in hepatocellular carcinoma were vascular endothelial growth factors 121 and 165. The expression of flt-1 and KDR/flk-1, both receptors for vascular endothelial growth factor, in hepatocellular carcinoma was also confirmed by RT-PCR. In hepatocellular carcinomas with hypervascularity, type IV collagen and laminin were present corresponding to basement membranes along the sinusoidal endothelial cells, which had few fenestrae. In hepatocellular carcinomas without hypervascularity, although type IV collagen was present along the sinusoidal endothelial cells that had a few fenestrae, laminin as well as basement membranes were rarely detected. Vascular endothelial growth factor expression in hepatocellular carcinomas with hypervascularity was stronger than in those not showing hypervascularity. In in vitro study, increased expression of vascular endothelial growth factor mRNA in hepatoma cells was observed under hypoxic conditions. These results suggest that vascular endothelial growth factor participates in the development of neovascularization and sinusoidal capillarization in hepatocellular carcinoma.

*Key words.* Hepatocellular carcinoma, Neovascularization, Sinusoidal capillarization, Vascular endothelial growth factor, Hypoxia

[1] The Second Department of Internal Medicine and Research Center for Innovative Cancer Therapy, Kurume University School of Medicine, 67 Asahi-machi, Kurume, Fukuoka 830-0011, Japan
[2] International Institute for Liver Research, 2432-3 Aikawa-machi, Kurume, Fukuoka 830-0011, Japan

# Introduction

In malignant neoplasms, angiogenesis is required for tumor growth and progression [1]. Angiogenesis is associated with necrotic hypoxic foci in tumors [2]. Recent data support the concept that hypoxia can alter the expression of genes encoding vascular cell growth and angiogenic factors [3]. Among several angiogenic factors, vascular endothelial growth factor (VEGF) is one of the main endothelial cell growth factors [4]. VEGF specifically stimulates the proliferation of endothelial cells through specific tyrosine kinase receptors flt-1 and KDR/flk-1 [5]. VEGF is a Mr.34 000–42 000 disulfide-bonded dimeric glycoprotein, expressed as four different isoforms due to alternative mRNA splicing [6]. The isoforms, VEGF121, VEGF165, VEGF189, and VEGF206 are composed of monomers containing 121, 165, 189, and 206 amino acids, respectively [6, 7]. VEGF121 and VEGF165 are secreted, while VEGF189 and VEGF206 are associated with heparin-bound proteoglycans in the extracellular matrix [7].

Hepatocellular carcinoma (HCC) is one of the most common malignant tumors in the tropics and the Far East, including Japan [8]. HCC develops multifocally in livers affected by chronic injury [9].

Although the portal blood supply to HCC is predominant in the early stage of hepatocarcinogenesis, the arterial blood supply increases with tumor enlargement. Arterialization in HCC is generally accompanied by hypervascularity. Hypervascularity is usually present in HCCs over 2 cm in diameter [10].

We have clarified the participation of VEGF in the arterialization and sinusoidal capillarization in HCC.

# Sinusoidal Capillarization in HCC

It has been reported that early in hepatocarcinogenesis, HCC does not usually have an abundant vasculature, showing hypo- or isovascularity on hepatic angiography [11].

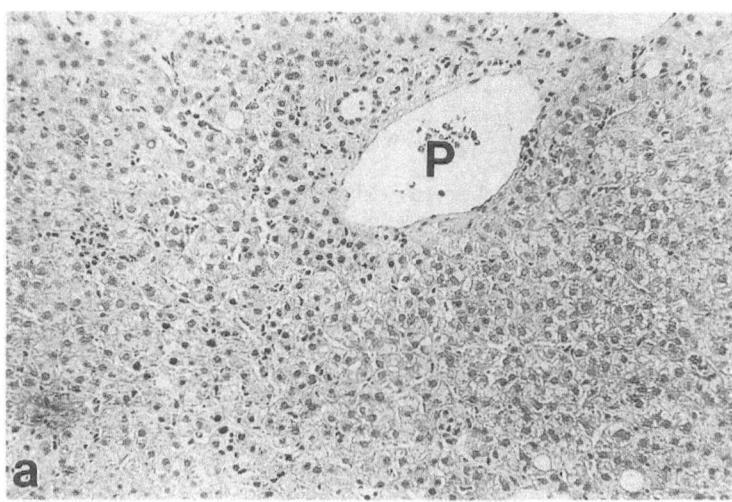

FIG. 1a–c. Light and electron microscopic analysis of portal vein and neoartery in HCC. **a** A portal vein in a well-differentiated small HCC without hypervascularity (<10 mm in diameter)

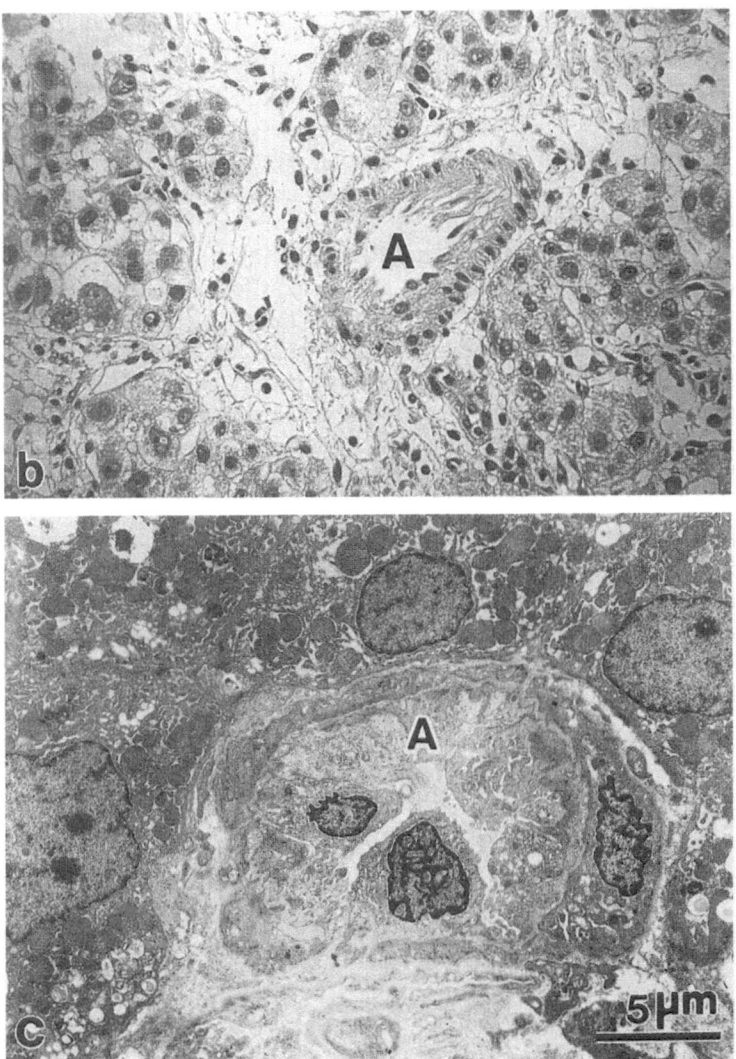

FIG. 1a–c. *Continued.* A neoartery observed by **b** light microscopy and **c** electron microscopy in moderately differentiated HCC with hypervascularity *P*, protal vein; *A*, artery (oringinal magnification: **a** ×320; **b** ×640)

At this stage, the portal blood supply to HCC is predominant (Fig. 1a) [12]. In HCC without hypervascularity, type IV collagen, a component of basement membranes, was detected continuously along the sinusoids, while laminin was rarely detected (Fig. 2a,b). Basement membranes were insufficiently developed, and a few fenestrae were observed in the sinusoidal endothelial cells in such cases of HCC (Fig. 3a).

With tumor enlargement, reduced portal blood flow and increased arterial blood

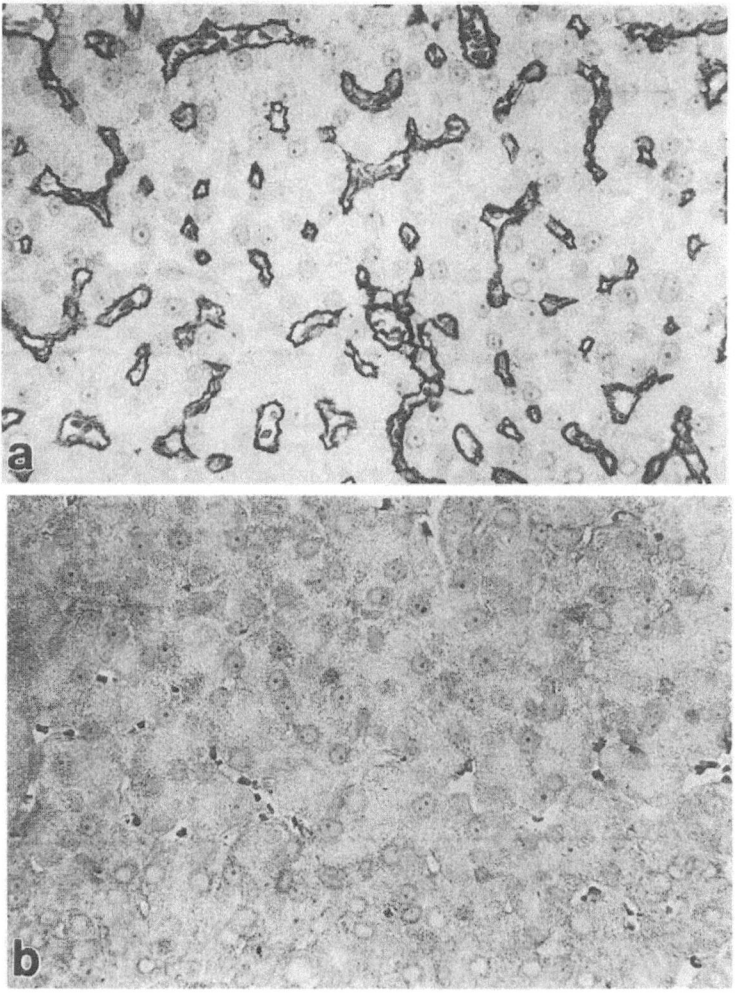

FIG. 2a–d. Immunohistochemical analysis of type IV collagen and laminin in HCC. **a** Immunoreactive products of anti-type IV collagen antibody detected along the sinusoid of well-differentiated small HCC without hypervascularity (<10 mm in diameter). **b** Immunoreactive products of anti-laminin antibody are not detected. Immunoreactive products of **c** anti-type IV collagen and **d** anti-laminin antibodies observed along the sinusoid of well-differentiated HCC with hypervascularity (original magnification: **a–d** ×640)

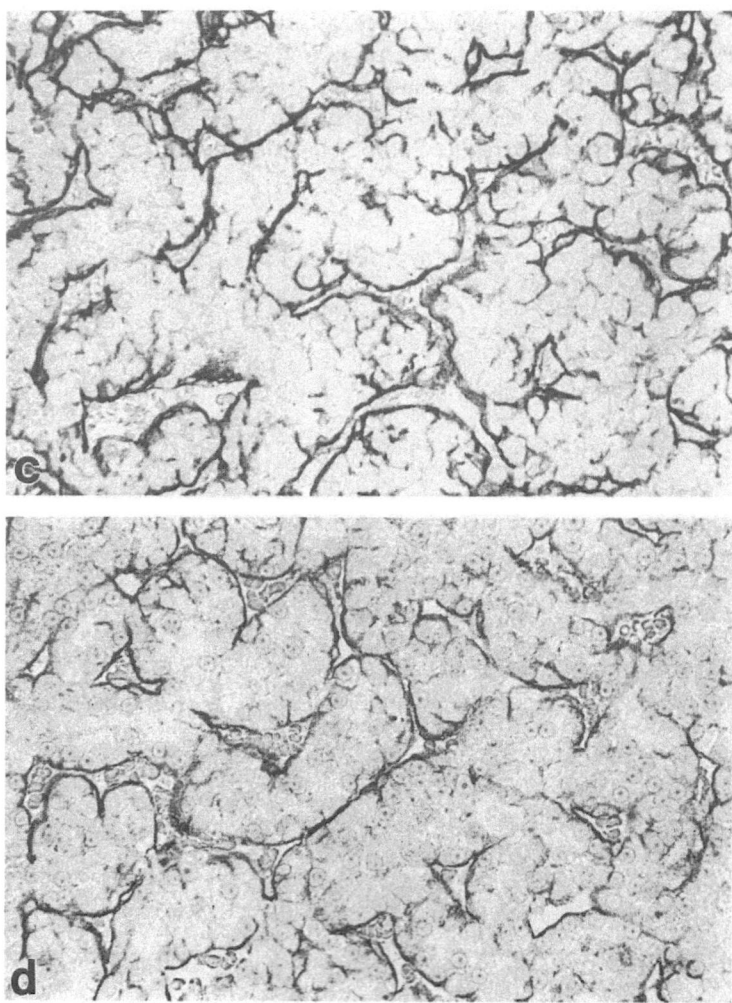

FIG. 2a–d. *Continued*

supply are observed in HCC [13]. In HCC more than 20 mm in diameter, arterialization (Fig. 1b,c) and hypervascularity are usually observed [10, 14]. In HCC with hypervascularity, type IV collagen and laminin were detected along the sinusoids (Fig. 2c,d). Basement membranes were observed on the basal sides of the sinusoidal endothelial cells, which had few fenestrae (Fig. 3b).

In small HCC, in which the arterial blood supply is not yet fully developed, the sinusoidal endothelial cells still do not have the morphology of capillaries. However, as the arterial blood supply increases, the internal pressure of the sinusoid seems to increase. The basement membrane formation and defenestration of sinusoidal endothelial cells appear to occur in order to preserve the sinusoidal structure from its own elevated internal pressure [15]. The development of arterialization seems to be a trigger for sinusoidal capillarization in HCC (Table 1).

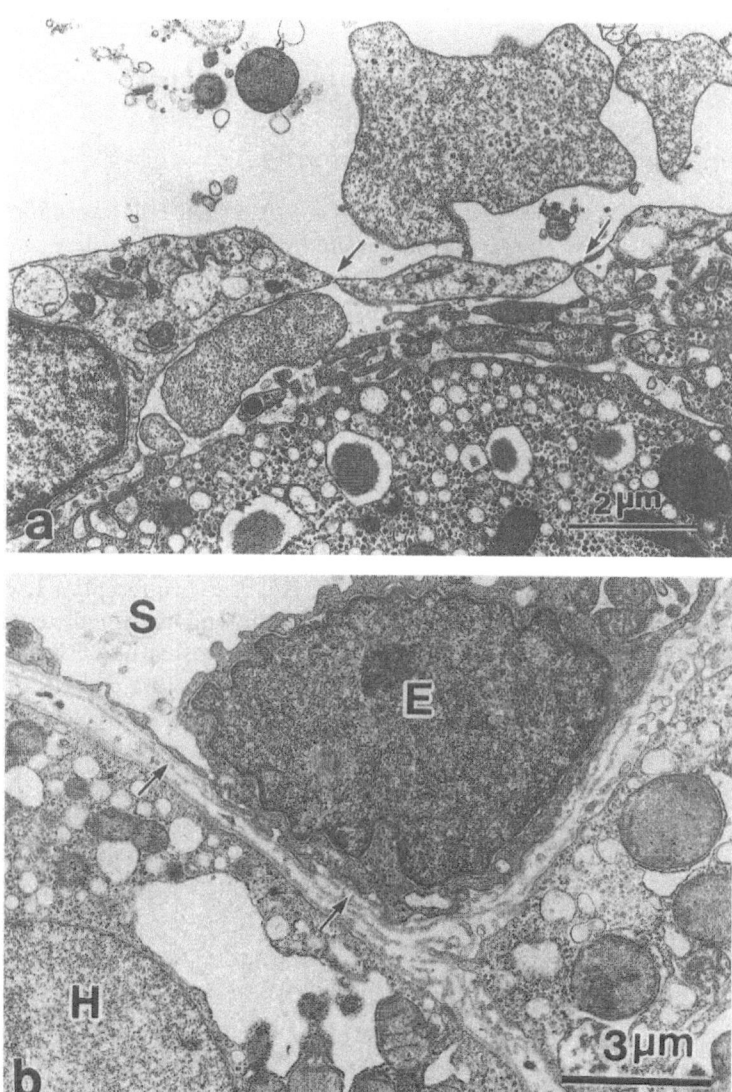

FIG. 3a,b. Electron microscopic analysis of HCC. **a** In HCC without hypervascularity, basement membranes are rarely detected. Sinusoidal endothelial cells have a few fenestrae (*arrows*). **b** In HCC with hypervascularity, basement membranes are clearly detected in the subendothelial space of a sinusoid (*arrows*). Sinusoidal endothelial cells have few fenestrae *S*, sinusoid; *E*, endothelial cell; *H*, hepatoma cell

TABLE 1. Semiquantitative analysis of laminin localization in HCC

|  |  | Laminin ($-$) | Laminin ($\pm$) | Laminin ($+$) |
|---|---|---|---|---|
| Hypervascularity | $-$ | 9/15 | 3/15 | 3/15 |
|  | $+$ | 2/25 | 3/25 | 20/25 |

# Expression of VEGF and its Receptors in HCC

## VEGF-Producing Cells and their Isoforms

The production of VEGF by hepatoma cells and hepatic stellate cells was confirmed by immunoelectron microscopy (Fig. 4) and in situ hybridization (Fig. 5).

Due to alternative mRNA splicing, VEGF consists of four different isoforms: two are diffusible (VEGF121, VEGF165), and two (VEGF189, VEGF206) are mostly bound to the extracellular matrix [6, 7]. By PCR analysis, VEGF121 and VEGF165 mRNA were found to be strongly expressed in HCC (Fig. 6). It seems that in HCC, hepatoma cells and hepatic stellate cells mainly produce diffusible VEGF.

## Expression of VEGF Receptors

Two receptors, flt-1 and KDR/flk-1, have been identified almost specifically in human endothelial cells that bind VEGF and mediate the proliferation of endothelial cells involved in the formation of new blood vessels [16]. The two receptors have been shown to be expressed preferentially in the proliferating endothelium of vessels [17]. A prerequisite for tumor angiogenesis, besides the expression of VEGF by tumor and stromal cells, is the expression of the VEGF receptors flt-1 and KDR/flk-1 in endothelial cells. By PCR analysis, flt-1 and KDR/flk-1 mRNAs were found to be expressed in HCC (Fig. 7). Thus, the VEGF–VEGF receptor system seems to participate in the angiogenesis of HCC.

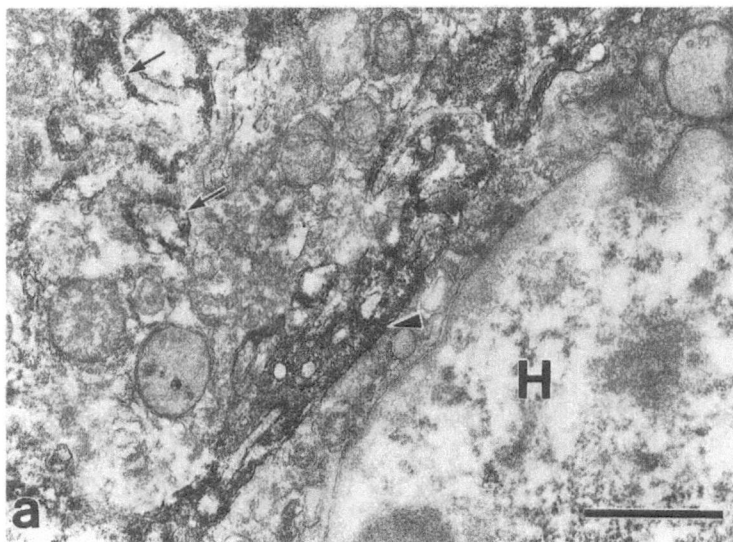

Fig. 4a,b. Immunoelectron microscopic analysis of VEGF in HCC. a Immunoreactive products of anti-VEGF antibody are detected in the cisternae of the rough endoplasmic reticula of a hepatoma cell (*arrows*) and in the intercellular spaces between hepatoma cells (*arrow head*) (bar, 1 μm)

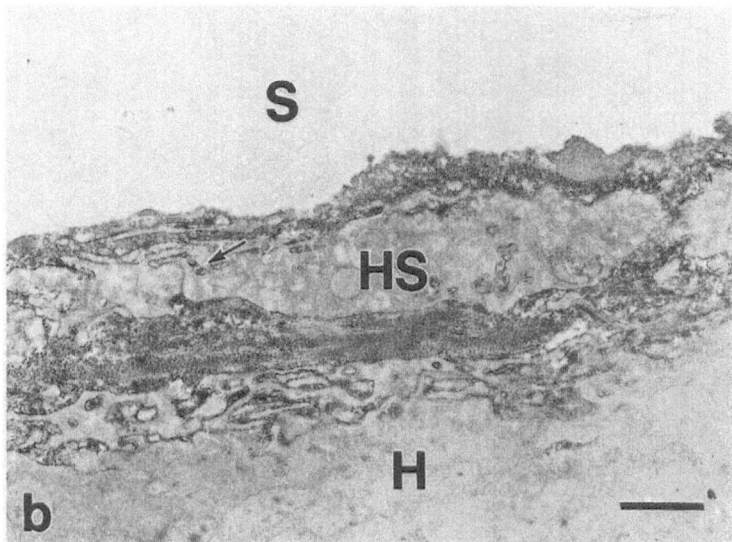

FIG. 4a,b. *Continued.* b These products are also detected in the cisternae of the rough endoplasmic reticula of a hepatic stellate cell (*arrow*) and the subendothelial space. *H*, hepatoma cell; *HS*, hepatic stellate cell; *S*, sinusoid

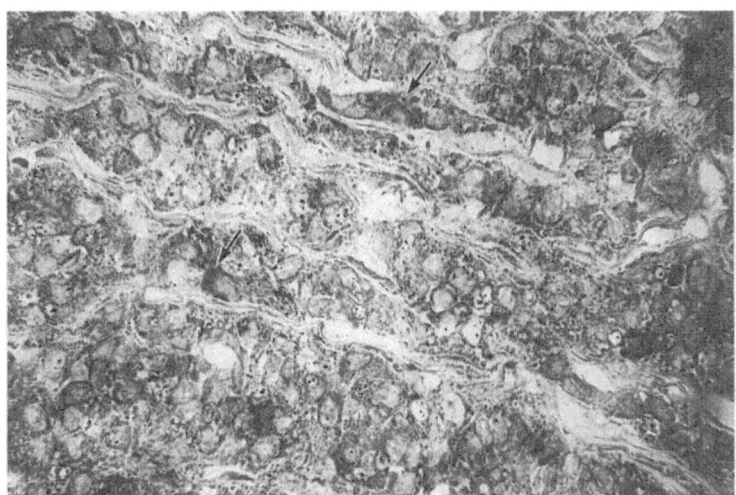

FIG. 5. Expression of VEGF mRNA in HCC. In moderately differentiated HCC, VEGF mRNA is strongly expressed in hepatoma cells (*arrows*) (original magnification: ×640)

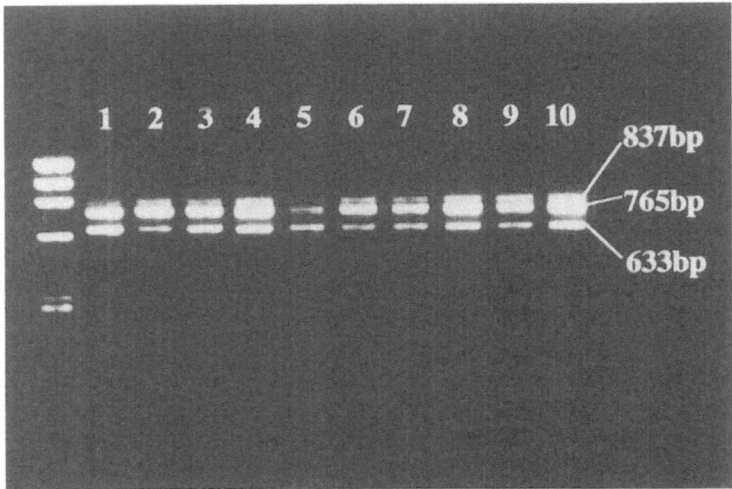

FIG. 6. Expression of VEGF isoform mRNAs in HCC by RT-PCR (reverse transcriptase-polymerase chain reaction. Ethidium-stained agarose gel shows representative products amplified from cDNA derived from HCC tissues (lanes 1–10). The calculated molecular weights of product bands are indicated. The sizes predicted for VEGF189, VEGF165, and VEGF121 are 837, 765, and 633 bp, respectively

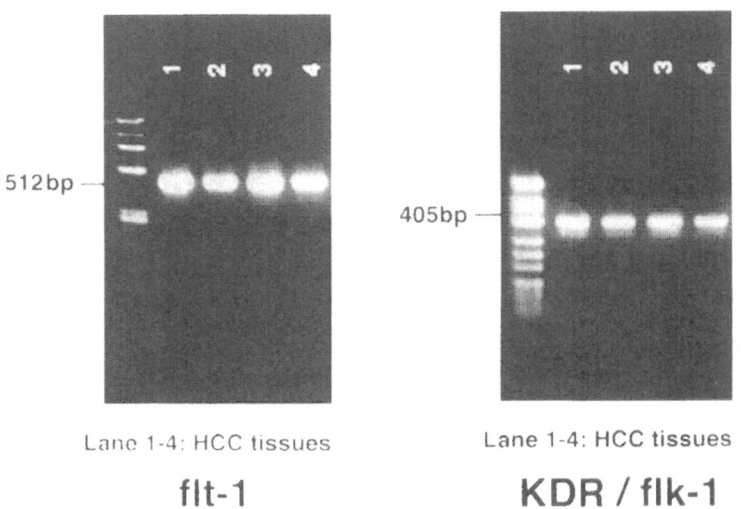

FIG 7. Expression of VEGF receptor mRNAs in HCC by RT-PCR. Ethidium-stained agarose gel shows representative products amplified from cDNA derived from HCC tissues (lanes 1–4). The calculated molecular weights of product bands are indicated. The sizes predicted for flt-1 and KDR/flk-1 are 512 and 405 bp, respectively

## Relationship Between VEGF Production and Tumor Differentiation

Most HCCs less than 10 mm in diameter consist solely of well-differentiated cancerous tissue. In larger HCCs, moderately or poorly differentiated HCC tissue is usually surrounded by well-differentiated HCC tissue. Furthermore, most advanced HCCs consist only of moderately to poorly differentiated HCC tissue [18]. HCC seems to originate as a well-differentiated tumor, becoming progressively less differentiated with enlargement.

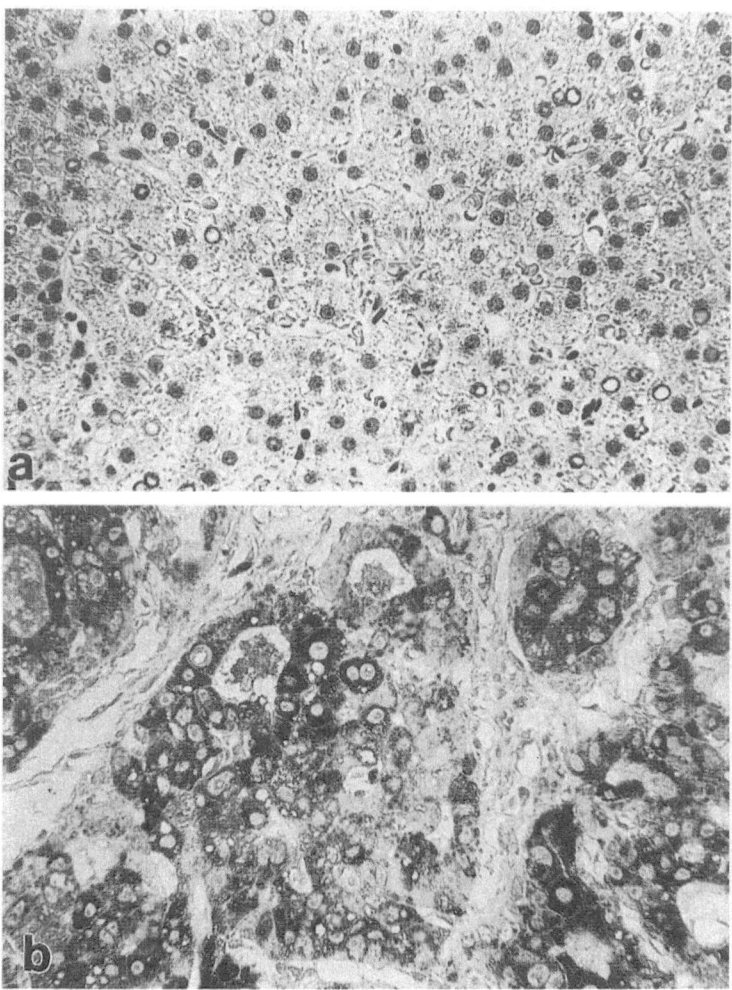

FIG. 8a,b. Immunohistochemical analysis of VEGF in HCC. a Immunoreactive products of anti-VEGF antibody are not detected in well-differentiated HCC, <10 mm in diameter. b Immunoreactive products of anti-VEGF antibody are strongly detected in hepatoma cells of moderately differentiated HCC (original magnification: a, b ×640)

TABLE 2. Immunostaining of VEGF in HCC

|  |  | Well diff. HCC (<10 mm) (n = 14) | Well diff. HCC (>10 mm) (n = 12) | Moderately diff. HCC (n = 12) | Poorly diff. HCC (n = 13) |
|---|---|---|---|---|---|
| VEGF | − | 13 | 4 | 1 | 2 |
|  | ± | 1 | 5 | 4 | 1 |
|  | + | 0 | 3 | 7 | 10 |

VEGF, vascular endothelial growth factor; diff., differentiated.
Degree of staining: +, positive staining; ± patchy staining; −, negative staining.
Immunostaining of VEGF was associated with tumor differentiation.
$P < 0.001$, Kruskal–Wallis test.

By immunohistochemistry, VEGF production was found to be lowest in well-differentiated small HCCs (tumors less than 10 mm in diameter) (Fig. 8a), followed by well-differentiated HCCs (tumors more than 10 mm in diameter), moderately differentiated HCCs (Fig. 8b), and poorly differentiated HCCs. VEGF production seems to increase with tumor dedifferentiation according to enlargement (Table 2).

## Relationship Between VEGF Production and Angiographic Findings

Early in hepatocarcinogenesis, HCCs do not usually have abundant vasculature, and show hypo- or isovascularity on hepatic angiography [11]. With tumor enlargement, increased arterial blood flow is observed [13]. In HCCs more than 20 mm in diameter, hypervascularity is usually detected [10, 14] (Table 3).

In small HCCs which do not show hypervascularity on hepatic angiography, little VEGF is produced. In contrast, in HCCs showing hypervascularity, abundant VEGF production is detected. VEGF seems to play a significant role in the development of arterialization and hypervascularity in HCC.

TABLE 3. Correlation between immunostaining of VEGF and tumor vascularity

|  |  | VEGF (−) | VEGF (±) | VEGF (+) |
|---|---|---|---|---|
| Hypervascularity | − (n = 22) | 16 | 6 | 0 |
|  | + (n = 29) | 4 | 5 | 20 |

VEGF, vascular endothelial growth factor.
Hypervascularity: (+), HCC showing hypervascularity by hepatic angiography; (−), HCC not showing hypervascularity.
Degree of staining: +, positive staining; ±, patchy staining; −, negative staining.
Immunostaining of VEGF was associated with tumor vascularity.
$P < 0.001$, Kruskal–Wallis test.

## Increased Expression of VEGF mRNA under the Condition of Hypoxia

In in vitro and in vivo studies, it has been proven that hypoxia is one of the most potent inducers of VEGF production [19]. In hepatoma cells, the mRNA levels of VEGF121 and VEGF165 increased significantly under hypoxic conditions (Fig. 9).

Recently, elevated levels of VEGF mRNA were found in tumor cells in the area adjacent to necrotic regions in HCC [20].

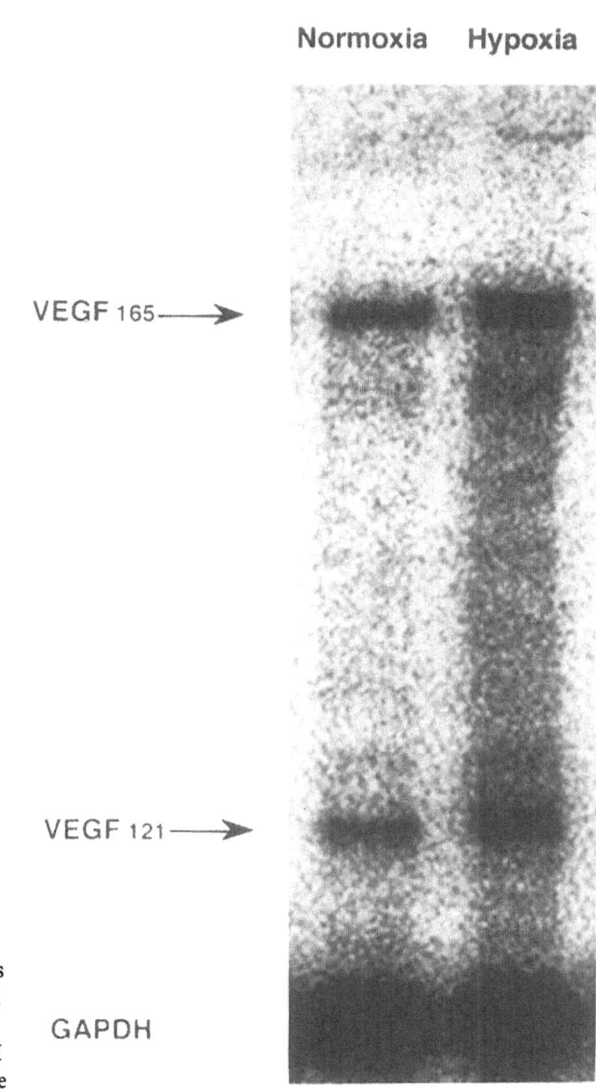

FIG. 9. Expression of VEGF mRNA in hepatoma cells (Huh-7) under hypoxic and normoxic conditions Up-regulation of VEGF121 and VEGF165 mRNAs under hypoxic conditions for 24h is observed in comparison with those under normoxic conditions. Levels of GAPDH mRNA are shown to compare RNA loading in two lanes

The rapid proliferation of hepatoma cells causes the comparative decrease of vessels in HCC. The hypoxic condition induced by the comparative decrease of vessels seems to be an inducer of VEGF production by hepatoma cells and hepatic stellate cells in HCC.

# Conclusions

We investigated the participation of VEGF in the development of neovascularization and sinusoidal capillarization in HCC.

Hepatoma cells and hepatic stellate cells produced mainly VEGF121 and VEGF165. The expression of flt-1 and KDR/flk-1 in HCC was also confirmed. In HCCs without hypervascularity, little VEGF production was detected. In those HCCs, sinusoidal capillarization was rarely observed. In contrast, in HCCs with hypervascularity, intense VEGF production was detected. Furthermore, sinusoidal capillarization was also observed in HCCs with hypervascularity. These findings indicate that VEGF plays an important role in neovascularization and sinusoidal capillarization in HCC.

## References

1. Folkman J (1990) What is the evidence that tumors are angiogenesis-dependent? Natl Cancer Inst 84:4–6
2. Senger DR, Van De Water L, Brown LF, et al. (1993) Vascular permeability factor (VPF, VEGF) in tumor biology. Cancer Metastasis Rev 12:303–324
3. Kourembanas S, McQuillan LP, Leung GK, et al. (1993) Nitric oxide regulates the expression of vasoconstrictors and growth factors by vascular endothelium under both normoxia and hypoxia. J Clin Invest 92:99–104
4. Leung DW, Cachianes G, Kuang W-J, et al. (1989) Vascular endothelial growth factor is a secreted angiogenic mitogen. Science (Washington, DC) 246:1306–1309
5. Walternberger J, Claesson-Welsh L, Seigbahn A, et al. (1994) Different signal transduction properties of KDR and flt-1, two receptors for vascular endothelial growth factor. J Biol Chem 269:26988–26995
6. Thischer E, Mitchell R, Hartman T, et al. (1991) The human gene for vascular endothelial growth factor. Multiple protein forms are encoded through alternative exon splicing. J Biol Chem 266:11947–11954
7. Park JE, Keller G-A, Ferrara N (1993) The vascular endothelial growth factor (VEGF) isoforms: Differential deposition into the subepithelial extracellular matrix and bioactivity of extracellular matrix-bound VEGF. Mol Biol Cell 4:1317–1326
8. Biscegli Am, Rustgo VK, Hoofnagle JM, et al. (1988) Hepatocellular carcinoma. Ann Intern Med 108:390–401
9. Oda T, Tsuda H, Scarpa A, et al. (1992) Mutation pattern of the p53 gene as a diagnostic marker for multiple hepatocellular carcinoma. Cancer Res 12:3674–3678
10. Bhattacharya S, Davidson B, Dhillon AP (1995) Blood supply of early hepatocellular carcinoma. Seminars Liver Dis 15:390–401
11. Kudo M, Tomita S, Kashida H, et al. (1991) Tumor hemodynamics in hepatic nodules associated with liver cirrhosis: Relationship between cancer progression and tumor hemodynamics change. Jpn J Gastroenterol 88:1554–1565
12. Tanaka S, Kitamura T, Fujita M, et al. (1992) Small hepatocellular carcinoma: Differentiation from adenomatous hyperplastic nodule with color Doppler flow imaging. Radiology 182:161–165

13. Mastui O, Kadoy M, Kameyama T, et al. (1991) Benign and malignant nodules in cirrhotic liver: Distinction based on blood supply. Radiology 178:493–497
14. Kondo F, Wada K, Nagato Y, et al. (1989) Biopsy diagnosis of well-differentiated hepatocellular carcinoma based on new morphologic criteria. Hepatology 9:751–755
15. Martinea-Hernandez A, Amenta PS (1983) The basement membrane in pathology. Lab Invest 48:656–677
16. Terman BI, Carrion ME, Kovacs E, et al. (1991) Identification of a new endothelial cell growth factor receptor tyrosine kinases. Oncogene 6:1677–1683
17. Hatva E, Kaipainen A, Mentule P, et al. (1995) Expression of endothelial cell-specific receptor tyrosine kinases and growth factors in human brain tumors. Am J Pathol 146:368–378
18. Kenmochi K, Sugihara S, Kojiro M (1987) Relationship of histologic grade of heaptocellualr carcinoma (HCC) to tumor size, and demonstration of tumor cells of multiple different grades in single small HCC. Liver 7:18–26
19. Shweiki D, Ifin A, Soffer D, et al. (1992) Vascular endothelial growth factor induced by hypoxia may mediate hypoxia-initiated angiogenesis. Nature 359:843–845
20. Suzaki K, Hayashi N, Niyamoto Y, et al. (1996) Expression of vascular permeability factor/vascular endothelial growth factor in human hepatocellular carcinoma. Cancer Res 56:3004–3009

# Natural Killer Cells in the Liver and Their Activators

Masatoshi Tanaka, Miki Shirachi, Masahiro Shimada, Yoshihiro Shimauchi, Ryoko Kuromatsu, Michio Sata, and Kyuichi Tanikawa

*Summary.* An impaired host defense mechanism is well known in patients with liver cirrhosis. To clarify the sight of natural resistance in the liver, we investigated hepatic natural killer (NK) activity, and a proportion of the NK cells in the hepatic sinusoids of normal and cirrhotic rats. Using a sinusoidal lavage method, liver-associated lymphocytes were obtained from normal and cirrhotic rats that were established using thioacetamide. NK activity was measured by $^{51}$Cr-release assay, and the NK cell count was measured by flow cytometric analysis using monoclonal antibodies. In addition, OK432 (a pharmaceutical preparation of $\alpha$-*Streptococcus pyrogens*), Sho-saiko-to (a Chinese herbal medicine), and interferon-$\alpha$ were administered to experimental rats and the subsequent changes in hepatic NK activity and the NK cell count were also observed. Not only hepatic NK activity, but also the proportion of hepatic NK cells were significantly lower in cirrhotic rats than in control rats. Hepatic NK activity and NK cell count in the liver increased significantly after the administration of NK cell activators such as OK432 and Sho-saiko-to. After the administration of interferon-$\alpha$, there was also as increase in the previously reduced hepatic NK activity and NK cell count of cirrhotic rats. The results of this study may lead to a clearer understanding of the host defense mechanism in cirrhotic patients.

*Key words.* Hepatic NK activity, NK cell, OK432, Sho-saiko-to, IFN-$\alpha$

## Introduction

Liver-associated lymphocytes are composed of T lymphocytes, B lymphocytes, and natural killer (NK) cells. NK cells account for about 20% of the lymphocytes in the liver, which is higher than their percentages in other organs [1]. Under light microscopy, hepatic NK cells appear in the form of large granular lymphocytes (LGLs), and under electron microscopy they are seen in their characteristic form as rod-cored vesicles [2] and electron-dense granules in the cytoplasm [3], known as "pit

The Second Department of Internal Medicine, Kurume University School of Medicine, 67 Asahi-machi, Kurume, Fukuoka 830-0011, Japan

cells." They are considered to protect the liver against the infiltration of metastatic tumor cells via the portal vein [4–7], and to eliminate hepatocytes infected by hepatitis viruses [8, 9]. In human studies, it has been reported that hepatic NK cells play an important role in cytotoxicity to autologous hepatocytes in the same manner as cytotoxic T lymphocytes in patients with chronic hepatitis [10, 11].

It is well known that various cytokines and biological response modifiers directly and indirectly activate NK cell activity in the blood and spleen. In this chapter, we describe changes in hepatic NK activity after the administration of OK432 (a type of bacterial pyrogen), Sho-saiko-to (a chinese herbal medicine), and interferon (IFN)-$\alpha$.

## Changes in Hepatic NK Activity after the Administration of OK432

OK432 (Chugai Pharmaceutical, Tokyo, Japan) is a pharmaceutical preparation of $\alpha$-*Streptococcus pyrogens*, and has been used clinically in cancer therapy as a biological response modifier [12]. 0.2 mg (2KE, Klinsche Einheit) of OK432 was injected into each experimental rat intravenously, and liver sinusoidal, blood, and splenic mononuclear cells of the rats were collected and examined [1]. Liver sinusoidal mononuclear cells were collected by the sinusoidal lavage method [13] with minor modifications. Three days after a single injection of OK432 (0.2 mg/rat), the number of cells in the hepatic sinusoids had increased approximately twofold, and the percentage of LGLs had increased 1.5-fold [1] (and the number of LGLs in the hepatic sinusoid had increased threefold). Subsets of liver sinusoidal lymphocytes were also analyzed. As shown in Fig. 1, OX-8-positive lymphocytes [14], which are rat cytotoxic

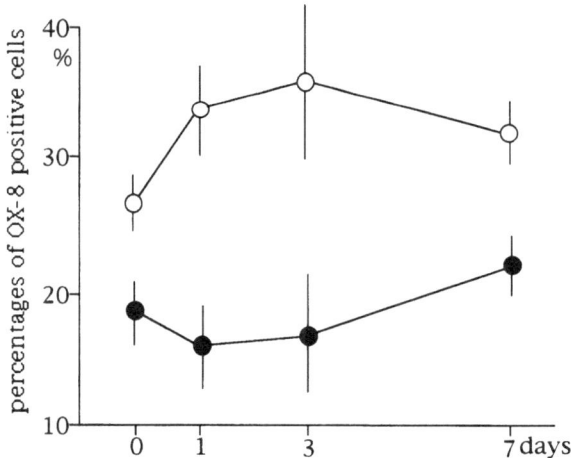

FIG. 1. Kinetics of OX-8-positive cell percentages in hepatic sinusoids and peripheral blood after intravenous injection of OK432 (0.2 mg/rat). The cell ratio was determined by flow cytometry. *Open circles* show the percentages of OX-8-positive cells in hepatic sinusoids, and *closed circles* show those in the peripheral blood. Data are expressed as mean $\pm$ SD of three experiments. (From [1])

TABLE 1. Natural killer activity in liver, peripheral blood, and spleen after administration of OK432 %specific lysis against YAC-1 (from [1] with minor modifications)

| | Sinusoidal lymphocytes (%) (n = 3) | PBL[a] (%) (n = 3) | Splenic lymphocytes (%) (n = 3) |
|---|---|---|---|
| Control | 57.2 ± 1.89 | 9.3 ± 2.61 | 7.4 ± 1.15 |
| 24 h after OK432 iv[b] | 63.9 ± 2.89 | 24.7 ± 0.55* | 20.4 ± 3.65* |
| 72 h after OK432 iv[b] | 69.3 ± 3.56* | 29.1 ± 6.10* | 27.1 ± 12.8* |
| 96 h after OK432 iv[b] | 75.2 ± 2.93** | 37.6 ± 1.05** | 40.4 ± 9.39** |

[a] peripheral blood lymphocytes.
[b] OK432 (0.2 mg/rat) was administered intravenously.
* $P < 0.02$ compared with control; ** $P < 0.005$ compared with control.
%specific lysis was studied by 4-h $^{51}$Cr release assay, and the effector target ratio was 20/1.
Data are expressed as mean ± SD.

T cells and NK cells, had increased in hepatic sinusoids at 1 day and 3 days after OK432 administration, while OX-8-positive cells had decreased in peripheral blood [1]. These data correspond to the increase in the proportion of LGLs in hepatic sinusoids.

NK activity was also analyzed using the results of a 4-h $^{51}$Cr release assay against YAC-1 cells. As shown in Table 1, hepatic NK activity was significantly higher than that in the blood and spleen in control rats. After OK432 administration, NK activity in the liver, blood, and spleen increased significantly, and hepatic NK activity was continuously higher than that in the peripheral blood and spleen [1]. OK432 is a pharmaceutical preparation of α-Streptococcus pyrogens, and activates NK cells directly [15] and indirectly through activated macrophages such as Kupffer cells [16]. We observed that Kupffer cells could digest OK432 directly in vivo and in vitro, and release cytokines such as tumor necrosis factor which could activate NK cells [17]. According to the present study, the NK activity increased serially after a single injection of OK432. This result might explain how activation of NK cell by OK432 in vivo could occur indirectly in the liver. Further investigation is necessary to clarify the mechanism of activation of hepatic NK cells after OK432 administration.

# Changes in Hepatic NK Activity after the Administration of Sho-saiko-to

Sho-saiko-to is a Chinese herbal medicine, and has been used clinically in Japan as an effective drug for chronic viral hepatitis [18]. We examined the effect of oral administration of Sho-saiko-to on hepatic NK activity [19]. Sho-saiko-to (Tsumura Pharmaceutical Co., Tokyo, Japan) was administered (500 mg/Kg/day) through a stomach tube for 5 days under ethylether anesthesia. Saline was given to control rats in the same way. The percentage of OX-8-positive lymphocytes, rat cytotoxic T lymphocytes, and NK cells in the hepatic sinusoids was 40% in control rats, and increased to 56% after the administration of Sho-saiko-to. Cytotoxic T lymphocytes and NK cells increased in cell number in hepatic sinusoids after oral administration of

Sho-saiko-to. Hepatic NK activity in Sho-saiko-to-treated rats was 37%, and was significantly higher than that in control rats (25%). After oral administration of Sho-saiko-to, significant increases were observed in hepatic NK activity and NK cell count in the liver of rats [20].

## Impaired Hepatic NK Activity in Cirrhotic Rats and its Activation by IFN-$\alpha$ Administration

In human studies, a reduction in peripheral blood NK activity in patients with liver cirrhosis (LC) has been reported [20–22]. Establishing a rat cirrhosis model using thiacetamide [23], we measured hepatic NK activity and also investigated NK cell numbers in the liver [24]. In this study, hepatic sinusoidal mononuclear cells isolated using sinusoidal lavage methods were divided into three fractions (low density (Fr.1), medium density (Fr.2), and high density (Fr.3)) on a discontinuous density gradient, as reported [7]. The Fr.1 fraction is rich in NK cells. As shown in Fig. 2, the hepatic NK activity of Fr.1 was significantly reduced in the LC rats (40.0 ± 3.8%) as compared with the control rats (48.4 ± 4.3%) ($P < 0.005$). Likewise, even in Fr.2 the hepatic NK activity of the LC rats was significantly reduced ($P < 0.01$). According to flow-cytometric analysis, there was a significant reduction in the percentage of CD3-8+ NK cells [25] in the LC rats in Fr.1 of the liver (Table 2). However, in all other fractions there was no difference in the percentage of NK cells in the control and LC rats. Using an immunohistochemical staining technique [24], we also observed a significant reduction in the absolute number of hepatic NK cells (MoAb 3.2.3+ NK cells [26]) in LC rats. If there is a reduction in hepatic NK activity in vivo, there are at least two possible explanations: a reduction in the function of individual hepatic NK cells, and/or a reduction in the absolute number of hepatic NK cells. Our results showed that the

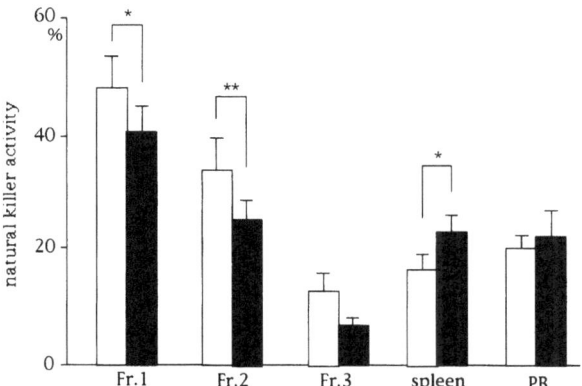

FIG. 2. Natural killer activity of lymphocytes obtained from hepatic sinusoids, spleen, and peripheral blood of control and LC rats. *Open columns* are data from control rats, and *closed columns* are data from LC rats. Fr.1, Fr.2, and Fr.3 are low-, medium-, and high-density lymphocytes, respectively, from hepatic sinusoids. Data are expressed as means ± SE. (From [24] with minor modifications)

TABLE 2. NK cell population in lymphocytes from liver, spleen, and peripheral blood of control and LC rats (from [24] with minor modifications)

| Cell surface marker | | Percentage positive cells | | | | |
|---|---|---|---|---|---|---|
| | | Fr.1[a] | Fr.2[a] | Fr.3[a] | Spleen | PBL[b] |
| 3.2.3+ | Control rats | 85.6 ± 4.9 | 29.9 ± 7.1 | 9.5 ± 3.6 | 15.4 ± 3.1 | 14.3 ± 1.6 |
| | LC rats | 73.1 ± 2.6 | 25.1 ± 2.2 | 5.8 ± 1.1 | 14.1 ± 3.0 | 18.9 ± 2.4 |
| P-value | | NS[c] | NS | NS | NS | NS |
| CD3-CD8+ | Control rats | 76.5 ± 3.8 | 30.3 ± 4.8 | 10.5 ± 2.5 | 10.4 ± 1.7 | 13.2 ± 1.2 |
| | LC rats | 62.7 ± 3.1 | 22.8 ± 1.6 | 8.5 ± 1.1 | 11.0 ± 2.0 | 15.6 ± 1.8 |
| P-value | | <0.05 | NS | NS | NS | NS |

[a] Fr.1, Fr.2, and Fr.3 are low-, medium-, and high-density lymphosites, respectively, from the liver.
[b] Peripheral blood lymphocytes.
[c] Not significant.
Data are expressed as mean ± SE.

hepatic NK activity of Fr.1 (NK-cell-rich fraction) of LC rats was significantly lower than that of control rats, and that the proportion of hepatic NK cells, as determined by flow-cytometric analysis (CD3-8+ NK cells for Fr.1), and the number of hepatic NK cells (MoAb 3.2.3+ NK cells) decreased in LC rats. Thus, both factors (a reduction in the individual function and the number of hepatic NK cells) may be involved in the reduction of hepatic NK activity in vivo. It has been reported previously that Kupffer cells play an important role in the differentiation and maturation process of NK cells [27], and that a reduction in the number and function of Kupffer cells had been observed in LC [28, 29]. When LC occurs, the reduction in the number of fenestra in endothelial cells in the liver sinusoids makes it impossible for Kupffer cells and NK cells to accumulate in the liver sinusoids, and this might also be a cause of the reduction in hepatic NK activity.

It has also been reported that IFN-$\alpha$ could enhance the NK activity of peripheral blood and normal liver [30–32]. LC rats were administered human recombinant IFN-$\alpha$ (INTRON A, Schering Plough, Tokyo, Japan). The dose was $5 \times 10^4 \text{IU}/100\,\text{g}$ body weight intravenously. Saline (0.2 ml/rat) was also administered as the control. NK activity 24 h after IFN-$\alpha$ administration was measured using a $^{51}$Cr-release assay. The NK activity of Fr.1 of the liver increased significantly 1.6-fold compared with that of the control rats (Fig. 3). In flow-cytometric analysis there was a significant increase in the percentage of CD3-8+ and MoAb3.2.3+ NK cells in Fr.1 of the liver and spleen after IFN-$\alpha$ administration. In Fr.2 of the liver, the percentage of CD3-8+ NK cells also increased (Table 3). After IFN-$\alpha$ administration, significant increases in NK activity and NK cell count were observed in LC rats.

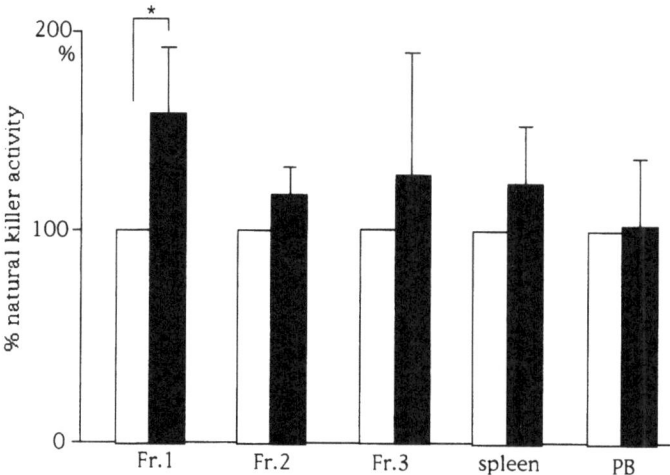

FIG. 3. Comparison of natural killer activity of lymphocytes obtained from hepatic sinusoids, spleen, and peripheral blood from IFN-$\alpha$- and saline-treated LC rats. The mean values from saline-treated LC rats were set as 100%. *Open columns* are data from saline-treated LC rats, and *closed columns* are data from IFN-$\alpha$-treated rats. Fr.1, Fr.2, and Fr.3 are low-, medium-, and high-density lymphocytes, respectively, from hepatic sinusoids. Data are expressed as means $\pm$ SE. (From [24] with minor modifications)

TABLE 3. NK cell population in lymphocytes from liver, spleen, and peripheral blood of LC rats injected with saline and IFN-$\alpha$ (from [24] with minor modifications)

| Cell surface marker | | Percentage positive cells | | | | |
|---|---|---|---|---|---|---|
| | | Fr.1[a] | Fr.2[a] | Fr.3[a] | Spleen | PBL[b] |
| 3.2.3+ | Saline-treated LC rats | 75.6 $\pm$ 3.4 | 24.6 $\pm$ 2.8 | 6.4 $\pm$ 2.1 | 14.1 $\pm$ 1.5 | 21.8 $\pm$ 1.8 |
| | IFN-$\alpha$-treated LC rats | 86.3 $\pm$ 2.1 | 25.2 $\pm$ 2.9 | 8.0 $\pm$ 3.1 | 19.3 $\pm$ 2.4 | 19.0 $\pm$ 2.5 |
| P-value | | <0.05 | NS[c] | NS | <0.05 | NS |
| CD3-CD8+ | Saline-treated LC rats | 59.0 $\pm$ 3.3 | 19.2 $\pm$ 2.3 | 9.1 $\pm$ 1.4 | 10.2 $\pm$ 2.3 | 15.4 $\pm$ 3.0 |
| | IFN-$\alpha$-treated LC rats | 68.3 $\pm$ 2.7 | 22.4 $\pm$ 2.2 | 8.9 $\pm$ 2.1 | 13.6 $\pm$ 2.2 | 14.1 $\pm$ 2.8 |
| P-value | | <0.01 | <0.05 | NS | <0.05 | NS |

[a] Fr.1, Fr.2, and Fr.3 are low-, medium-, and high-density lymphosites, respectively, from the liver.
[b] Peripheral blood lymphocytes.
[c] Not significant.
Data are expressed as mean + SE.

# Conclusion

In human studies, a reduction in peripheral blood NK activity has been reported in patients with liver cirrhosis [20-22]. The results obtained in our studies may contribute to a better understanding of the impaired host defence mechanism, and provide a clue to the development of new strategies to prevent infections and carcinomas occurring in patients with chronic liver disease.

## References

1. Tanaka M, Ogata H, Yoshimoto K, et al. (1989) Harvest of liver sinusoidal large granular lymphocytes (pit cells) and augmentation of natural killer activity by the administration of OK432. Cells Hepatic Sinusoid 2:451-455
2. Kaneda K, Dan C, Wake K (1983) Pit cells as natural killer cells. Biomed Res 4:567-576
3. Wisse E, Noordende JM, van der Meulen J, et al. (1976) The pit cells: description of a new type of cell occurring in rat liver sinusoids and peripheral blood. Cell Tissue Res 173:423-435
4. Wiltrout RH, Mathieson BJ, Talmadge JE, et al. (1984) Augmentation of organ-associated natural killer activity by biological response modifiers. J Exp Med 160:1431-1449
5. Budzynski W, Chirigos M, Gruy E (1987) Augmentation of natural cell activity in tumor-bearing and normal mice by MVE-2. Cancer Immunol Immunother 24:253-258
6. Vanderkerken K, Bowens L, Van dBK, et al. (1993) Origin and differentiation of hepatic natural killer cells (pit cells). Hepatology 22:919-925
7. Vanderkerken K, Bowens L, Wisse E (1990) Characterization of a phenotypically and functionally distinct subset of large granular lymphocytes (pit cells) in rat liver sinusoids. Hepatology 12:70-75
8. Bukowski JF, Wada BA, Habu S, et al. (1983) Natural killer cell depletion enhances virus synthesis and virus-induced hepatitis in vivo. J Immunol 131:1531-1538
9. Welsh RM, Brubaker JO, Vargas CM, et al. (1991) Natural killer (NK) cell response to virus infections in mice with severe combined immunodeficiency. The stimulation of NK cells and the NK cell-dependent control of virus infections occur independently of T and B cell function. J Exp Med 173:1053-1063
10. Liaw YF, Lee CS, Tai SL, et al. (1995) T cell-mediated autologous hepatocytotoxicity in patients with chronic hepatitis C virus infection. Hepatology 22:1368-1373
11. Poralla T, Hutteroth TH, Meyer BK (1984) Cellular cytotoxicity against autologous hepatocytes in acute and chronic non-A, non-B hepatitis. Gut 25:114-120
12. Uchida A, Micksche M (1983) Intrapleural administration of OK432 in cancer patients. Int J Cancer 31:1-5
13. Bouwens L, Remels L, Baekeland M, et al. (1987) Large granular lymphocytes or "pit cells" from rat liver: isolation, ultrastructural characterization and natural killer activity. Eur J Immunol 17:37-42
14. Reynolds C, Sharrow S, Ortaldo J, et al. (1981) Natural killer activity in the rat. II. Analysis of surface antigen on LGL by flow cytometry. J Immunol 127:2204-2208
15. Uchida A, Micksche M (1981) In vitro augmentation of natural killing activity by OK432. Int J Immunopharmacol 3:365-375
16. Kawaguchi T, Suematsu M, Koizumi M, et al. (1983) Activation of macrophage function by intraperitoneal administration of the streptococcal antitumor agent OK432. Int J Immunopharmacol 6:177-189
17. Shimauchi Y, Tanaka M, Yoshitake M, et al. (1993) Functional differences between rat Kupffer cells and splenic macrophages. Cells Hepatic Sinusoid 4:198-200

18. Oka H, Yamamoto S, Kuroki T, et al. (1995) Prospective study of chemoprevention of hepatocellular carcinoma with Sho-saiko-to. Cancer 76:743–749
19. Shimada M, Tanaka M, Shimauchi Y, et al. (1993) Oral administration of Sho-saiko-to (TJ-9, Japanese herbal medicine) enhanced liver-associated natural killer activity. Cells Hepatic Sinusoid 4:536–537
20. Carpentier B, Franco D, Paci L, et al. (1984) Deficient natural killer cell activity in alcoholic cirrhosis. Clin Exp Immunol 58:107–115
21. Chuang WL, Liu HW, Chang WY (1990) Natural killer cell activity in patients with hepatocellular carcinoma relative to early development and tumor invasion. Cancer 65:926–930
22. Laso FJ, Madruga JI, Gioron JA, et al. (1997) Decreased natural killer cytotoxic activity in chronic alcoholism is associated with alcoholic liver disease but not active ethanol consumption. Hepatology 25:1096–1100
23. Zimmermann T, Muller A, Machnik G, et al. (1987) Biochemical and morphological studies on production and regression of experimental liver cirrhosis induced by thioacetamide in Uje: WIST rats. Z Versuchstierkd 30(5–6):165–180
24. Shirachi M, Sata M, Miyajima I, et al. (1998) Liver-associated natural killer activity in cirrhotic rats. Microbiol Immunol 42:117–124
25. Bouwens L, Wisse E (1987) Immuno-electron microscopic characterization of large granular lymphocytes (natural killer cells) from rat liver. Eur J Immunol 17:1423–1428
26. Luo D, Vanderkerken K, Bouwens L, et al. (1995) The number and distribution of hepatic natural killer cells (pi cells) in normal rat liver: an immunohistochemical study. Hepatology 21:1690–1694
27. Vanderkerken K, Bowens L, De NW, et al. (1993) Origin and differentiation of hepatic natural killer cells (pit cells). Hepatology 18:919–925
28. Arii S, Monden K, Itai S, et al. (1990) Depressed function of Kupffer cells in rats with CCL4-induced liver cirrhosis. Res Exp Med Berl 190:173–182
29. Lough J, Rosenthall L, Arzoumanian A, et al. (1987) Kupffer cell depletion associated with capillarization of liver sinusoids in carbon tetrachloride-induced rat liver cirrhosis. J Hepatol 5:190–198
30. Actis G, Ponzetto A, D'Urso N, et al. (1991) Chronic active hepatitis B. Interferon-activated natural killer-like cells against a hepatoma cell line transfected with the hepatitis B virus nucleic acid. Liver 11:106–113
31. Amagai T, Kita M, Imanishi J, et al. (1983) Augmentation of natural killer activity of human peripheral blood lymphocytes by human leukocytes by human leukocyte interferon: characterization of the augmented activity. Gann (Jpn J Cancer Res) 74:887–895
32. Castilla A, Camps-Bansell J, Civeira M, et al. (1993) Lymphoblastoid alpha-interferon for chronic hepatitis C: a randomized controlled study. Am J Gastroenterol 88:233–239

# Modulation of Hepatic Sinusoidal Cell Function by Transduction of Genes in the Liver: Gene Therapy for Hepatic Micro-Metastasis

YASUSHI SHIRATORI[1], FUMIHIKO KANAI[1], HIROFUMI HAMADA[2], HIROSHI MORIYAMA[3], YOKO HIKIBA[4], MAKOTO NAITO[3], and MASAO OMATA[1]

*Summary.* The immune defense system in the liver is known to consist of Kupffer cells, pit cells, lymphocytes, neutrophils, and other infiltrating immune responsive cells. In the liver, Kupffer cells as well as pit cells play an important role in tumor defense and the immune surveillance system. Activation of these cells could contribute to cytotoxicity against tumor cells. In an experimental model of hepatic metastasis of colon carcinoma, biological response modifiers potentially activate these immune responsive cells and reduce hepatic metastasis of tumor cells. Since the activation of pit cells may be induced by interleukin-2 (IL-2), the local tumor surveillance system of the liver can be activated by gene transduction of IL-2 cDNA in hepatocytes using adenovirus vector. Local production of IL-2 may enhance the natural killer (NK) activity of pit cells, leading to a reduction of hepatic metastasis of colon carcinoma. The modulation of sinusoidal cells by gene transduction (gene therapy) may provide a tool to change the pathophysiology of the liver, leading to a clinical treatment for liver diseases.

*Key words.* Hepatic large granular lymphocytes (pit cells), Interleukin-2 (IL-2), Biological response modifier (BRM), Gene therapy, Tumor surveillance system in the liver

## Role of the Immune Surveillance System in the Liver

The immune defense system in the liver (Fig. 1) is known to consist of Kupffer cells, pit cells, lymphocytes, neutrophils, and other infiltrating immune responsive cells. Pit cells are known to be organ-associated natural killer (NK) cells in the liver [1]. A

[1] Department of Internal Medicine (II), Faculty of Medicine, The University of Tokyo, 7-3-1 Hongo, Bunkyo-ku, Tokyo 113, Japan
[2] Department of Molecular Biotherapy Research, Cancer Chemotherapy Center, Cancer Institute, Tokyo, Japan
[3] Second Department of Pathology, Niigata University School of Medicine, 757 Asahimachi-dori Ichibancho, Niigata 951-8122, Japan
[4] Division of Gastroenterology, Institute of Adult Disease, Asahi Life Foundation, Tokyo, Japan

FIG. 1. Immune surveillance system in the liver. *HC*, hepatocyte; *EC*, endothelial cells; *PC*, pit cells; *Tc*, cytotoxic T-cells; *PMNs*, polymorphonuclear cells; *Mo*, macrophages

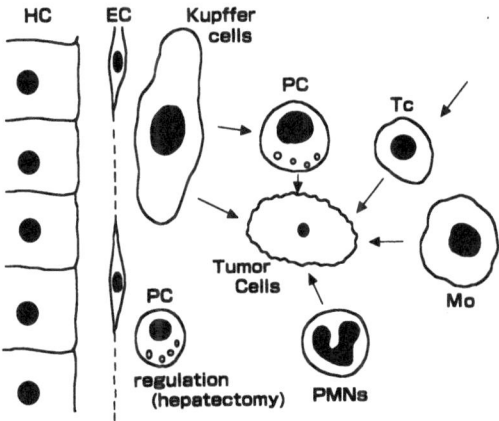

recent study revealed that not only Kupffer cells but also pit cells in the liver play an important role in tumor defense and the immune surveillance system [2]. Activation of these cells could contribute to cytotoxicity against tumor cells, and biological response modifiers (BRMs) have the potential to activate these immune responsive cells.

## Tumor Defense System in the Liver and Biological Response Modifier (Fig. 2)

### Kupffer Cells

Kupffer cells showing an enhanced phagocytic function contribute to the cytotoxicity of tumor cells. Kupffer cells activated in vitro by lipopolysaccharide or lymphokines have been shown to have high cytotoxic activity against several kinds of tumor cells [3], but tumor cell destruction by activated macrophages is nonselective [4, 5]. Stimulation of Kupffer cells in vivo by agents such as glucan is reported to inhibit hepatic metastasis and enhance long-term survival by increasing the number of

FIG. 2. Immune surveillance in the liver. Tumor defense system and biological response modifier (*BRM*). *KC*, Kupffer cells; *MDP*, muramyl dipeptide; *Mo*, macrophages; *IFN*, interferon; *PGs*, prostaglandins; *NK*, natural killer, *NC*, natural cytotoxicity

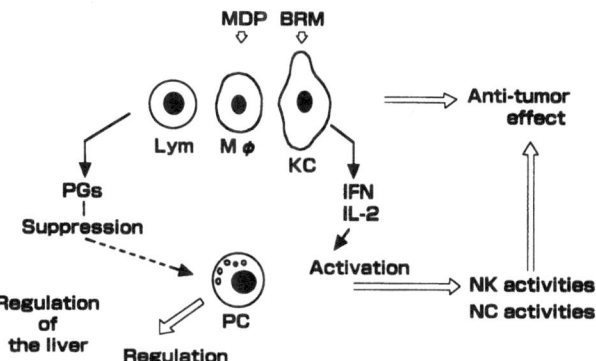

activated Kupffer cells [6]. Furthermore, stimulation of Kupffer cells by liposomal-muramyl dipeptide (MDP) enhances phagocytic or tumoricidal activity in macrophages, indicating that the action of liposomes could be important [7]. On the other hand, inhibition of Kupffer cell function results in an enhancement of liver metastasis.

## Organ-Associated Lymphocytes (Natural Killer Cells) and Pit Cells

Nonadherent, nonparenchymal liver cells have been reported to exert cytotoxicity against YAC-1 tumor cells [8]. NK activity has been attributed to cells having a morphology of large granular lymphocytes (LGL) [9, 10]. An increase in mononuclear cells in the liver after BRM administration is reported to correspond to an increase in LGL number and NK activity, and the major effect is considered to be the result of increased lymphocyte infiltration into the liver [10], although local division of hepatic LGL could also contribute to the numerical increase of hepatic LGL after BRM administration [11].

## Experimental Study on the Tumor Defense System in the Liver

In our previous study, colon 38 adenocarcinoma (dimethylhydrazine-induced colon carcinoma) originating from a single strain of mice was used, and was maintained in the flanks of mice in vivo. Colon 38 adenocarcinoma is a differentiated carcinoma, in contrast to the undifferentiated cell type of colon 26 adenocarcinoma [7], and is known to be sensitive to lymphokine-activating killer cells or tumor-infiltrating lymphocytes [TIL] in combination with interleukin-2 (IL-2). In addition, tumor cells were inoculated into the superior mesenteric vein, from where they stream into the liver to establish metastasis in the liver. Many hepatic metastasis in experimental animals are found to be located preferentially at or near the surface of the target organs. This surface preference is often so marked that a reliable estimation of the number of metastasis in an organ can be made by examining it from the outside.

In previous experiments [12], male specific pathogen-free C57BL/6 strain mice, aged 6–7 weeks, were used. The mice received an i.v. injection of 0.1 mg killed streptococcal preparation (OK 432; Chugai Pharmaceutical Tokyo, Japan) on day $-2$ as a BRM. An administration of OK432 enhanced the NK activity of hepatic mononuclear cells (Fig. 3), and reduced the number of hepatic metastasis of colon carcinoma (Fig. 4). The enhanced NK activity of these cells was completely stopped by treatment with anti-asGM$_1$ serum plus complement in vitro. Administration of this serum in vivo reduced the NK activity of hepatic mononuclear cells and increased the number of hepatic metastasis of tumor cells. Since colon 38 adenocarcinoma cells are difficult to maintain in culture, cytotoxic activity against the tumor cells was examined by in vivo neutralizing assay. In vivo tumor-neutralization assay revealed that tumor growth was completely inhibited when the tumor cells were mixed with hepatic mononuclear cells of the OK432-treated mice at a ratio of 1:5 (Fig. 5). Among these hepatic sinusoidal cells, asGM$_1$-positive hepatic mononuclear cells play an important role in neutralizing colon tumor cells in vivo.

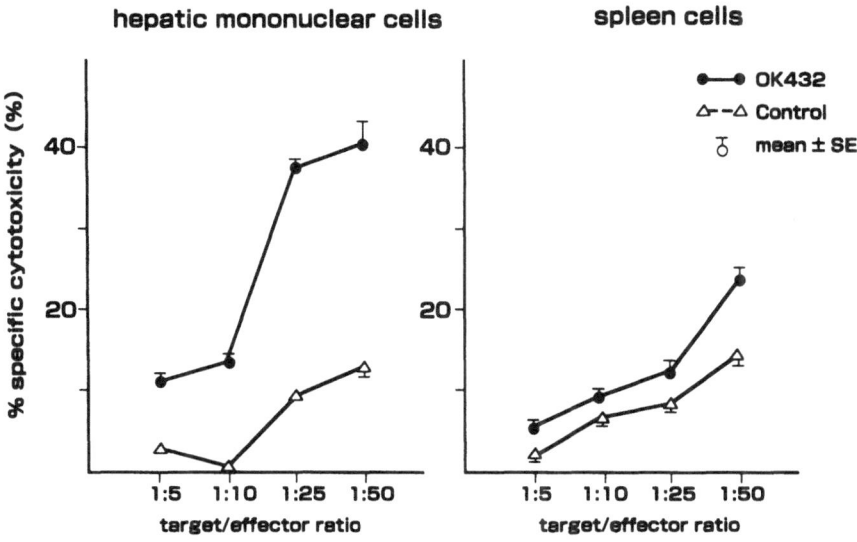

FIG. 3. Natural killer activity of hepatic mononuclear cells and spleen cells

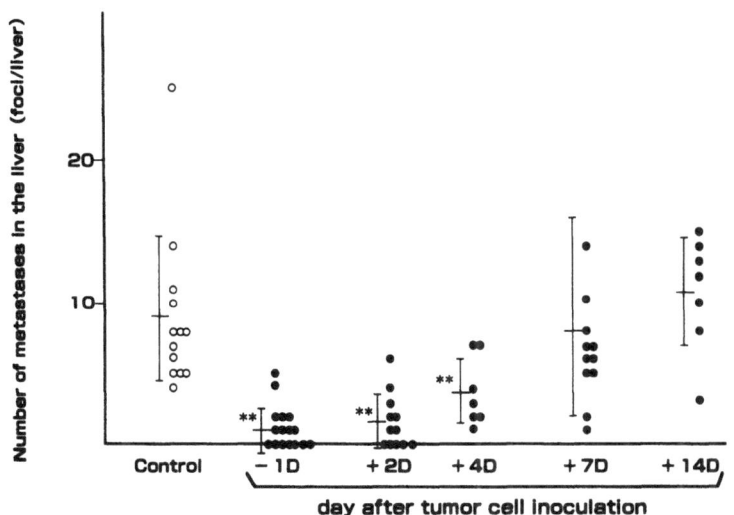

FIG. 4. Inhibition of hepatic metastases of colon 38 adenocarcinoma by OK432 (BRM)

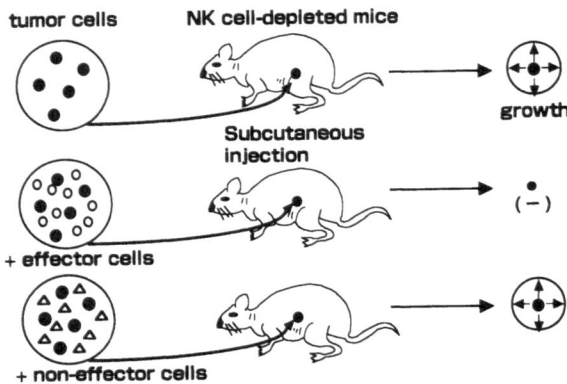

**tumor cells     NK cell-depleted mice**

**Subcutaneous injection**

growth

**+ effector cells**

( − )

**+ non-effector cells**

Fɪɢ. 5. In vivo tumor neutralization assay

## Heterogeneity of Hepatic Large Granular Lymphocytes

Recent studies have reported that rat hepatic LGL are heterogenous in the expression of asGM$_1$ antigen, and that some parts of rat hepatic NK cells are resistant to anti-asGM$_1$ antibody [13, 14]. In our previous study, the NK activity of hepatic mononuclear cells in sham- or splenectomy-operated mice was enhanced by the asGM$_1$-OK432 treatment, but their enhanced NK activities were only partially reduced by the treatment with anti-asGM$_1$ serum plus complement in vitro, indicating that asGM$_1$-negative cells exert NK activity against YAC-1 cells when asGM$_1$-positive cells are completely depleted in a body [15].

# Immunomodulation Therapy for Cancer

IL-2 is a growth factor of LGL/NK cells, and is known to be a potent stimulator for cytotoxic T-lymphocytes (CTL). Previous study revealed that an enhancement of cell mediated cytotoxicity was observed after 6h stimulation by IL-2 in vitro, and that this enhancement was more significant after 24–72h of culture with rIL-2. IL-2 induces NK cells which are highly cytotoxic against tumor cells. Many of these activated killer cells adhere to plastic, and adherent lymphokine-activated killer (LAK) (A-LAK) cells are more potently cytotoxic against tumor cells. The results obtained from immunotherapy with IL-2 in combination with LAK cells showed a dramatic reduction in the number of established metastatic lesions in several experimental animal models [16]. IL-2-stimulated adoptively transferred A-LAK cells are found to make contact with the metastatic tumor cells. Recent studies have revealed the migration of A-LAK cells into the infiltrating area or metastatic lesions of tumors. Other work showed that A-LAK cells migrated to the lung and then subsequently migrated to the liver and spleen 2–6h following i.v. injection, and that an increased number of LAK cells was then found in the malignant lesion [17, 18]. However, the infiltration of LAK cells into the tumor lesions seemed very heterogeneous after i.v. injection. Significant infiltration of liver metastasis was seen only after intraportal injection of A-LAK cells, indicating impaired traffic of intravenous-injected A-LAK cells through the lung capillaries.

Earlier research also showed the pathological toxicity induced by repeated intravenous or intraperitoneal injection of recombinant IL-2, and IL-2 administration may lead to damage to the endothelial lining cells [19]. However, systemic administration of IL-2 showed a mild inhibitory effect of hepatic metastasis of colon carcinoma (unpublished observation), and Bouwens et al. [19] demonstrated an accumulation of LGL and Kupffer cells in the liver of rats treated with a continuous infusion of IL-2.

In addition, it has been shown that tumor targets appear to be more susceptible to anti-CD-3-activated T-cells than LAK cells, and that anti-CD-3 treatment enhanced activated T-lymphocytes and reduced the number of hepatic metastasis [20]. However, the mechanism of activation induced by anti-CD-3 treatment has not yet been clarified.

# Gene Therapy for Metastatic Cancer in the Liver

Gene therapy for cancer is of four types (Fig. 6) [21–24]: (1) genetic immunomodulation (i.e., insertion of a cytokine gene into tumor cells, or in situ injection of plasmid carrying an HLA gene into a tumor mass that is negative for the injected HLA gene); (2) virus-directed enzyme prodrug therapy (insertion of a suicide gene into tumor cells in situ with subsequent activation of the suicide mechanism); (3) gene replacement therapy (the use of tumor suppressor genes and/or anti-oncogene); (4) protection of host cells from anticancer drugs (the use of a multiresistant (MDR) gene to protect bone marrow cells to allow higher-dose chemotherapy).

## Methodology of Gene Transfer

A variety of methods are used to increase the efficacy of DNA uptake by the cells. The procedure can broadly be divided into three types: biological, chemical, and physiological techniques. Among these procedures, viral vectors are the most efficient means for the transfer of genes into target cells, and are therefore preferred over physical methods.

## Gene Delivery into the Liver

The development of strategies for gene therapy in the liver is a challenging task because this organ is involved in the manifestation of numerous genetic and malig-

1 ) *Genetic immunomodulation*
        **cytokine gene**
        **HLA gene**

2 ) *Drug targeting*
        *Virally directed enzyme prodrug therapy*
        **suicide gene  -   thymidine kinase        GCV**
        **                        cytosine deaminase    5-FC**

3 ) *Gene replacement*
        **tumor suppressor gene**
        **p53, RB, WT1, NF1, E-cadherin, nm23, JE/MCP1**
        **GCF, rap1A**

4 ) *Normal tissue protection*
        **MDR 1**

FIG. 6. Cancer gene therapy

|                                          | Adenovirus vector              | Retrovirus vector        |
| ---------------------------------------- | ------------------------------ | ------------------------ |
| Size of the gene to be transferred       | 7.5 kbp                        | 8 kbp                    |
| Titer                                    | $10^{11}$-$10^{12}$ cfu/ml     | $10^6$-$10^8$ cfu/ml     |
| Duration of transgene expression         | transient                      | indefinite               |
| Expression level                         | high                           | low                      |
| Repeated administration in vivo          | hampered by immune response    |                          |
| Indications for liver-directed gene therapy | Yes                         | No                       |
| Risks                                    | inflammatory response          | insertional mutagenesis  |

FIG. 7. Adenovirus vector vs. retrovirus vector

nant diseases. Most of the available techniques for gene transfer are also applied to hepatocytes ex vivo. Retroviral and adenoviral vectors have been studied with regard to hepatocyte-directed gene transfer in vivo and in vitro [25–27]. Attempts to retransplant retrovirally transduced hepatocytes back to patients have shown the limit of the ex vivo approach.

The obvious alternative would be the development of suitable techniques for gene transfer in vivo using adenovirus vector, and the comparative data using adenovirus or retrovirus vector are summarized in Fig. 7. Hepatocytes can be targets for clinical adenovirus infection because the respiratory epithelium and the liver share the same embryonic origin. The merits of the adenovirus vector system are organ specificity (hepatocytes), the extent of expression, the chronicity of expression, and the safety of recombinant adenovirus vector.

## Genetic Immunomodulation of Cancer

The strategy in recent antitumor gene therapy by genetic immunomodulation is to use the vector of genes encoding for cytokines which induce cytotoxic T-cell activity [28–30]. An application of cytokines has already been shown to be a promising method in cancer treatment. However, it reveals a severe problem resulting from the requirement to apply systemically high doses of the cytokines; application of therapeutically effective concentrations is often accompanied by toxic side-effects. This problem may be circumvented by "tumor cell targeted cytokine gene therapy": the tumor cells are genetically engineered to produce a given cytokine in vitro and upon injection into mice provide a locally enhanced cytokine concentration. This makes use of a more physiological mode of action by the cytokine eventually to attract effector cells chemotactically and/or induce a tumor-specific immune response. Additionally, upon destruction of the tumor cells, the source for the cytokine production is eliminated.

In cytokine gene therapy protocol, the cell type engineered to produce the cytokine is crucial. In most gene immunomodulation therapy, the transfection of pleiotropic

FIG. 8. Strategy of gene therapy
for hepatic metastasis of colon
carcinoma

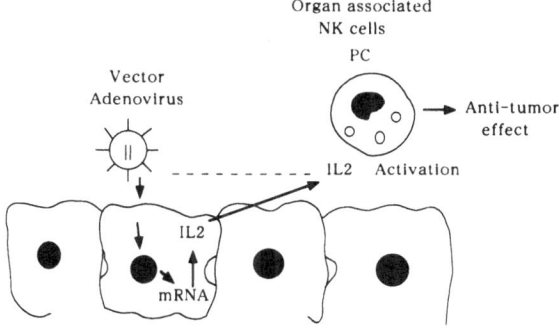

cytokine genes into the immune cells of the host in addition to tumor cells, and the
antitumor response, can be enhanced by cytotoxic T-cells, i.e., macrophages which
can in turn be induced by the expression of appropriate cytokines by the cells. The
best characterized model so far has been the transfection of the TNF gene into tumor-
infiltrating lymphocytes (TIL) [31].

There already exist liver-associated lymphocytes in the liver, and it is possible that
specific delivery of cytokine genes into the liver might attract and activate
neighboring lymphocyte and NK cell activity in the liver. Adenovirus vector is known
to be specifically targeted into the liver, especially in hepatocytes [25–27]. Thus,
cytokines for enhanced NK activity encoded in adenovirus vector might provide
a new strategy for an enhanced immune surveillance system in the liver (Fig. 8)
[32].

## Genetic Immunomodulation by IL-2

IL-2 is a growth factor that stimulates the proliferation of cytotoxic T-cells, NK cells,
and LAK cells, all of which can participate in the antitumor response. In the mouse,
systemic administration of IL-2 induces the expansion and long-term persistence of
adoptively transferred tumor-specific T-cells. However, systemic administration of
cytokine IL-2 into experimental animals has been used, but with an increased frequency of a variety of adverse events. Since locally secreted cytokines were also able
to influence the generation of antitumor immune responses, adenoviral vector could
be used to introduce the IL-2 gene. By using the host immune system, the
immunocompetent cells accumulated in some tumors, probably as a part of an immune attack on the tumor (tumor-infiltrating lymphocytes, TIL) via antitumor functions. A modified induction of paracrine antitumor immunoreactivity might be a
potential gene therapy for cancer.

Since pit cells show characteristic features of NK cells that could be activated by IL-
2, this study has been conducted to introduce the transduction of the IL-2 gene into
hepatocytes using adenovirus vector to produce IL-2 which might enhance the NK
activity of pit cells in the neighborhood, leading to inhibition of hepatic metastasis of
colon carcinoma in vivo [32].

A recombinant adenovirus vector (Adex1CAmIL2) was constructed by inserting an
expression unit composed of CAG promotor (cytomegalovirus enhancer plus chicken

## Adex1CAmIL2

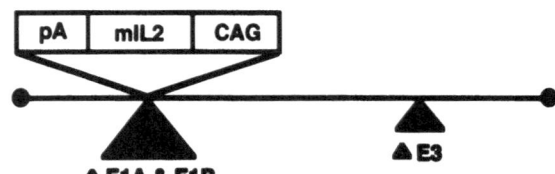

FIG. 9. Construct of IL-2 cDNA encoded adenovirus vector (Adex1CAmIL2)

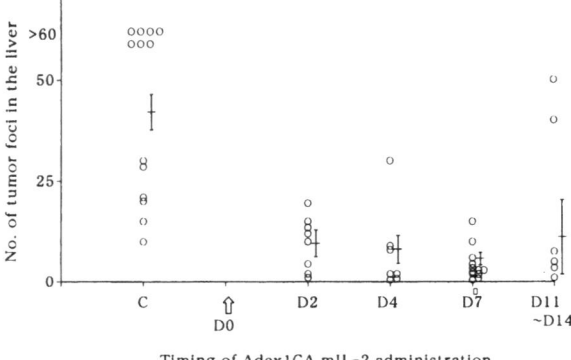

Timing of Adex1CA miL-2 administration after tumor inoculation

FIG. 10. Inhibition of hepatic metastases of colon 38 adenocarcinoma by Adex1CAmIL2

beta-actin promotor), murine IL-2 cDNA, and rabbit beta-globin polyadenylation signal (Fig. 9).

After administration of Adex1CAmIL2, IL-2 mRNA expression was found to be markedly enhanced in hepatocytes by analysis with northern blotting and by immunostaining, and an enhanced expression was demonstrated until the 7th day. Serum IL-2 activities were also markedly increased after Adex1CAmIL2 for 7 days, with systemic administration of $4 \times 10^7$ p.f.u. per animal. The NK activity of hepatic mononuclear cells was also markedly enhanced after administration of Adex1CAmIL2, and persisted for 7–10 days. Although micrometastatic foci were established at 4–7 days after tumor cell inoculation, hepatic metastasis of colon 38 tumor cells was inhibited by administration of Adex1CAmIL2 until the 7th day after tumor cell inoculation (Fig. 10).

## Conclusion

The potential immunotherapeutic treatment of liver metastasis with IL-2 is of great interest, and local treatment of IL-2 should be performed to reduce the side-effects. In these circumstances, IL-2 gene transduction using adenovirus vector made CTL more potent in the liver in vivo. Expression of the IL-2 gene in the CTL enhanced their antitumor activity in vivo. In these cases, systemic IL-2 concentration in serum was relatively low, but local concentration of IL-2 in the liver might be increased. Since local production of IL-2 may be important, this study was conducted using adenovirus vector to express the transducted cytokine gene in the liver.

Gene transduction using adenovirus was demonstrated in hepatocytes only. Local expression and production of IL-2 in the liver enhanced the NK activity of neighboring liver-associated lymphocytes (pit cells), which subsequently had some cytotoxicity against tumor cells. Thus, the number of hepatic metastases was reduced in the mice receiving Adex1CAmIL2. This gene therapy is only effective within 7 days after tumor cell inoculation, during which time the tumor foci remain small. This procedure may have clinical potential for the inhibition of hepatic metastasis of colon carcinoma by enhancing the activity of liver-associated lymphocytes (pit cells). In addition to these possibilities, gene therapy for specific targeting and an adequate on–off switching system might provide further progress in developing gene therapy in vivo.

## References

1. Kaneda K, Dan C, Wake K (1983) Pit cells as natural killer cells. Biomed Res 4:567–576
2. Wiltrout RH, Herberman R, Zhang SR, et al. (1985) Role of organ-associated NK cells in decreased formation of experimental metastases in lung and liver. J Immunol 134:4267–4275
3. Xu Z, Fidler IJ (1984) The in situ activation of cytotoxic properties in murine Kupffer cells by the systemic administration of whole *Mycobacterium bovis* organisms or muramyl tripeptide. Cancer Immunol Immunother 18:118–122
4. Gardner C, Wasserman AJ, Laskin DL (1987) Differential sensitivity of tumor targets to liver macrophage-mediated cytotoxicity. Cancer Res 47:6686–6691
5. Fogler WE, Fidler IJ (1985) Nonselective destruction of murine neoplastic cells by syngeneic tumoricidal macrophages. Cancer Res 45:14–18
6. Williams DL, Sherwood ER, McNamee RB, et al. (1985) Therapeutic efficacy of glucan in a murine model of hepatic metastatic disease. Hepatology 5:198–206
7. Phillips NC, Rioux J, Tsao M (1988) Activation of murine Kupffer cell tumoricidal activity by liposomes containing lipophilic muramyl dipeptide. Hepatology 8:1046–1050
8. Cohen SA, Salazar D, von Muenchhausen W, et al. (1985) Natural antitumor defense system of the murine liver. J Leukocyte Biol 37:559–569
9. Zarcone D, Prasthofer EF, Malavasi F, et al. (1987) Ultrastructural analysis of human natural killer cell activation. Blood 69:1725–1736
10. Trinchieri G, Perussia B (1984) Human natural killer cells: Biologic and pathologic aspects. Lab Invest 50:489–513
11. Wiltrout RH, Mathieson BJ, Talmadge JE, et al. (1984) Augmentation of organ-associated natural killer activity by biological response modifiers. Isolation and characterization of large granular lymphocytes from the liver. J Exp Med 160:1431–1449
12. Shiratori Y, Nakata R, Okano K, et al. (1992) Inhibition of hepatic metastasis of colon carcinoma by asialo GM1-positive cells in the liver. Hepatology 16:469–478
13. Bouwens L, Wisse E (1987) Immune-electron microscopic characterization of large granular lymphocytes (natural killer cells) from rat liver. Eur J Immonol 17:1423–1428
14. Bouwens L, Remels L, Baekeland M, et al. (1987) Large granular lymphocytes or "Pit cells" from rat liver: Isolation, ultrastructural characterization and natural killer activ-

ity. Eur J Immunol 17:37–42

15. Shiratori Y, Kawase T, Nakata R, et al. (1995) Effect of splenectomy on hepatic metastasis of colon carcinoma and natural killer activity in the liver. Dig Dis Sci 40:2398–2406

16. Smithson G, Bittick TH, Chervenak R, et al. (1991) The role of NK cells in the regulation of experimental metastasis in a murine lymphoma system. J Leukocyte Biol 49:621–629

17. Basse P, Herberman RB, Nannmark U, et al. (1991) Accumulation of adoptively transferred adherent, lymphokine-activated killer cells in murine metastases. J Exp Med 174:479–488

18. Felgar R, Hiserodt JC (1990) In vivo migration and tissue localization of highly purified lymphokine-activated killer cells (A-LAK cells) in tumor-bearing rats. Cell Immunol 129:288–298

19. Bouwens L, Marinelli A, Kuppen PJK, et al. (1990) Electron microscopic observations on the accumulation of large granular lymphocytes (Pit cells) and Kupffer cells in the liver of rats treated with continuous infusion of interleukin-2. Hepatology 12:1365–1370

20. Gallinger S, Hoskin DW, Mullen JBM, et al. (1990) Comparison of cellular immunotherapies and anti CD-3 in the treatment of MCA-38-LD experimental hepatic metastases in C57BL/6 mice. Cancer Res 50:2476–2480

21. Strauss M (1994) Liver-directed gene therapy: Prospective and problems. Gene Ther 1:156–164

22. Li Q, Kay MA, Finegold M, et al. (1993) Assessment of recombinant adenoviral vectors for hepatic gene therapy. Hum Gene Ther 4:403–409

23. Gutierrez AA, Lemoine NR, Sikora K (1992) Gene therapy for cancer. Lancet 339:715–721

24. Gore ME, Collins MK (1994) Gene therapy for cancer. Eur J Cancer 30A: 1047–1049

25. Jaffe HA, Danel C, Longenecker G, et al. (1992) Adenovirus-mediated in vivo gene transfer and expression in normal rat liver. Nat Genet 1:372–378

26. Kass-Eisler A, Falck-Pedersen E, Elfenbein DH, et al. (1994) The impact of developmental stage, route of administration and the immune system on adenovirus-mediated gene transfer. Gene Ther 1:395–402

27. Kozarsky K, Wilson JM (1993) Gene therapy: Adenovirus vectors. Curr Opinion Genet Dev 3:499–503

28. Chen SS, Chen XHL, Wang Y, et al. (1995) Combination gene therapy for liver metastasis of colon carcinoma in vivo. Proc Natl Acad Sci USA 92:2577–2581

29. Nakamura Y, Wakimoto H, Abe J, et al. (1994) Adoptive immunotherapy with murine tumor-specific T lymphocytes engineered to secrete interleukin 2. Cancer Res 54:5757–5760

30. Gansbacher B, Zier K, Daniels B, et al. (1990) Interleukin 2 gene transfer into tumor cells abrogates tumorigenicity and induces protective immunity. J Exp Med 172:1217–1224

31. Balnkenstein T, Qin Z, Uberla K, et al. (1991) Tumor suppression after tumor cell-targeted tumor necrosis factor alpha gene transfer. J Exp Med 173:1047–1052

32. Shiratori Y, Kanai F, Hamada H, et al. (1998) Gene therapy for hepatic micro-metastasis of murine colon carcinoma. J Hepatol 28:886–895

# Morphological Aspects of Hepatic Sinusoidal Walls in Reperfusion Injury after Liver Preservation for Liver Transplantation

Takafumi Ichida

*Summary.* Bleb formation in hepatocytes, activated Kupffer cells, and phenotypic changes in sinusoidal endothelial cells occurred during the preservation and reperfusion period of liver to be used for liver transplantation. Current morphological studies have revealed that sinusoidal endothelial cells lost their viability, and positive staining for markers of capillary endothelial cells occurred with basement membrane formation. Kupffer cells swell, ruffle, and degranulate, releasing a number of inflammatory mediators, cytokines, and superoxide radicals. In spite of the changes in sinusoidal cells, hepatocyte structure recovered after reperfusion. Activated Kupffer cells and sinusoidal endothelial cells with phenotypic changes were able to interact with inflammatory cells, producing a disturbance of the microcirculation.

Phenotypic and morphologic changes in sinusoidal endothelial cells occurred within 12 h after harvesting of the donor liver. This indicates that sinusoidal capillarization during reperfusion might be due to cytoprotection under cold and ischemic conditions.

*Key words.* Reperfusion injury, Liver transplantation, Activated Kupffer cell, Sinusoidal endothelial cell injury

## Introduction

Liver transplantation has become a widely accepted treatment for end-stage liver diseases, and long-term survival has approached 58% for adult and 71% for pediatric recipients in 7-year survival studies [1]. Both acute and chronic rejection can occur following liver transplantation. Most recipients show some evidence of mild acute cellular rejection, occurring from post-operative day 5 to day 28, which can be controlled with immunosuppressants. Although poor function of transplanted liver grafts initially occurred in 10–25% of recipients [2], primary graft nonfunction led to graft failure and re-transplantation was conducted in 5–10% of cases [3, 4]. Approximately 40% of re-transplantations in a Pittsburgh study were due to primary graft

Department of Internal Medicine III, Niigata University School of Medicine, 757 Asahimachi-dori-Ichibancho, Niigata 951-8122, Japan

nonfunction [5]. Conversely, no evidence of primary graft nonfunction was reported by the Japanese Study Group of Living Donor Liver Transplantation in 522 Japanese recipients of living related-donor liver transplants, including 462 children and 60 adults, until the middle of August 1997.

Consequently, we suspect that the incidence of primary graft failure and poor initial function is strongly dependent on the durations of warm and cold storage, and is thus related to injury associated with graft harvesting, storage, and reperfusion. Inadequately preserved livers usually fail 1–2 days after transplantation, whereas immunological rejection does not begin for about a week.

Our aim is to illustrate and review the morphological aspects of reperfusion injury occurring after cold ischemic storage, and to describe the hepatic sinusoidal cells involved in this event, based on our experience. A prospective study was carried out at Pittsburgh University after obtaining informed consent. Twenty patients undergoing liver transplantation were eligible for the study. Twenty biopsy samples were taken from each of the back-table donor livers and the reperfused livers after transplantation.

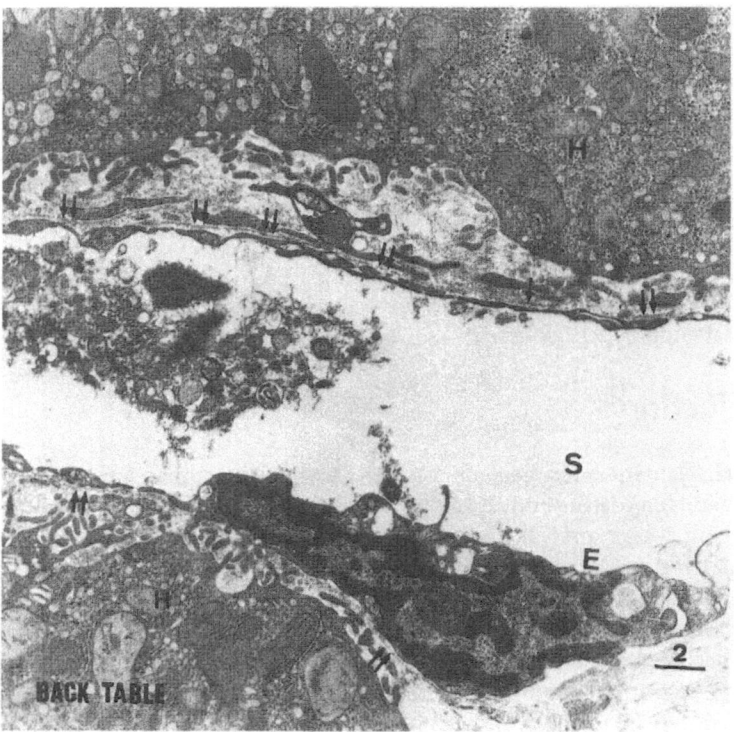

FIG. 1. Back-table biopsy showing degenerated sinusoidal endothelial cells (*E*) and basement membrane formation (*double arrows*) in the space of Disse. *S*, sinusoidal space; *H*, hepatocyte

# Damage to and Phenotypic Changes in Sinusoidal Endothelial Cells

The polarity of the sinusoidal endothelial cells was the same as that of normal liver sinusoids in both the back-table and reperfused liver biopsies. However, some of the sinusoidal endothelial cells in the reperfused biopsies revealed multilayering and had developed autovacuoles and large lysosomes in their cytoplasm (Fig. 1). No marked bleb formation could be observed in sinusoidal endothelial cells, but incomplete formation of the sieve plate and a diminished number of pores [6] with basement membrane formation beneath these cells in the space of Disse (Figs. 1 and 2) were striking findings in these biopsies. Basement membrane formation was often

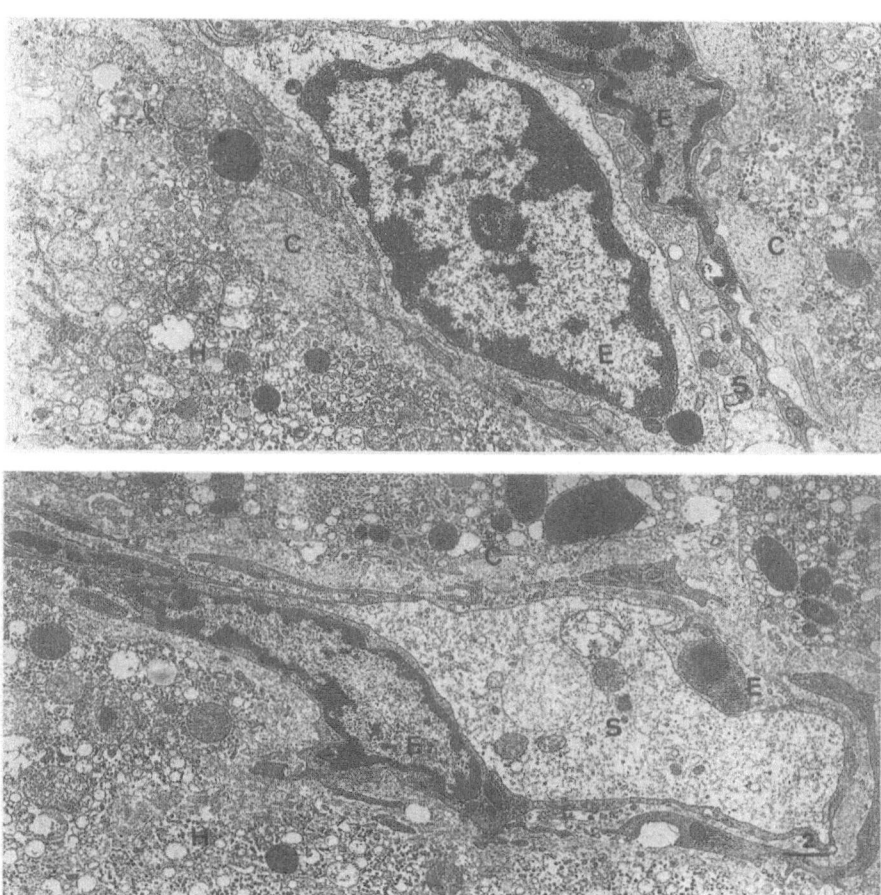

FIG. 2. Multilayered sinusoidal endothelial cells (*E*) with a diminished number of pores. Numerous collagen bundles (*C*) are also marked in the space of Disse. *S*, sinusoidal space; *H*, hepatocyte

observed in patients with pathological conditions such as liver cirrhosis [7], hepatocellular carcinoma [8], and alcoholic liver injury [9]. Although the sinusoidal endothelial cells exhibited a tendency toward degeneration and loss of the properties of the sieve plate, Weibel–Palade bodies [10] seldom appeared in their cytoplasm during the study period. Furthermore, without any specific heterogeneity, interactions between neutrophils, lymphocytes, thrombocytes, and sinusoidal endothelial cells were distinguished in the sinusoidal space.

In human biopsy materials, OKM-5 is a histological marker for sinusoidal endothelial cells that is stained under normal condition [11]. This staining becomes fainter as fibrogenesis progresses, and cirrhotic liver tissue shows marked loss of OKM-5 staining [12]. In addition, both factor VIII-related antigen [13] and ulex europaeus agglutinin 1 lectin (UEA-1) [14] are markers for capillary endothelial cells. Staining of

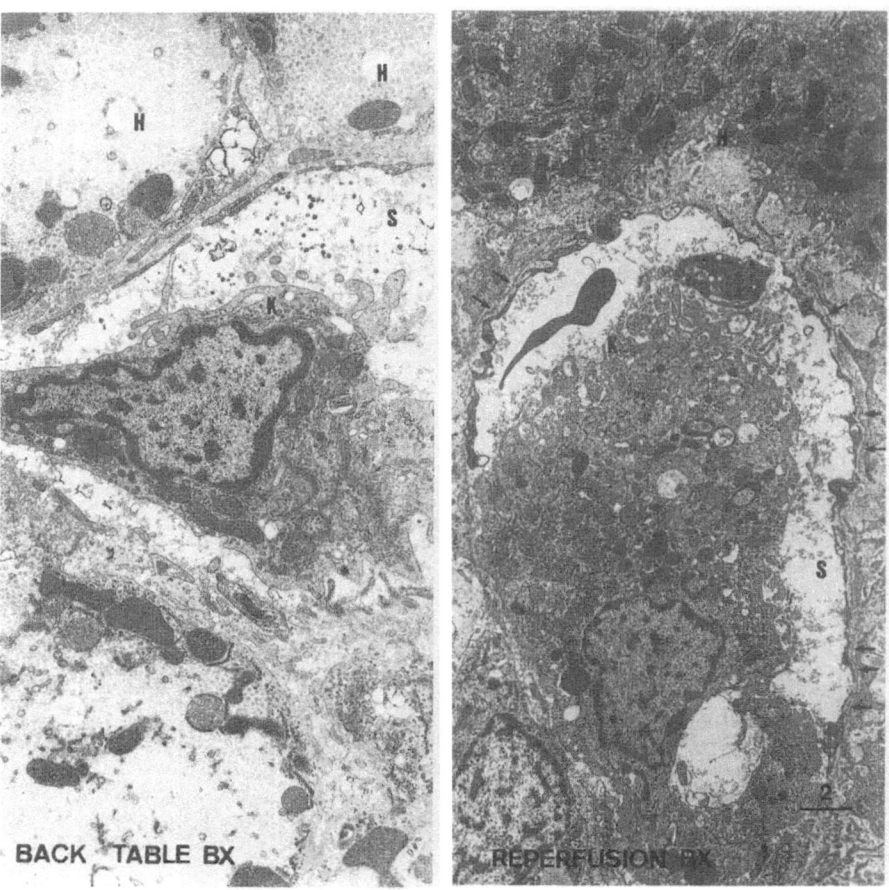

Fig. 3. A Kupffer cell (K), possessing numerous ruffles and spikes on its surface, located in the sinusoidal space (S) and causing a blockage of the blood stream. Large lysosomes and multiple organelles can be observed. These characteristics are typical of activated Kupffer cells. H, hepatocyte; *arrow*, basement membrane

these markers can be in areas of piecemeal necrosis during chronic active hepatitis, and in the peripheral areas of regenerative nodules in liver cirrhosis and hepatocellular carcinoma [15].

An immunohistochemical study of these endothelial cell markers revealed that approximately half of the biopsies with preservation and reperfusion injuries exhibited a loss of positivity for OKM-5, while one-third showed the appearance of positivity for factor VIII-related antigen and UEA-1. This major loss of property of sinusoidal endothelial cells is a key phenomenon indicative of ischemia/reperfusion injury of the liver after liver transplantation.

It takes more than 24 h for the loss of viability of Kupffer cells to become apparent, but the death of virtually all the sinusoidal endothelial cells occurred within minutes. This situation leads to the denudation of hepatic sinusoids [16–20].

## Kupffer Cell Activation

The majority of Kupffer cells showed numerous ruffles, degranulation, and spikes, with many lysosomes in their cytoplasm (Fig. 3). Some of the Kupffer cells migrated into the sinusoidal space, thus tending to block the sinusoidal stream

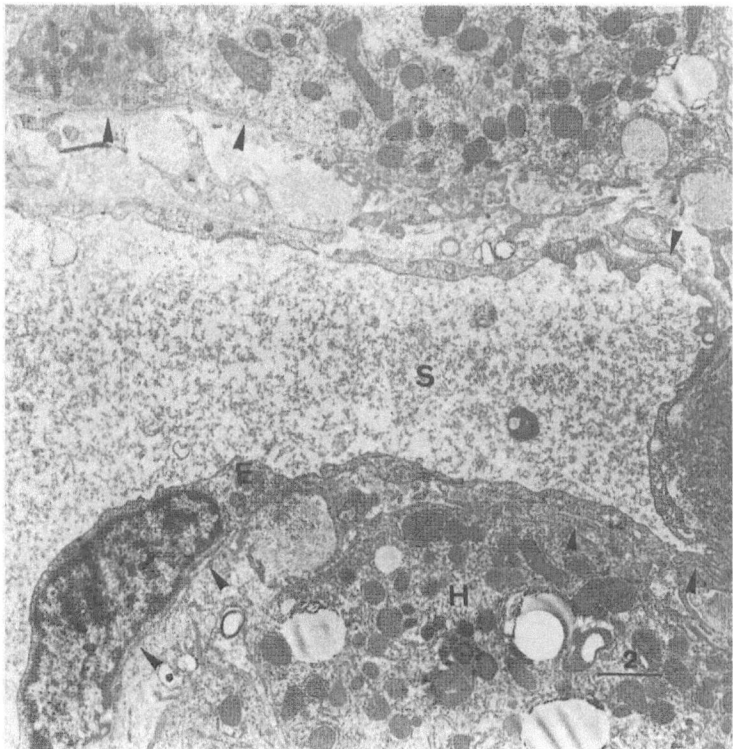

FIG. 4. Basement membrane formation (*arrowheads*) in the space of Disse can be detected with defenestrated sinusoidal endothelial cells (*E*) in reperfusion biopsy. *S*, sinusoidal space; *H*, hepatocyte

and the circulation. These ultrastructural characteristics were recognized as typical of activated Kupffer cells [20, 21], and corresponded with up-regulated function. Activated Kupffer cells release numerous inflammatory mediators, including radicals, tumor necrosis factor-α interleukins 1 and 6, prostaglandins, and nitric oxide. Thus, Kupffer cell activation may precipitate a "cytokine storm" after transplantation [20].

## Hepatic Sinusoidal Capillarization

Although the precise medical details of the donors were not known, the function and morphological condition of the donor livers was judged to be almost normal, and the donors were selected as being suitable for liver transplantation. However, it might have been difficult to determine accurately whether any of the donors had been a

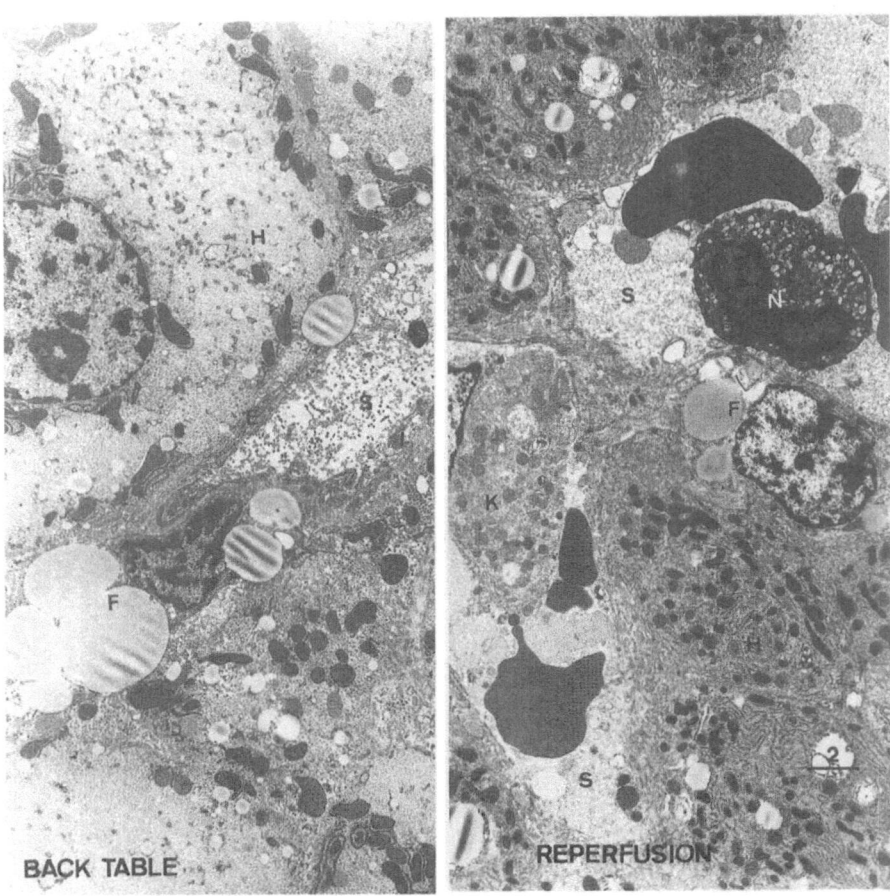

FIG. 5. Fat-storing cells (F) with enlarged fat droplets in their cytoplasm were grouped around these collagen bundles in both back-table biopsy (*left panel*) and reperfusion biopsy (*right panel*). H, hepatocyte; S, sinusoidal space; E, sinusoidal endothelial cell

habitual drinker. In spite of these factors, hepatic sinusoidal capillarization was confirmed by electron microscopy in 12 of the 20 patients (Figs. 1 and 4). Generally continuous, but sometimes discontinuous, basement membrane formation was observed beneath the sinusoidal endothelial cells in the space of Disse with monolayered sinusoidal endothelial cells, and basement membrane was also located near the surface of the hepatocytes.

In addition, several collagen bundles were distributed in the space of Disse. Fat-storing cells with enlarged fat droplets in their cytoplasm were grouped around these collagen bundles (Fig. 5). This fine structure indicates the activation of fat-storing cells and potential blocking of the microcirculation in the space of Disse.

Type IV collagen, a representative type of collagen, was apparent in the sinusoidal walls in 18 of the 20 patients (90%), and laminin, a representative noncollagenous

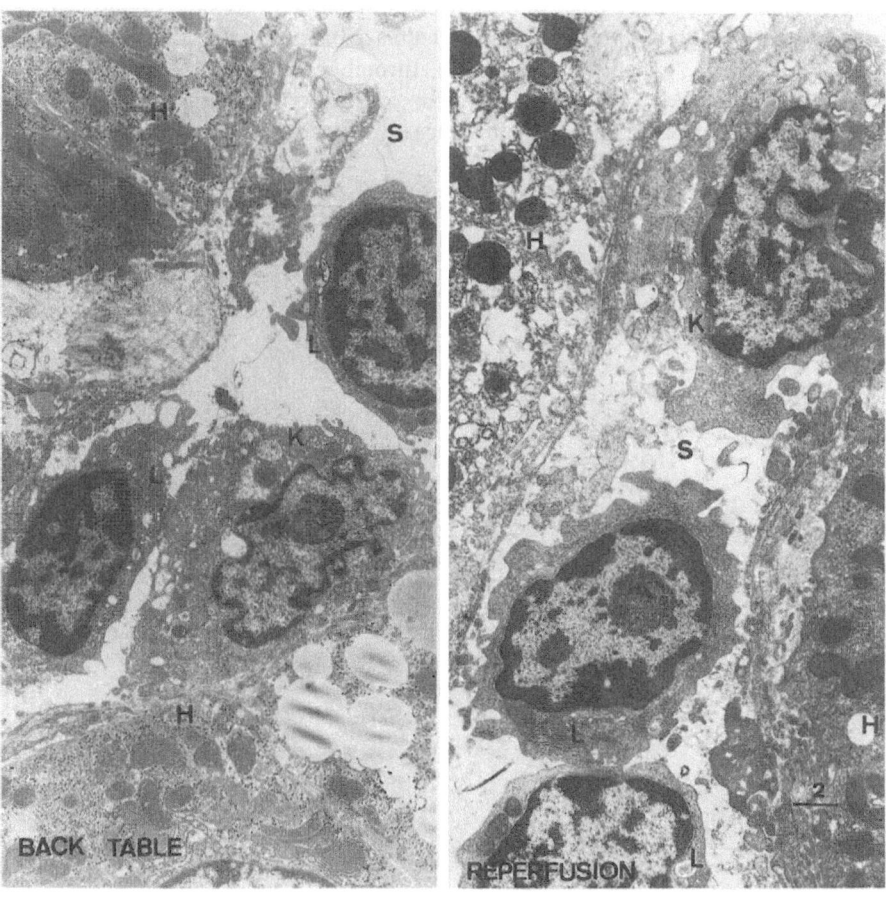

FIG. 6. Cellular adhesion in the simusoidal wall. In the sinusoidal space (S), activated Kupffer cells (K) and lymphocytes (L) were distributed in close contact, and degenerative changes such as mild bleb formation were observed in the sinusoidal endothelial cells in both back-table biopsy (*left panel*) and reperfusion biopsy (*right panel*). H, hepatocyte

protein of the basement membrane [22, 23], was detected in the sinusoidal walls in six patients (33%). These proportions corresponded to the degree of basement membrane formation in both the back-table and reperfusion biopsies. These results support the theory that hepatic sinusoidal capillarization occurs after ischemia/ reperfusion injury.

## Cellular Adhesion in the Sinusoidal Wall (Fig. 6)

We suspect that translocation of bacterial cell wall products across the gut mucosa [24], which occurs frequently in cadaveric donors, may produce lipopolysaccharides. These lipopolysaccharides are powerful stimulants of Kupffer cell activation, releasing tumor necrosis factor (TNF)-$\alpha$. TNF-$\alpha$ expression and synthesis of intercellular adhesion molecules increased after reperfusion. Increased expression of intercellular adhesion molecules (ICAMs) indicates an enhanced capacity for adhesion between lymphocytes (Fig. 7), neutrophils (Fig. 8), thrombocytes (Fig. 6), and sinusoidal endothelial cells [25]. Such adhesion leads to phenotypic changes in sinusoidal endothelial cells and promotes disturbance of the microcirculation in the both sinusoids and the space of Disse.

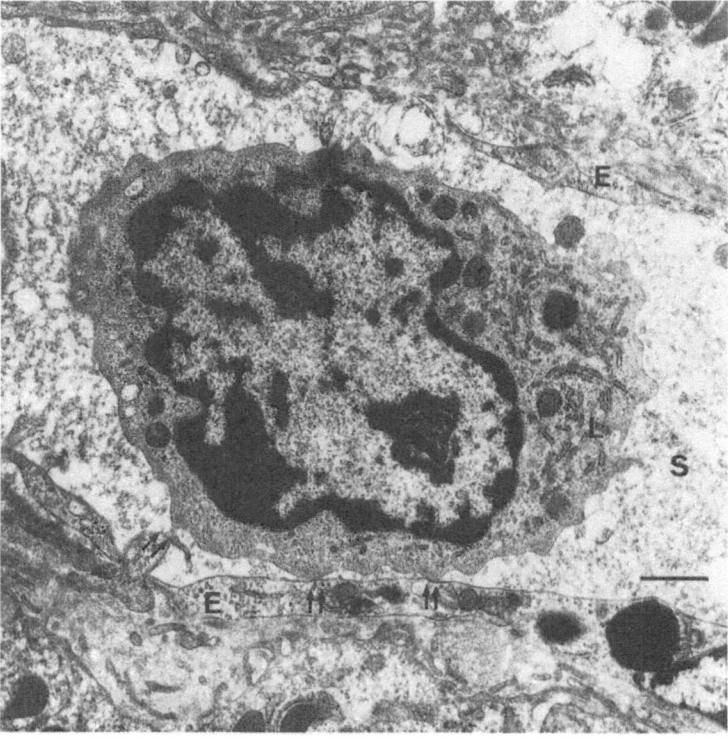

FIG. 7. A lymphocyte (L) attaches to a sinusoidal endothelial cell (E) with point attachment (*double arrow*) in reperfusion biopsy. S, sinusoidal space

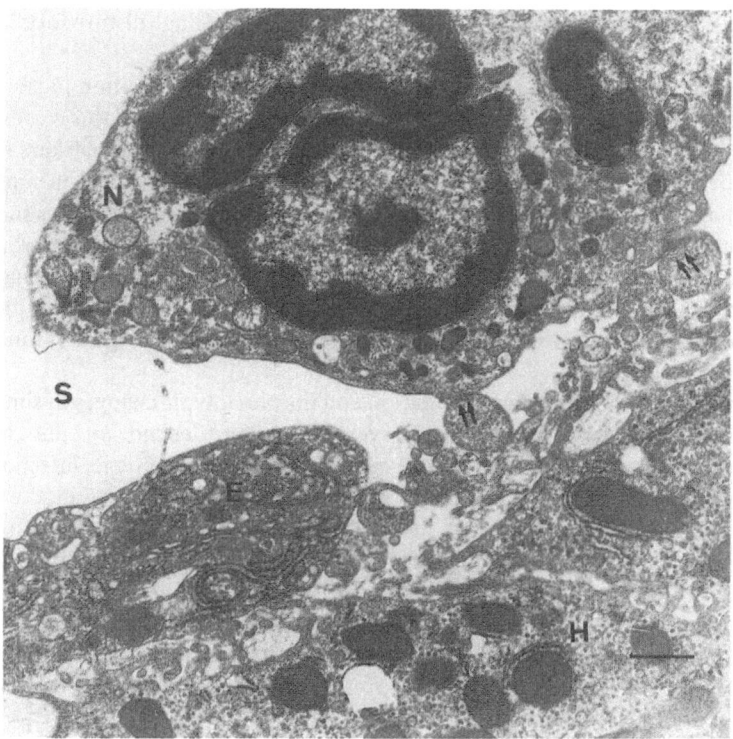

FIG. 8. A neutrophile (*N*) attaches to degenerated sinusoidal endothelial cells (*E*) in the sinusoidal space (*S*). Arrows, attachment site; *H*, hepatocyte

Our observations revealed interactions between inflammatory cells and sinusoidal endothelial cells. Degenerative changes such as mild bleb formation were observed in the sinusoidal endothelial cells that interacted and stuck to these inflammatory cells. An immunohistochemical study demonstrated positive staining for CD54 in the sinusoidal walls in seven of the 11 patients with ischemia/reperfusion injury, and staining on the hepatocyte surface in four of the 11.

## Discussion

During storage in cold UW solution [26], both hepatocyte and sinusoidal cells were injured in the cold fluid and ischemic situation, leading to preservation injury. Bleb formation in hepatocytes and some rounding of both Kupffer cells and sinusoidal endothelial cells occurred during the preservation period. After reperfusion of the blood supply, sinusoidal endothelial cells lose their viability, and positive staining for markers of capillary endothelial cells occurs with basement membrane formation. Kupffer cells swell, ruffle, and degranulate, releasing a number of inflammatory mediators, cytokines, and superoxide radicals. In spite of the changes in the sinusoidal cells, hepatocyte structure recovers after reperfusion.

Activated Kupffer cells and sinusoidal endothelial cells with phenotypic changes were able to interact with inflammatory cells, producing disturbance of the microcirculation.

After reperfusion, the up-regulation of type IV collagen and laminin in sinusoidal endothelial cells reflects the formation of basement membranes, and this corresponds with the loss of OKM-5 and the acquisition of capillary endothelial markers (Factor VIII-related antigen and UEA-1). Phenotypic and morphologic changes in sinusoidal endothelial cells occur within 12 h after harvesting of the donor liver. This indicates that sinusoidal capillarization during reperfusion might be due to cytoprotection under cold and ischemic conditions. In general, basement membrane formation is observed in liver cirrhosis and alcoholic liver damage, and these diseases progress toward a terminal state. However, reperfused liver did not progress to a nonfunctional state in our study.

Whether basement membrane formation and the phenotypic changes in sinusoidal endothelial cells are reversible or irreversible might depend on the dose of immunosuppressant administered, the grade of any opportunistic infection, the degree of any fatty changes in the donor's liver, the initiation of rejection, the degree of activation of Kuppfer cells, and the disturbance of the microcirculation in the sinusoids. In fact, excessive expression of both type IV collagen and laminin has been detected in the sinusoidal walls in livers that failed due to primary nonfunction [27]. It is still unclear how the reversibility of sinusoidal endothelial cell damage is regulated. Further studies will need to be carried out to address this question in the light of the development of more extensive preservation solutions containing calcium blockers, pentoxifylline and antioxidants.

## References

1. Belle SH, Beringer KC, Detre KM (1997) Recent findings concerning liver transplantation in the United States. In: Cecka JM, Terasaki PI (eds) Clinical transplants 1996. UCLA Tissue Typing Laboratory, Los Angeles, pp 15–29
2. Ploeg RJ, D'Alessandro AM, Knechtle SJ, et al. (1993) Risk factors for primary dysfunction after liver transplantation—A multivariate analysis. Transplantation 55:807–813
3. Greig PD, Woolf GM, Sinclair SM, et al. (1989) Treatment of primary liver graft nonfunction with prostaglandin E1. Transplantation 48:447–453
4. Furukawa H, Todo S, Imventarza O, et al. (1991) Effect of cold ischemia time on the early outcome of human hepatic allografts preserved with UW solution. Transplantation 51:1000–1004
5. Doyle HR, Morelli F, McMichael J, et al. (1996) Hepatic retransplantation. Analysis of risk factors associated with outcome. Transplantation 61:1499–1505
6. Wisse E, De Zanger RB, Charels K, et al. (1985) The liver sieve: Considerations concerning the structure and function of endothelial fenestrae, the sinusoidal wall and the space of Disse. Hepatology 5:683–692
7. Schaffner F, Popper H (1963) Capillarization of hepatic sinusoids in man. Gastroenterology 44:239–242
8. Ichida T, Hata K, Yamada S, et al. (1990) Subcellular abnormalities of liver sinusoidal lesions in human hepatocellular carcinoma. J Submicrosc Pathol 22:221–229
9. Taguchi K, Asano G (1988) Neovascularization of pericellular fibrosis in alcoholic liver disease. Acta Pathol Jpn 38:615–626
10. Weibel ER, Palade GE (1964) New cytoplasmic components in arterial endothelia. J Cell Biol 23:101–112

11. Nagura H, Koshizawa T, Fukuda Y, et al. (1988) Hepatic vascular endothelial cells heterogeneously express surface antigens associated with monocyte, macrophages and T lymphocytes. Virchow Arch (Pathol Anat) 409:407–416

12. Ichida T, Hata K, Yamada S, et al. (1991) Alteration of liver sinusoidal endothelial cells in liver diseases. In: Tsuchiya M (ed) Frontiers of mucosal immunology. Elsevier, Amsterdam, pp 201–204.

13. Hoyler LW, De Los Santos PR, Hoyer JR (1973) Antihemophilic factor antigen: Localization in endothelial cells by immunofluorescent microscopy. J Clin Invest 52:2737–2744

14. Petrovic LM, Burrough A, Scheuer PJ (1989) Hepatic sinusoidal endothelium: *Ulex* lectin binding. Histopathology 14:233–243

15. Ichida T, Sugitani S, Satoh T, et al. (1996) Localization of hyaluronan in human liver sinusoids: A histochemical study using hyaluronan-binding protein. Liver 16:365–371

16. Caldwell-Kenkel JC, Thurman RG, Lemasters JJ (1988) Selective loss of non-parenchymal cell viability after cold ischemic storage of rat livers. Transplantation 45:834–837

17. McKeown CMB, Edwards V, Phillips MJ, et al. (1988) Sinusoidal lining cell damage: The critical injury in cold preservation of liver allografts in the rat. Transplantation 46:178–182

18. Momii S, Koga A (1990) Time-related morphological changes in cold-stored rat livers. Transplantation 50:745–750

19. Clavien PA, Harvey PRC, Strasberg SM (1992) Preservation and reperfusion injuries in liver allografts. Transplantation 53:957–978

20. Lemasters JL, Thurman RG (1997) Reperfusion injury after liver preservation for transplantation. Annu Rev Pharmacol Toxicol 37:327–338

21. Noguchi K, Sakisaka S, Tanikawa K (1989) Morphological and functional characteristics of activated Kupffer cell. In: Wisse E, Knook DL, Decker K (eds) Cells of the hepatic sinusoids. vol 2. Kupffer Cell Foundation, The Netherlands, pp 147–148

22. Hahn E, Wick G, Pencev D, et al. (1980) Distribution of basement membrane proteins in normal and fibrotic human liver: Collagen type IV, laminin and fibronectin. Gut 21:63–71

23. Martinez-Hernandez A (1985) The hepatic extracellular matrix. II. Electron immunohistochemical studies in rats with $CCL_4$-induced cirrhosis. Lab Invest 53:166–186

24. Van Goor H, Rosman C, Grond J, et al. (1994) Translocation of bacteria and endotoxin in organ donors. Arch Surg 129:1063–1066

25. Takei Y, Gao W, Hijioka T, et al. (1991) Increase in survival of liver grafts after rinsing with warm Ringer's solution due to improvement of hepatic microcirculation. Transplantation 52:225–230

26. Todo S, Nery J, Yanaga K, et al. (1989) Extended preservation of human liver grafts with UW solution. JAMA 261:711–714

27. Noguchi K, Iwaki Y, Kobayashi M, et al. (1993) Capillarization of the hepatic sinusoid in failed liver graft. In: Knook DL, Wisse E (eds) Cells of the hepatic sinusoids. vol 4. Kupffer Cell Foundation, The Netherlands, pp 362–364

# Ultrastructural and Functional Alteration in Hepatic Sinusoidal Cells in Cold-Preserved Rat Liver

S. Arii, M. Niwano, Y. Takeda, T. Moriga, A. Mori, K. Hanaki, and M. Imamura

*Summary.* Tissue damage during cold preservation of a liver graft is a crucial problem in attempts to obtain better results in liver transplantation. This chapter describes the morphological and functional changes in sinusoidal endothelial cells (SEC), Kupffer cells, and those of fatty liver during cold preservation. We found apoptotic changes in SEC in cold-preserved liver, which seem to be one of the causative mechanisms of damage, in addition to the participation of activated Kupffer cells as described below. An enhancement of TNF-$\alpha$-producing activity and asialo GM-1 expression was also observed, indicating Kupffer cell activation. In an experiment using $GdCl_3$, a potent inhibitor of Kupffer cell function, activated Kupffer cells were found to be strongly involved in SEC injury. This ultrastructural study with both SEM and TEM showed a prominent string-like appearance and detachment of the SEC processes after 24 h preservation, whereas the SEC was better preserved in the $GdCl_3$-pretreated group. A study with microvascular casting also revealed that $GdCl_3$ contributed to the maintenance of SEC compared with the corresponding control, which showed an impairment in the radial arrangement and discontinuity of the sinusoid. These morphological changes may have a causative role in the microcirculatory disturbances in the liver, possibly inducing primary nonfunctioning graft. Furthermore, we clarified that SECs in fatty liver were very fragile and were progressively destroyed. Interestingly, we also found that fatty droplets expanded with an increase in the length of cold preservation.

*Key words.* Ultrastructure, Hepatic sinusoidal cells, Fatty liver, Apoptosis, Cold preservation

## Introduction

Liver transplantation was established as a treatment for end-stage liver disease in the 1980s. However, several problems remain to be resolved in order to obtain better results. Crucial among current issues is tissue damage during cold preservation [1, 2].

First Department of Surgery, Kyoto University, School of Medicine, 54 Kawara-cho, Shogoin, Sakyo-ku, Kyoto 606-8507, Japan

Recently, much attention has been directed toward the pathogenetic role of hepatic sinusoidal cells in this type of injury.

In this chapter, we describe the morphological and functional changes in hepatic sinusoidal cells, most notably endothelial cells and Kupffer cells, during cold preservation of liver tissue, and we then clarify the preventive role of Kupffer cell blockade on simusoidal endothelial injury.

Furthermore, considering the shortage of donor livers, it is a serious waste to discard fatty liver grafts because of the high risk of primary nonfunction [3, 4]. We therefore also report our ultrastructural observations of cold-preserved fatty liver, which indicate rapid and severe changes in both hepatocytes and sinusoidal endothelial cells.

## SEC (Sinusoidal Endothelial Cell)

Although the exact mechanism of cold-preservation injury is still unknown, recent investigations have shown that sinusoidal endothelial damage precedes parenchymal injury. McKowen et al. [1] showed that sinusoidal endothelial cells became progressively more damaged during cold preservation, whereas parenchymal cells maintained a relatively normal appearance. To describe these changes in detail, they demonstrated that sinusoidal endothelial cells degenerated and partially disappeared after 4 h cold preservation in 0.9% NaCl and 2 mmol/l $CaCl_2$. The injury is still reversible at this point, but after 8 h cold preservation the endothelial cells had almost completely disappeared. Hepatic parenchymal cells, however, maintained an almost normal appearance, although slight bleb formation was observed. After 4 h cold preservation in Euro-Collins solution, a sieve plate of endothelial cells exhibited mesh-like degeneration and the cell cytoplasmas were swollen. After 8 h preservation, sieve

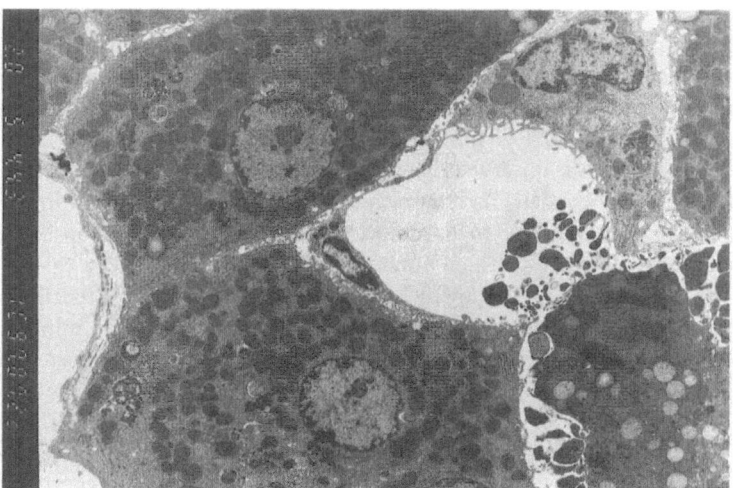

Fig. 1. Transmission electron micrograph (TEM) of a 24-h cold-preserved liver. Apoptotic changes were seen in SECs

plates were completely destroyed, and endothelial cells were detached from the sinusoidal wall.

However, the causative mechanism of SEC injury remains to be resolved. As mentioned above, Kupffer cell activation, by which tissue-toxic mediators were massively secreted, is probably involved in this injury. In addition to the participation of Kupffer cells, we found apoptotic changes in SECs in cold-preserved liver tissue, as shown in Fig. 1.

Therefore, not only Kupffer cell blockade but also suppression of apoptosis in SECs may be possible new strategies to avoid hepatic injury during cold preservation.

## Kupffer Cells

Some morphological studies have demonstrated the activation of Kupffer cells during cold preservation. Caldwell-Kenkel et al. [2] revealed rounding, ruffling, polarization, vacuolization, degranulation, and an appearance like dense worm holes in their electron microscope observations, and concluded that Kupffer cells were activated. Based on this evidence, we studied the function of Kupffer cells in cold preservation. It was found that cold preservation enhanced TNF-$\alpha$ producing activity in Kupffer cells, and an increased expression of asialo GM-1 antigen was also demonstrated [5].

### Involvement of Kupffer Cells in Sinusoidal Endothelial Injury During Cold Preservation/Reperfusion

As mentioned earlier, sinusoidal endothelial damage precedes parenchymal injury. The activation of Kupffer cells has been shown to be closely involved in the pathogenesis of SEC injury. Kupffer cells are known to produce monokines, oxygen radicals, proteases, prostanoids, and other mediators, as well as to have phagocytic ability. Therefore, the activation of Kupffer cells in cold preservation with subsequent reperfusion may stimulate the release of a large quantity of tissue-toxic mediators, which lead to sinusoidal endothelial injury or malfunction. We have already reported that the expression of TNF-$\alpha$ mRNA increased in cold-preserved liver, and that further enhancement was observed following reperfusion. We also demonstrated that anti-TNF-$\alpha$ antibody partially but significantly ameliorated reperfusion injury.

Based on these findings, we focused on the ultrastructure of SECs in cold-stored liver tissue pretreated with $GdCl_3$, a potent Kupffer cell inhibitor. The exact mechanism of the effect of $GdCl_3$ on Kupffer cells has yet to be resolved. Husztik et al. [6] suggested that $GdCl_3$ blocked the phagocytosis of Kupffer cells by inhibiting the surface attachment phase. Koudstaal et al. [7] speculated that $GdCl_3$ injected intravenously forms aggregates at neutral pH in the blood stream which are taken up by Kupffer cells. Subsequently, the colloidal particles dissolve again at pH 5.0 in the endosomal–lysosomal compartment of the cell and attach to the components of this compartment. This recycling of $GdCl_3$ probably leads to cellular disintegration. As for the hepatic toxicity of $GdCl_3$, no significant change in ultrastructural morphology was seen, although $GdCl_3$-injected rats exhibited a slight elevation in serum transaminase level.

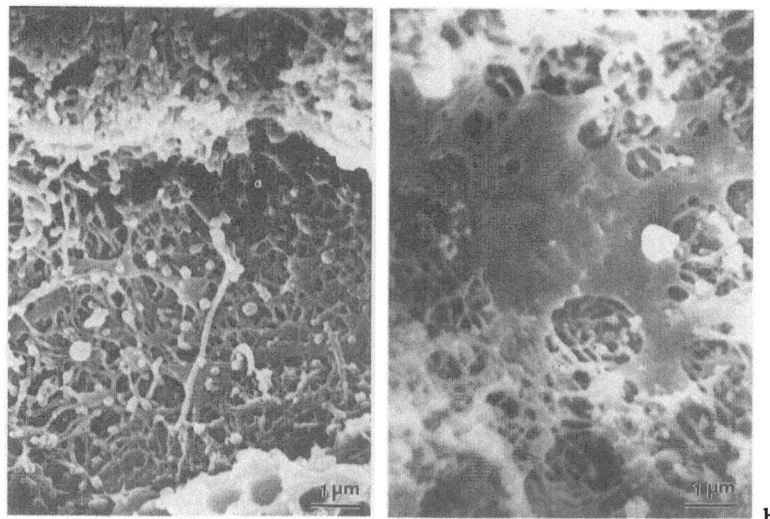

FIG. 2. Scanning electron micrograph (SEM) of a hepatic sinusoid of a 24-h cold-preserved liver. **a** Control; **b** with GdCl$_3$-pretreatment

Morphological studies on SECs after 24 h preservation showed a prominent string-like appearance of the processes in the control group, whereas the SECs were better preserved in the GdCl$_3$-pretreated group (Fig. 2). Furthermore, after 36 h preservation, the sinusoid frame was destroyed and the microvilli of the hepatocytes had disappeared in the control group, whereas the SEC processes and the microvilli of the hepatocytes were preserved in the GdCl$_3$-pretreated group. A TEM study after 24 h preservation revealed detachment of the sinusoidal epithelia in the control group; in contrast, this change was observed only slightly in the GdCl$_3$-pretreated group (Fig. 3).

Studies of the control group using microvascular casting showed impairment in the radial arrangement of the sinusoids and significant dilatation of the sinusoidal caliber after 24 h preservation, and a discontinuity of the sinusoids with nonfilling and extravasation of the casting material after 36 h preservation (Figs. 4 and 5). These changes were not seen in the GdCl$_3$-pretreated group. These studies therefore showed that Kupffer cells were strongly involved in the morphological integrity of SECs and sinusoids [8].

Leucocyte adhesion to SECs may also have a causative role in reperfusion injury. We therefore studied the expression of the adhesion molecule ICAM-1 on cold-preserved SECs [9]. SECs were isolated from cold-preserved liver using an elutriation rotor, and the expression of ICAM-1 was determined using a flow cytometer. ICAM-1 was found to be strongly enhanced during cold preservation. An ex-vivo reperfusion experiment using liver tissue and a leucocyte suspension found that coincident with the enhancement of ICAM-1 expression, there was an increase in the number of accumulated leucocytes. Interestingly, both ICAM-1 expression and leucocyte accumulation were strongly suppressed to nearly normal levels by pretreatment not only

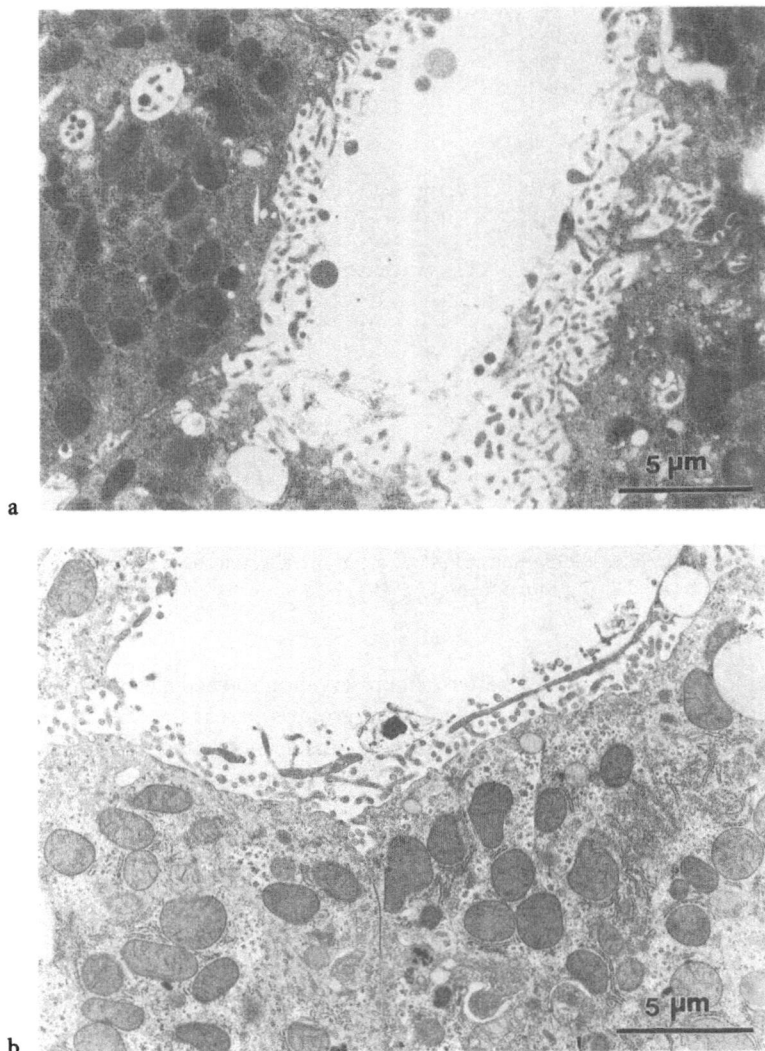

FIG. 3. TEM of 24-h cold-preserved liver. **a** Control; **b** with GdCl₃-pretreatment

with anti-ICAM-1 antibody, but also with GdCl₃. Furthermore, glutamate oxaloacetate transaminase and lactate dehydrogenase levels in the perfusate were significantly reduced in association with the suppression of leucocyte accumulation. Scanning electron microscopy showed that in cold-preserved liver following GdCl₃ pretreatment, the SECs showed an almost normal structure concomitant with the adherence of relatively few leucocytes. In tissue without GdCl₃ pretreatment, the sinusoidal structure was destroyed and a massive accumulation of leucocytes was noted. These findings imply that communication occurs between Kupffer cells and SECs in the

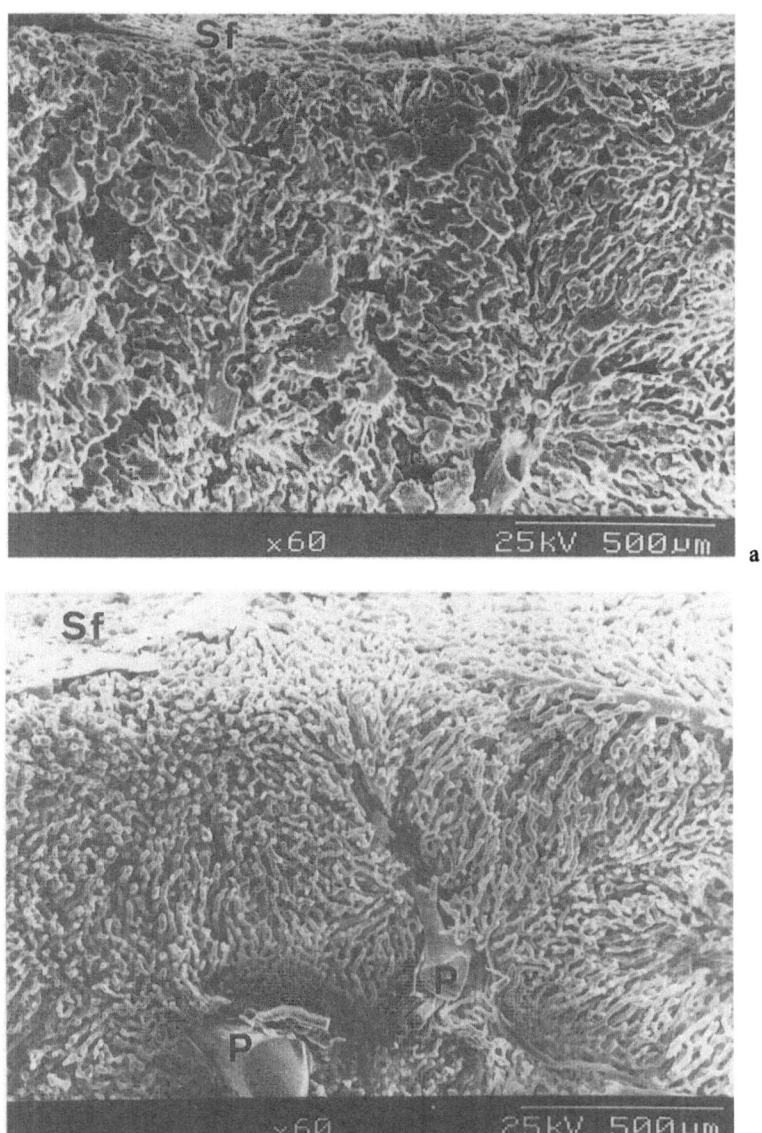

FIG. 4. Vascular casting of a hepatic sinusoid of 24-h cold-preserved liver. **a** Control; **b** with GdCl$_3$-pretreatment. *Sf*, superficial area; *P*, portal vein. *Arrows* indicate a leakage of resin

hepatic sinusoid through cytokines such as TNF-$\alpha$ and interleukin-1 secreted by Kupffer cells, because these cytokines enhance ICAM-1 expression on the vascular endothelium. Leukocyte adherence to the sinusoidal endothelium would probably disturb sinusoidal microcirculation. Furthermore, leucocytes release oxygen radicals, collagenase, elastase, and other factors, all of which may result in tissue damage.

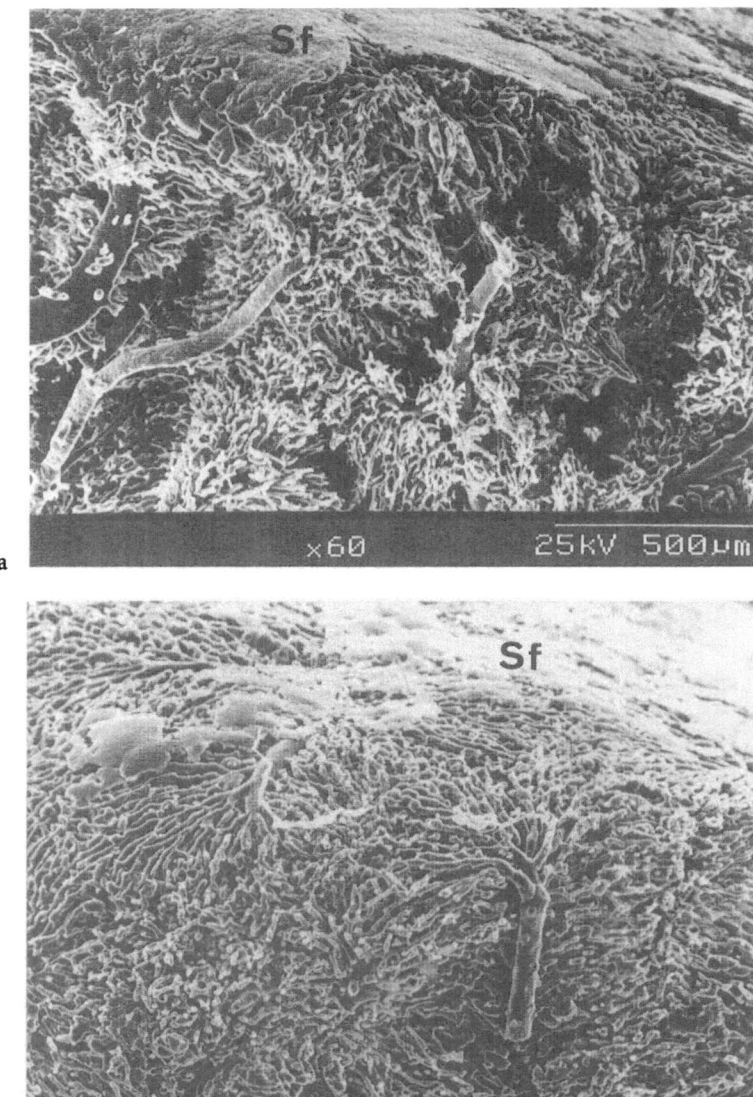

FIG. 5. Vascular casting of a hepatic sinusoid of 36-h cold-preserved liver. **a** Control; **b** with GdCl₃-pretreatment. *Sf,* superficial area

## Fatty Liver

We used fatty livers from male Wistar rats weighing 200–250 g body weight which were fed a choline-deficient diet. The fatty droplets in hepatocytes expanded during cold preservation in a time-dependent manner, and oppressed intracellular organelles to the cellular margin during 24 h cold preservation. Furthermore, the

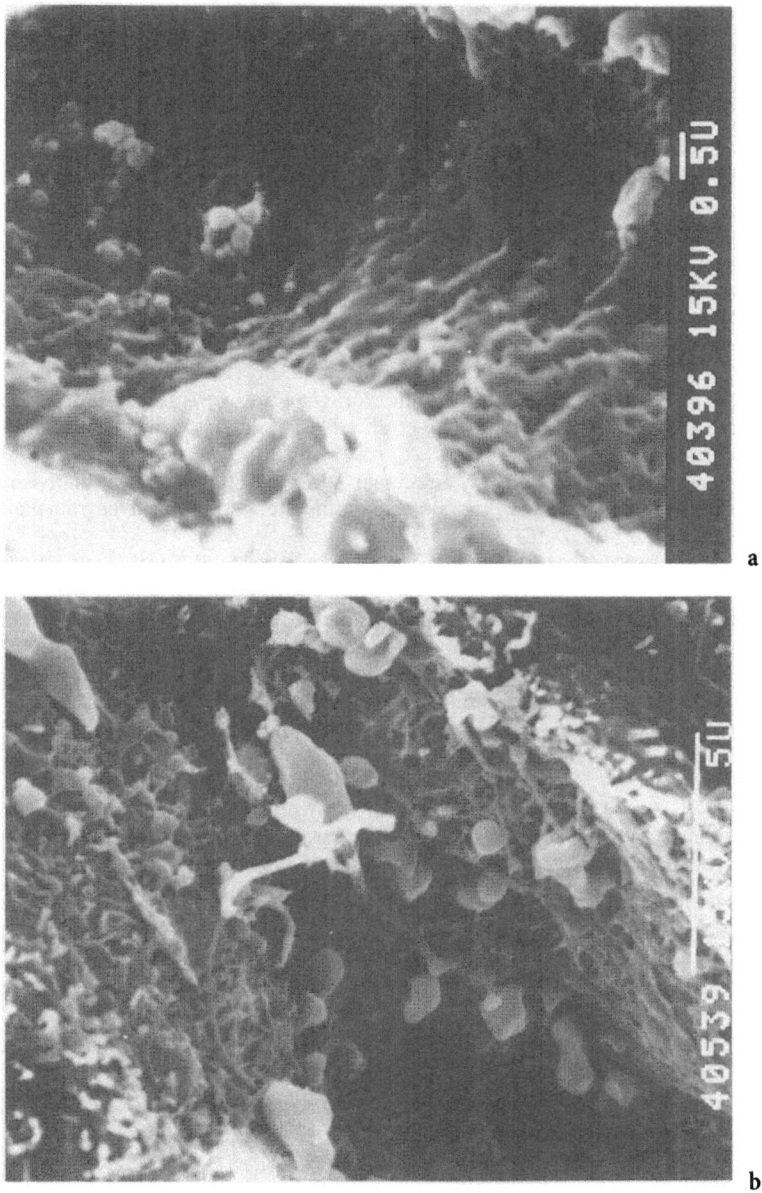

FIG. 6. SEM of a hepatic sinusoid of 4-h cold-preserved fatty liver. a Nonfatty liver; b fatty liver

expansion of fatty droplets appeared to cause a disarrangement in the sinusoidal architecture and a narrowness of the sinusoidal caliber.

SECs were more vulnerable in fatty liver than in nonfatty liver, even without cold preservation. In 4-h cold preservation of nonfatty liver, SECs were slightly damaged and a few gaps were seen which resulted from the fusion of fenestrae, microvilli originating from hepatocytes, and blebs detached from the tips of microvilli. However, SECs in fatty liver exhibited a string-like appearance with an increase in blebs and enlarged gaps (Fig. 6). Thus, SECs in cold-preserved fatty liver were considered to be more fragile than those in nonfatty liver. These changes may be closely associated with microcirculatory disturbances, which could possibly lead to primary nonfunction of a fatty liver graft, although further studies are needed to resolve the precise mechanism which accounts for cold-preservation injury of fatty liver.

## References

1. McKowen CMB, Edwards V, Phillips MJ, et al. (1988) Sinusoidal lining cell damage: the critical injury in cold preservation of liver allografts in the rat. Transplantation 46:178–191
2. Caldwell-Kenkel JC, Currin RT, Tanaka Y, et al. (1989) Reperfusion injury to endothelial cells following cold ischemic storage of rat livers. Hepatology 10:292–299
3. Teramoto K, Bowers JL, Khettry U, et al. (1993) A rat fatty liver transplant model. Transplantation 55:737–741
4. D'alessandro AM, Kaloyogln M, Sollingehr W, et al. (1991) The predictive value of donor liver biopsies for the primary nonfunction after orthotopic liver transplantation. Transplantation 51:157–163
5. Arii S, Monden K, Adachi Y, et al. (1994) Pathogenic role of Kupffer cell activation on the reperfusion injury of cold-preserved liver. Transplantation 58:1072–1077
6. Husztik E, Lazar G, Parducz A (1980) Electron microscopic study of Kupffer cell phagocytosis blockade induced by gadolinium chloride. Br J Exp Pathol 61:624–630
7. Koudstaal J, Dijkhuis FWJ, Hardonk MJ (1991) Selective depletion of Kupffer cells after intravenous injection of gadolinium chloride. Cells of the hepatic sinusoid, vol 3. p 58
8. Niwano M, Arii S, MondenK, et al. (1997) Amelioration of sinusoidal endothelial cell damage by Kupffer cell blockade during cold preservation of rat liver. J Surg Res 72:36–48
9. Monden K, Arii S, Ishiguro S, et al. (1995) Involvement of ICAM-1 expression on sinusoidal endothelial cell and neutrophil adherence of the reperfusion injury of cold-preserved liver. Transplant Proc 27:759–761

# Cholestasis and Hepatic Sinusoidal Cells

Kazunori Noguchi, K. Sasatomi, Ryukichi Kumashiro,
T. Kawahara, Shotaro Sakisaka, Michio Sata,
and Kyuichi Tanikawa

*Summary.* The aim of this study was to evaluate the morphological and functional changes in Kupffer cells and sinusoidal endothelial cells in cholestasis. Under an electron microscope, Kupffer cells in cholestasis were seen to be markedly enlarged and contained electron-dense material and distorted mitochondria. A clinical clearance study with chondroitin sulfated iron showed that the endocytic function of the Kupffer cells was significantly reduced in the cholestatic condition. In an in vitro study, the endocytic function of cultured Kupffer cells was decreased by two kinds of bile acid, taurochenodeoxycholate and taurocholate. However, tauroursodeoxycholate did not affect the endocytic activity of Kupffer cells.

With immunohistological staining, lipid A was clearly observed in the endotoxin in Kupffer cells from a normal rat, but it was scarcely detectable in the Kupffer cells from a cholestatic rat. The expression of the membrane CD14 on the Kupffer cells was sparse in a cholestatic patient compared with that in a control patient. ICAM-1 was markedly expressed on the sinusoidal endothelial cells of a cholestatic rat model. These findings suggested that the endocytic function of the Kupffer cells seems to be impaired by the application of bile acids to the plasma membrane and by a reduction in cell activity resulting from a low expression of membrane CD14. Furthermore, the function of sinusoidal endothelial cells seems to be altered in association with Kupffer cell dysfunction. These results support the theory that cholestatic patients have an increased risk of sepsis and endotoxemia, with potential morbidity and mortality.

*Key words.* Cholestasis, Kupffer cell, Sinusoidal endothelial cell, Endotoxin, Primary biliary cirrhosis

## Kupffer Cell Function in Cholestasis

Kupffer cells are mononuclear cells resident in the hepatic sinusoid. They are strategically situated at the confluence of portal venous drainage and bear the major responsibility for sequestering and eliminating foreign bodies delivered from the gut

The Second Department of Internal Medicine, Kurume University School of Medicine, 67 Asahimachi, Kurume, Fukuoka 830-0011, Japan

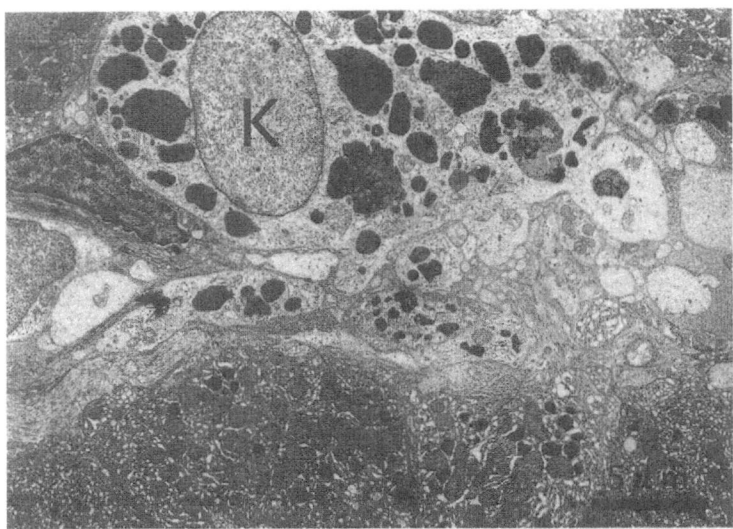

FIG. 1. Electron micrograph of a Kupffer cell (*K*) from a patient with obstructive jaundice. The Kupffer cell is markedly enlarged with a flattened cell membrane, and contains electron-dense material and distorted mitochondria in the cytoplasm

into the portal circulation. Kupffer cells are the major component of the reticuloendothelial system (RES), and have a key role in the defense mechanisms of a living being. Cholestasis accompanies an accumulation of bile constituents such as bile material, cellular debris, and abundant lysosomes in the blood. A decrease in the secretion of bile acids and immunoglobulin A from the liver to the intestine may allow excessive growth of enteric bacterial flora and increased production of endogenous endotoxin. It has been reported that the intestinal absorption of endotoxin is increased because of the permeability of the intestinal mucosa in cholestatic conditions [1]. Therefore, in cholestasis the Kupffer cells would have to handle greater amounts of bile constituents, bacteria, and endotoxins than in a normal state.

## Morphological Aspects of Kupffer Cells in Cholestasis

Electron microscopy shows that Kupffer cells in patients with obstructive jaundice are markedly enlarged, with a flattened cell membrane, and contain electron-dense material and distorted mitochondria (Fig. 1). This suggests that the dysfunction of the Kupffer cells in cholestasis results morphologically from an overload, which is led by endocytosis of a large amount of foreign materials in the hepatic sinusoidal circulation.

## Clearance Activity of Kupffer Cells in Cholestasis

In clinical study, the colloidal chondroitin sulfated iron (CSFe) clearance test was used to evaluate the endocytic function of Kupffer cells in patients with extrahepatic ob-

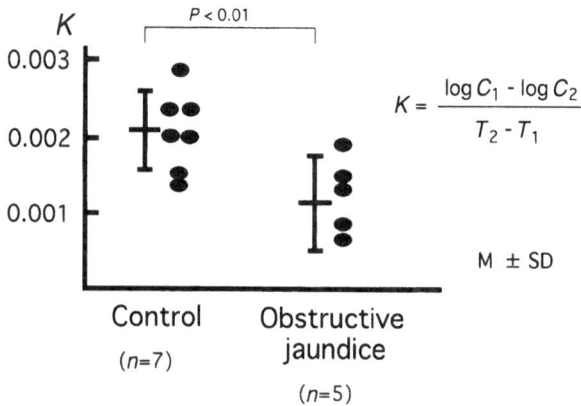

FIG. 2. Colloidal chondroitin sulfated iron (CSFe) clearance in patients with obstructive jaundice compared with controls. The clearance rate $(K)$ is significantly low in patients with obstructive jaundice. $T_1$ and $T_2$ indicate the time after CSFe injection of 2 mg/kg body weight. $C_1$ and $C_2$ represent the serum concentration of iron at times $T_1$ and $T_2$

structive jaundice. CSFe was injected into the antecubital vein at a dose of 2 mg/kg body weight in the early morning. Five and 20 min after injection, the concentration of serum iron was determined and the clearance rate was calculated. Seven healthy subjects served as controls. The clearance rate $(K)$ of CSFe in patients with obstructive jaundice was 0.0011 ± 0.0005 (mean ± SD), and was significantly lower than that of healthy controls (0.0023 ± 0.00075), as shown in Fig. 2. This clinical study clearly showed that Kupffer cells are functionally altered in the cholestatic condition.

It has also been reported that cultured Kupffer cells isolated from rats with bile duct ligation showed a change in receptor-mediated endocytic function [2]. These cultured cells showed that distribution of Fc receptor on the plasma surface of the Kupffer cell became sparse in cholestatic rat compared to the control one [2]. The effect of bile acid on the endocytosis of Kupffer cells was tested by adding three kinds of taurin-conjugated bile acids to the culture medium. Taurochenodeoxycholate (TCDCA), taurocholate (TCA), and tauroursodeoxycholate (TUDCA) were added to the culture medium of Kupffer cells isolated from normal rats in a final concentration of 500 μm/l. After preincubation with each bile acid for 30 min, an endocytosis study was performed using CSFe. The results indicated that certain bile acids added into the culture medium cause a reduction in the endocytosis of CSFe by Kupffer cells (Fig. 3). Taurochenodeoxycholate at 500 μm/l caused a reduction in endocytosis of more than 50%. Taurocholate also depressed endocytosis significantly, but tauroursodeoxycholate did not impair the endocytic activities of Kupffer cells. Bile acids which accumulate in the serum in cholestasis are known to have a direct effect on the cell membrane [3]. The plasma membrane of Kupffer cells is exposed to the relatively higher levels of bile acid during long-term cholestasis. The cleansing properties of bile acids vary with the number and site of the hydroxyl groups and the form of conjugation [3]. Generally, the cleansing property becomes stronger when the number of hydroxyl groups decreases. Depression of endocytosis was more evident

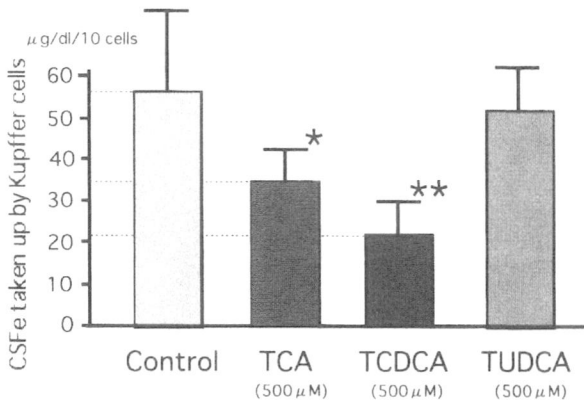

FIG. 3. Effect of bile acids on the endocytosis of colloidal iron by cultured Kupffer cells isolated from a normal rat. Endocytosis of colloidal iron was inhibited by taurochenodeoxycholate (*TCDCA*) and taurocholate (*TCA*), but not by tauroursodeoxycholate (*TUDCA*). All data are presented as mean ± SD. *$P < 0.05$; **$P < 0.01$

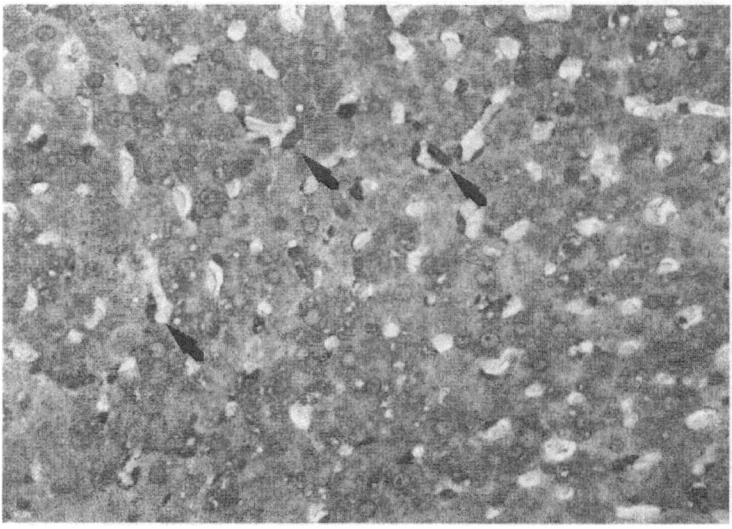

FIG. 4. Light micrography of the distribution of endotoxin lipid A in the hepatic sinusoid of a control rat 5 min after injection of 0.5 mg lipopolysaccharide into the portal vein. Immunohistological staining with an anti-lipid A antibody shows that Kupffer cells (*arrows*) contain endotoxin lipid A in their cytoplasm. ×400

with TCDCA and TCA in this study. These two bile acids are the dominant ones in cholestatic serum. Although ursodeoxycholate has less effect than other bile acids, it is a minor fraction in the serum. If the percentage of ursodeoxycholate in the serum became high, the more active bile acids would be replaced and the membrane damage might be reduced [4].

## Endotoxin Clearance by Kupffer Cells in Cholestasis

The initial uptake of endotoxin by the liver is mediated by the Kupffer cells [5]. Most studies have indicated that endotoxin uptake in Kupffer cells is not receptor-mediated [6]. Endotoxin is derived from the gut and is a normal constituent of portal venous plasma. However, systemic endotoxemia occurs in 25%–85% of patients with obstructive jaundice [7, 8]. Therefore, an experimental study was performed to estimate the endotoxin uptake by Kupffer cells in control rats with a sham operation and in cholestatic rats with bile duct ligation for 7 days. Liver specimens were obtained from rats 5 min after the injection of 0.5 mg lipopolysaccharide (LPS) into the portal vein. The distribution of endotoxin in the liver was examined by light and confocal laser scanning microscopy with immunohistological staining using a murine anti-lipid A monoclonal IgM antibody (supplied by Pfizer Pharmaceuticals Inc., New York) as the primary antibody against LPS and a biotinylated or FITC-conjugated anti-mouse IgM antibody as the secondary antibody. Lipid A, an important part of endotoxin, was clearly detected in the cytoplasm of Kupffer cells of control rats under both a light microscope (Fig. 4) and a confocal laser microscope (Fig. 5a). However, endotoxin lipid A was scarce in Kupffer cells in cholestatic rats (Fig. 5b). These findings suggest that Kupffer cells in cholestasis may have a decreased ability to clear endotoxin from portal blood, and jaundiced patients with long-term cholestasis have an increased risk of systemic endotoxemia or Gram-negative sepsis, with potential morbidity and mortality [9–13].

## Reduced Activation of Kupffer Cells in Cholestasis

Membrane CD14 has been identified as a receptor which promotes the cell activation system of peritoneal macrophages and monocytic cells [14]. This protein is one of the binding proteins for endotoxin complexes with septin or lipopolysaccharide-binding protein [15, 16]. Therefore, the expression of membrane CD14 on Kupffer cells was studied using a human liver specimen biopsied operatively from a patient with obstructive jaundice. The localization of CD14 on the Kupffer cells was examined by confocal laser scanning microscopy with immunohistological staining using an anti-CD14 antibody and a FITC-conjugated antibody. A biopsied liver specimen from a patient with non-active HCV hepatitis served as the control. Confocal laser microscopic analysis showed that the membrane CD14 of Kupffer cells in a cholestatic patient was sparsely expressed compared with that in the control patient (Fig. 6).

Activation of the Kupffer cells by endotoxin or its complexes is probably a physiological phenomenon because a small amount of endotoxin is derived from the gut every time a meal is taken. Our study indicates that most Kupffer cells in a cholestatic condition could not express CD14 on the cell membrane and could not promote their own activity. This would probably result in a cytokine network centering around the

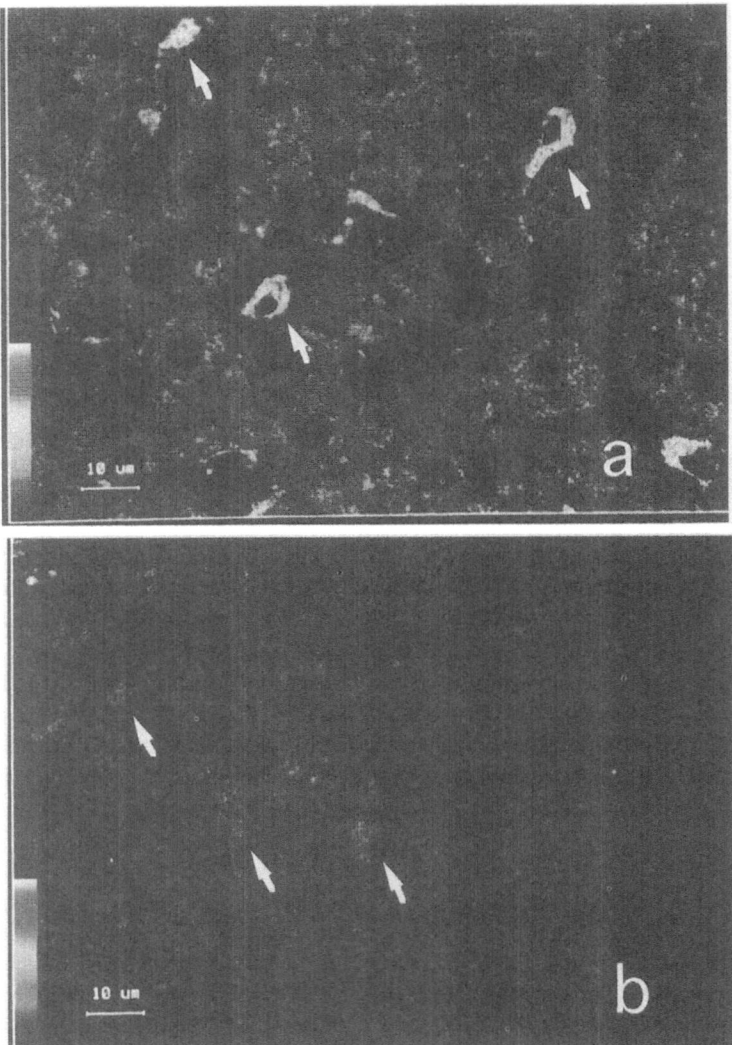

FIG. 5. Confocal laser scanning micrographs of Kupffer cells (*arrows*) with immunohistological staining using an anti-lipid A antibody. a Kupffer cells (*arrows*) in the same control rat as in Fig. 4 clearly contain a large amount of endotoxin lipid A. b Kupffer cells (*arrows*) in a cholestatic rat 7 days after bile duct ligation. Endotoxin lipid A is very low in these Kupffer cells compared with those in the control rat

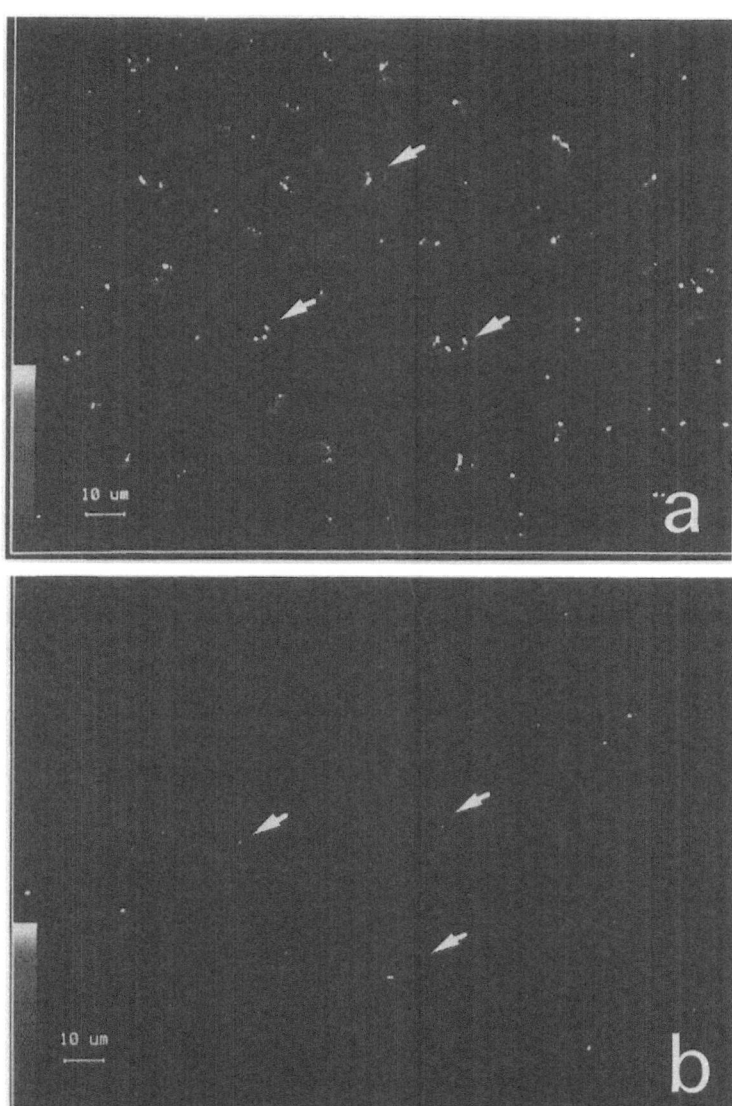

FIG. 6. Confocal laser scanning micrographs of the localization of membrane CD14 on Kupffer cells (*arrows*) using an immunohistological staining method. The expression of membrane CD14 on Kupffer cells in a cholestatic patients (**b**) is sparse compared with that in a control patient (**a**)

Kupffer cell and impairing the defense mechanism of the liver RES. However, the mechanism of this reduction of expressed CD14 remains obscure. It might result from cell membrane damage or from the high dose of endotoxin present in the sinusoidal circulation, because a large dose of endotoxin suppresses the endocytic activity of Kupffer cells [17].

## Sinusoidal Endothelial Cells in Cholestasis

Whereas endotoxin appears to be taken up selectively by Kupffer cells, many other nonparticulate macromolecules are taken up by sinusoidal endothelial cells as well [18–20]. This finding reveals that the sinusoidal endothelial cell is also, at least in part, a component of the liver RES. In fact, sinusoidal endothelial cells contain a large number of foreign bodies in their cytoplasm under cholestatic conditions such as primary biliary cirrhosis (PBC) [21]. This morphological change is sinusoidal cells might alter their characteristic fenestration and induce the hepatocyte injury found in cholestasis [21]. On the other hand, ICAM-1 was strongly expressed in the sinusoidal endothelial cells of a cholestatic rat model (Fig. 7). ICAM-1 expression in the sinusoidal endothelium by TNF-α or IL-1 has been well documented in an in vitro study [22], and these cytokines are mainly produced in macrophages in the spleen activated by endotoxin [23]. Thus, a functional change in sinusoidal endothelial cells might handle cell infiltration and adhesion in the hepatic sinusoid in cholestasis [24].

Receptors of Fc and C3b have been identified on Kupffer cells [25]. Sinusoidal endothelial cells, however, have an Fc receptor on their surface but not a C3b receptor [25, 26]. This finding suggests that the sinusoidal endothelial cells may be unable to

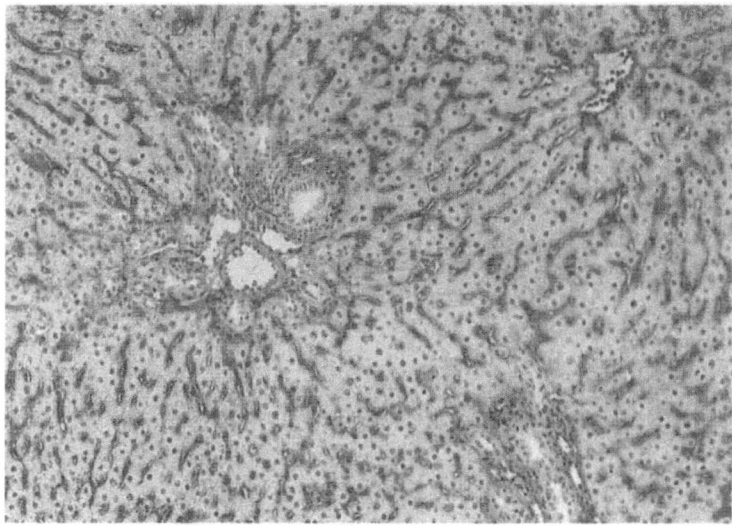

FIG. 7. Expression of IACM-1 in a rat liver lobule 4 days after bile duct ligation, with immunohistological staining using an anti-rat ICAM-1 antibody. ×100

clear IgM-immune complexes from the circulation. It is known that the serum level of IgM is significantly elevated in patients with PBC, and this elevated IgM is associated with anti-lipid A antibody [21]. Although the endocytosis of sinusoidal endothelial cells seems to be strongly enhanced to compensate for Kupffer cell dysfunction in PBC, the elevation of serum IgM may be due to Kupffer cell dysfunction in C3b receptor-mediated endocytosis. Thus, morphological and functional alterations in hepatic sinusoidal cells seem to be an important key in the pathogenesis of cholestasis.

## References

1. Tanikawa K, Noguchi K, Sasatomi K (1996) Role of cytokines and adhesion molecules in the pathogenesis of biliary liver diseases. In: Berg PA, Leuschner U (eds) Bile acids and immunology. Kluwer, Dortrecht, pp 86–93
2. Tanikawa K, Sata M, Kumashiro R, et al. (1989) Kupffer cell function in cholestasis. In: Wisse E, Knook DL, Decker K (eds) Cells of the hepatic sinusoid, vol 2. Kupffer Cell Foundation, pp 288–292
3. Hoffman AF (1990) Bile acid hepatotoxicity and the rationale of UDCA therapy in chronic cholestatic liver disease. In: Paumgartner G, Stiehl A, Barbara L, Roda E (eds) Some hypotheses. Strategies for the treatment of hepatobiliary diseases. Kluwer, Lancaster, pp 43–56
4. Guldutuna S, Zimmer G, Imhof M, et al. (1993) Molecular aspects of membrane stabilization by ursodeoxycholate. Gastroenterology 104:1736–1744
5. Fox ES, Thomas P, Broitman S, et al. (1990) Hepatic mechanisms for clearance and detoxification of bacterial endotoxin. J Nutr 1:620–628
6. Toth CA, Thomas P (1992) Liver endocytosis and Kupffer cells. Hepatology 16:255–266
7. Bailey ME (1976) Endotoxin, bile salts and renal function in obstructive jaundice. Br J Surg 63:774–778
8. Ingoldby CJ, McPherson GAD, Blumgart LH (1984) Endotoxemia in human obstructive jaundice. Am J Surg 147:766–771
9. Pain JA (1987) Reticuloendothelial function in obstructive jaundice. Br J Surg 4:1091–7094
10. Ding JW, Anderson R, Norgren L, et al. (1992) The influence of biliary obstruction and sepsis on reticuloendothelial function in rats. Eur J Surg 158:157–164
11. Clements WDB, Halliday M, McCaigue MD, et al. (1993) The effect of extrahepatic obstructive jaundice on Kupffer cell clearance capacity (KCCC). Ann Arch 128:200–205
12. Scott-Conner CE, Grogan JB (1994) The pathophysiology of biliary obstruction and its effect on phagocytic and immune function. J Surg Res 57:316–336
13. Ding JW, Anderson R, Soltesz V, et al. (1994) Obstructive jaundice impairs reticuloendothelial function and promotes bacterial transolcation in the rat. J Surg Res 57:238–245
14. Wright SD, Ramos RA, Tobias, et al. (1990) CD14. A receptor for complexes of lipopolysaccharide (LPS) and LPS binding protein. Science 249:1431–1433
15. Lei MG, Stimpson ST, Morrison DC (1991) Specific endotoxic lipopolysaccharide-binding receptors on murine splenocytes. III. Binding specificity and characterization. J Immunol 147:1925–1932
16. Gallay P, Carrel S, Glauser MP, et al. (1993) Purification and characterization of murine lipopolysaccharide-binding protein. Infect Immun 61:378–383
17. Keller GA, West MA, Cerra FB, et al. (1985) Multiple systems organ failure. Modulation

of hepatocyte protein synthesis by endotoxin activated Kupffer cells. Ann Surg 201:87–96

18. Blomhoff R, Eskild W, Berg T (1984) Endocytosis of formaldehyde-treated serum albumin via scavenger pathway in liver endothelial cells. Biochem J 2:81–86

19. Kindberg GM, Tooleshaug H, Gjøen T, et al. (1991) Lysosomal and endosomal heterogeneity in the liver: a comparison of the intracellular pathway of endocytosis in rat liver cells. Hepathology 13:254–259

20. Tanabe D, Kamimoto Y, Kai M, et al. (1996) Effects of biliary obstruction on the endocytic activity in hepatocyte and liver sinusoidal endothelial cell in rats. Eur Surg Res 28:201–211

21. Noguchi K, Ide T, Sata M, et al. (1991) Ultrastructural features of hepatic sinusoidal cells in patients with primary biliary cirrhosis. In: Wisse E, Knook DL, McCuskey RS (eds) Cells of the hepatic sinusoid, vol 3. Kupffer Cell Foundation, pp 118–121

22. Ohira H, Ueno T, Shakado S, et al. (1994) Cultured rat hepatic sinusoidal endothelial cells express intercellular adhesion molecule-1 (ICAM-1) by tumor necrosis factor α or interleukin-1 α stimulation. J Hepatol 20:729–734

23. Tanikawa K (1995) Cytokines and adhesion molecules in the liver. In: Gerok W, Decker K, Andiso T, Gross V (eds) Cytokine and the liver. Kluwer, Dortrecht, pp 37–45

24. Ohtsuka M, Miyazaki M, Kondo Y, et al. (1997) Neutrophil-mediated sinusoidal endothelial cell injury after extensive hepatectomy in cholestatic rats. Hepatology 25:636–641

25. Van Bossuny H, Bouwens L, Wisse E (1988) Isolation, purification and culture of sinusoidal cells. In: Bioulac-Sage P, Balabaud C (eds) Sinusoids in human liver: health and disease. Kupffer Cell Foundation, pp 1–16

26. Muro H, Shirasawa H, Maeda M, et al. (1987) Fc receptor of sinusoidal endothelium in normal rats and humans. Gastroenterology 93:1078–1085

# Congenital Lipidosis

SHOTARO SAKISAKA, MASARU HARADA, MOTONARI KAWAGUCHI,
EITAROH TANIGUCHI, and KYUICHI TANIKAWA

*Summary.* We studied livers from patients with cholesterol ester storage disease and Gaucher's disease by light and electron microscopy, and present their morphological features. A 57-year-old male with a complaint of right hypochondrial pain was diagnosed with gallstones and cholecystitis. He then underwent cholecystectomy. Although his serum lipid profiles indicated no marked abnormality, his liver appeared orange–yellow. Light microscopy (LM) showed marked lipid accumulation in hepatocytes and Kupffer cells. Electron microscopy (EM) revealed numerous membrane-bound lipid droplets and crystalline-like cholesterol in hepatocytes, as well as in Kupffer cells. Liver lipid analysis revealed a markedly high content of cholesterol ester and triglyceride. Liver lipid analysis and morphology, especially ultrastructural features, led to the diagnosis of cholesterol ester storage disease. A 23-year-old female was admitted because of nose-bleeding and pancytopenia. Radiographic examination revealed marked hepatosplenomegaly and an ovarian tumor. When she had an operation for the ovarian tumor, liver and spleen biopsy was done because metabolic disease was suspected. Liver and spleen specimens showed many large macrophages which contained abundant amorphous deposits. EM revealed that numerous large macrophages occupied the liver sinusoids and spleen. The accumulated substance was in long tubules, which on cross section showed rectangular or circular profiles. These morphological findings and biochemical data confirmed Gaucher's disease. Collectively, EM study is a very useful approach for diagnosis of congenital disorders of the lipid metabolism.

*Key words.* Cholesterol ester storage disease, Gaucher's disease, Electron microscopy, Ultrastructure

The Second Department of Internal Medicine, Kurume University School of Medicine, 67 Asahi-machi, Kurume, Fukuoka 830-0011, Japan

# Introduction

Congenital lipidosis affecting the liver is caused mainly by the congenital defect of lysosomal enzymes in hepatocytes and in liver macrophages (Kupffer cells). Diseases of this type include Fabry's disease, Gaucher's disease, and Nieman Pick's disease. However, leukodystrophies, such as Wolman's disease and cholesterol ester storage disease (CESD), are also characterized by the accumulation of lipids in the liver.

In this study, we consider cases of CESD and Gaucher's disease in relation to the ultrastructure of the liver.

# Cholesterol Ester Storage Disease

Wolman's disease was named after its discoverer, and was first described in 1956 [1]. Since that time, more than 40 cases have been reported [2]. Wolman's disease and CESD, a milder form of Wolman's disease, are autosomal recessive diseases. These are caused by a deficiency of lysosomal acid lipase, characterized by tissue accumulation of esterified cholesterol and triglycerides. CESD was first reported by Fredrickson in 1963 [3] and more than 27 cases have been reported [2].

## *Case Presentation*

*Case.* The patient was a 57-year-old male.
*Chief Complaint.* The patient complained of right hypochondrial pain.
*Present Illness.* The right hypochondrial pain had persisted for some time before the patient was admitted to our hospital.
*Physical Examination.* No abnormal findings were noted in the vital signs. Neither anemia nor jaundice was detected. Heart and breathing appeared normal. The liver was palpable by two finger breadths under the right costal margin. The liver was elastic and firm, without tenderness. The spleen was palpable by one finger breadth under the left costal margin.
*Laboratory Data.* Hematology: WBC 4800/mm$^3$; RBC 405 × 10$^4$/mm$^3$. Blood chemistry: total bilirubin 1.2 mg/dL; direct bilirubin 0.5 mg/dL; alanine aminotransferase 54 KU; aspartate aminotransferase 34 KU; lactate dehydrogenase 172 KU; alkaline phosphatase 10.8 KAU; total cholesterol 228 mg/dL; total protein 7.0 g/dL; albumin 4.0 g/dL; indocyanine green 13.5%. Radiographic examination revealed gallstones. The patient underwent cholecystectomy for the treatment of gallstones and liver biopsy for diagnosis of the liver disease. The liver was enlarged and appeared orange–yellow.
*Light-Microscopic Findings.* Light microscopy (LM) showed that hepatocytes as well as Kupffer cells were markedly enlarged and contained lipid-like material. There were no marked inflammatory reactions such as inflammatory cell infiltration or cell necrosis. Lipid infiltration in hepatocytes was seen throughout the liver lobule. The diagnosis was abnormal fat infiltration in the liver (Fig. 1).
*Electron-Microscopic Examination.* Electron microscopy (EM) showed crystalline-like cholesterol and round lipid deposits in hepatocytes and in Kupffer cells (Fig. 2).

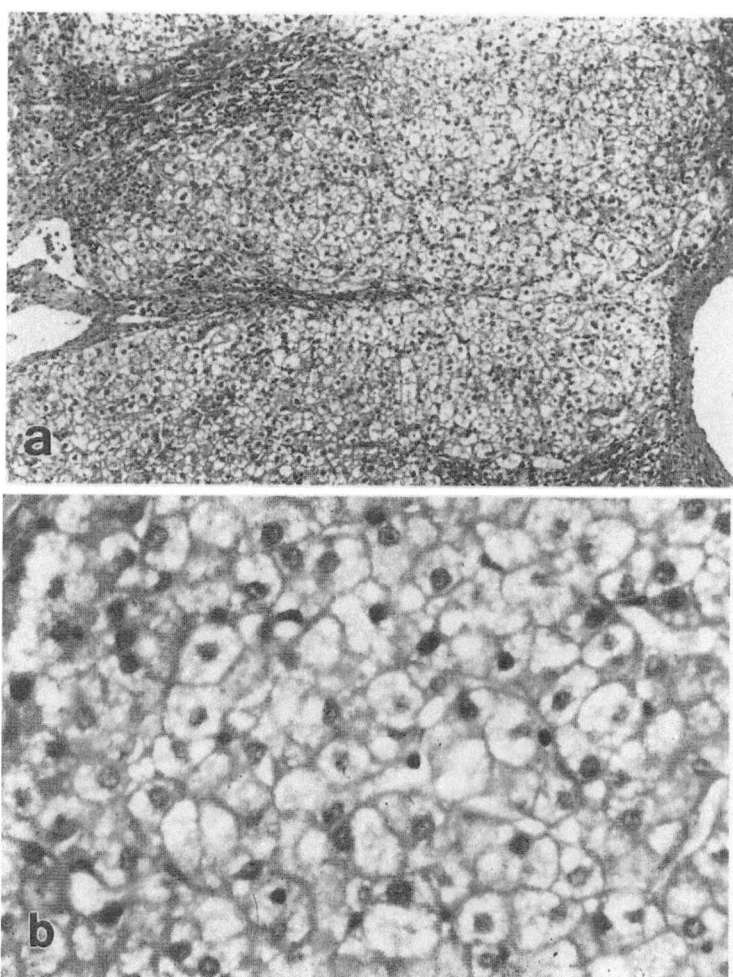

FIG. 1a,b. Light micrograph of the liver of a patient with CESD. **a** Lipid infiltration in hepatocytes can be seen throughout the liver lobule. **b** Hepatocytes as well as Kupffer cells are markedly enlarged and contain lipid-like materials. Hematoxylin and eosin stain. **a** ×150; **b** ×450

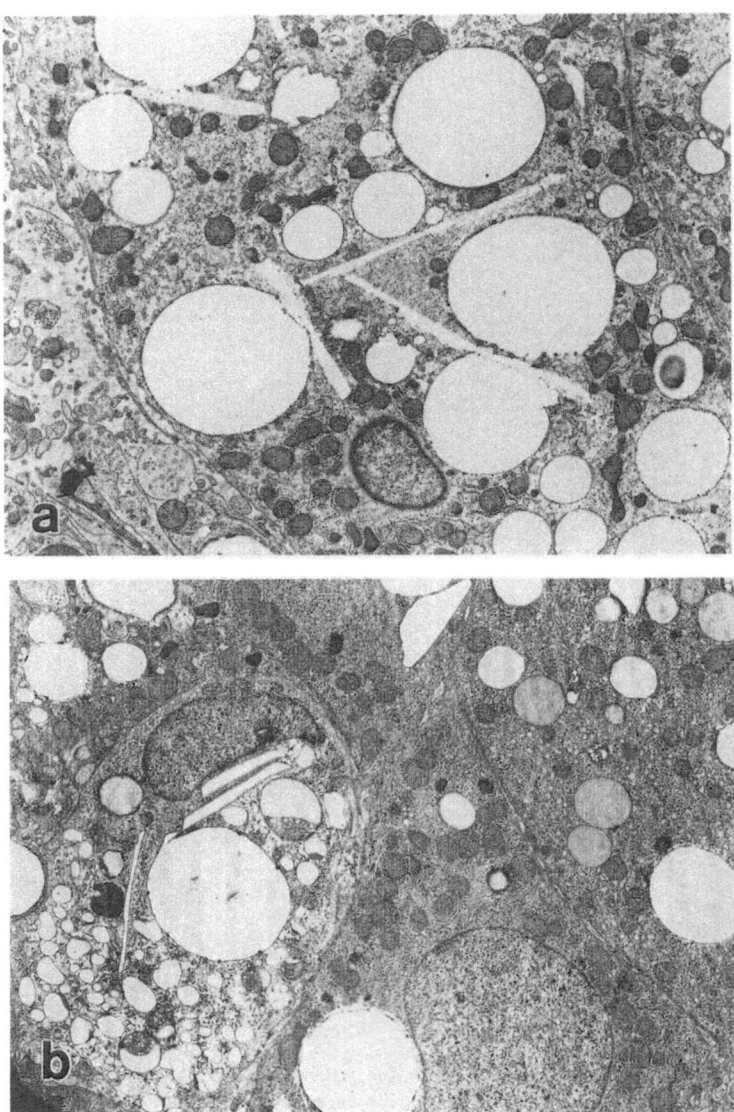

FIG. 2a–c. Transmission electron micrographs of the liver of a patient with CESD. Crystalline-like cholesterol and round lipid deposition can be seen in **a** hepatocytes and **b, c** Kupffer cells. **a** ×4300; **b** ×4300; **c** ×3400

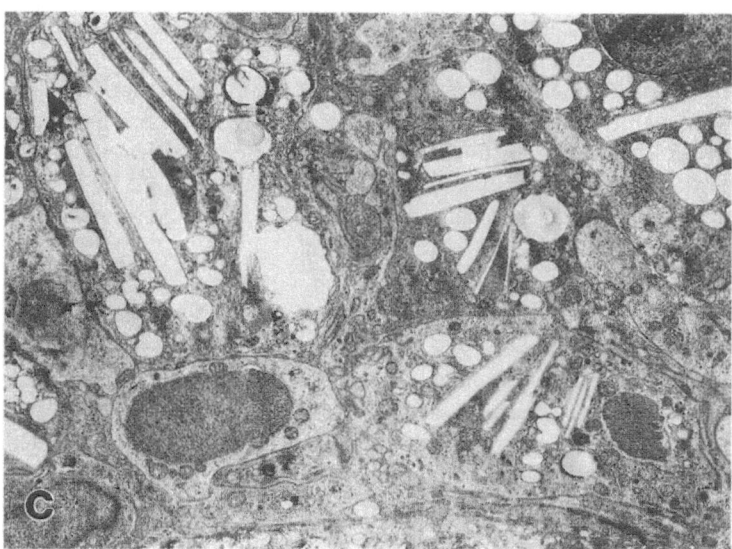

FIG. 2a–c. *Continued*

TABLE 1. Lipid composition of the liver

| Lipids (mg/g wet weight) | Normal liver | Patient's liver |
|---|---|---|
| Total cholesterol | 3.8 | 24.1 |
| Free cholesterol | 2.9 (76.3) | 4.1 (17) |
| Esterified cholesterol | 0.9 (23.7) | 20.0 (83) |
| Triglyceride | 3.5 | 91.0 |
| Phospholipids | 11.7 | 8.7 |

Figures in parentheses are percentages.

*Biochemical Analysis.* Biochemical analysis of the homogenate of the biopsy liver revealed an enormous deposition of esterified cholesterol and triglyceride in the liver (Table 1).

## Discussion

The findings of the liver lipid analysis and EM study suggested the presence of CESD. Both CESD and Wolman's disease are characterized by a congenital defect of acid lipase A. The gene locus responsible for these diseases is localized in chromosome 10q23 [2]. In CESD, esterified cholesterol accumulates in the liver, the intestine, and around the blood vessels. We have not checked the latter two lesions. EM demonstrated characteristic cholesterol deposition in hepatocytes and in Kupffer cells, which causes hepatomegaly. Generally, CESD is recognized in childhood or soon after, and progression is slow. In contrast, Wolman's disease is characterized by rapid progression and in most cases is fatal within 6 months.

The present case shows late onset and mild clinical manifestation, which are compatible with symptoms of CESD. The disease, which affects both liver and spleen, frequently results from deposition in macrophages and Kupffer cells. CESD should always be considered in the diagnosis of diseases characterized by hepatomegaly. Histological examination, especially by EM, could be a useful diagnostic tool.

# Gaucher's Disease

Gaucher's disease, an autosomal recessive disease that was first described in 1882, mainly affects Ashkenazi Jews, and it is the most common lysosomal storage disorder [2, 4]. Gaucher's disease is characterized by a defect in lysosomal β-glucocerebrosidase, so that the substrate b-glucocerebroside accumulates in the reticuloendothelial system throughout the body, particularly in the liver, bone marrow, and spleen.

## Case Presentation

*Case.* The patient was a 23-year-old female.
*Chief Complaint.* The patient complained of nose-bleeding.
*Present Illness.* When the patient visited the doctor because of nose-bleeding, pancytopenia and hepatosplenomegaly were noted. The patient was transferred to our department for further examination.
*Physical Examination.* No abnormal findings were noted in the vital signs. Anemia was apparent without jaundice. Heart and breathing appeared normal. The liver was palpable by four finger breadths under the right costal margin. The liver was elastic and firm, without tenderness. The spleen was palpable by five finger breadths under the left costal margin. No lymphadenopathy was observed. No neurological abnormality was seen.
*Laboratory Data.* Hematology: WBC 2800/mm$^3$; RBC 304 × 10$^4$/mm$^3$; Platelets 66 000. Blood chemistry: aspartate aminotransferase 54 KU; alanine aminotransferase 32 KU; lactate dehydrogenase 263 KU; alkaline phosphatase 9.5 KAU; total protein 8.6 g/dL; albumin 3.2 g/dL; indocyanine green 13.5%; prothrombin time 48%; hepaplastin test 57%; IgG 3589 mg/dL; IgA 405 mg/dL; IgM 405 mg/dL; erythrocyte sedimentation rate 60 mm/h; acid phosphatase 57 KU (normal range, 1.0–4.0); angiotensin converting enzyme (ACE) 87.8 IU/L (normal range, 8.3–21.4); β-glucocerebrosidase in WBC 1.1 nmol/mgP/h (normal range, 4.1–9.7). Radiographic examination revealed a greatly enlarged liver and spleen and an ovarian tumor. Liver and spleen biopsy was done during an operation for the ovarian tumor.
*Light-Microscopic Findings of the Biopsy Liver and Spleen.* The hepatic sinusoids were occupied by many large cells (70–80 μm in diameter) with pale cytoplasm. Many similar cells were also observed in the spleen (Fig. 3).
*Electron-Microscopic Examination.* EM revealed greatly enlarged macrophages, which are typical of Gaucher's cells, with material accumulated in the cytoplasm of the cells. These cells occupied the liver sinusoids. High-magnification EM showed numerous tubules (40–60 nm in diameter) surrounded by single membranes in the cytoplasm. These cells were also observed in the spleen (Fig. 4).

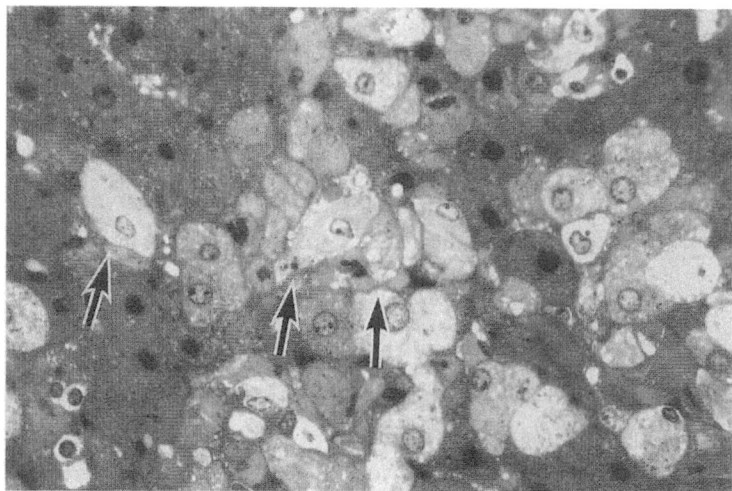

FIG. 3. Light micrograph of the liver of a patient with Gaucher's disease. Markedly enlarged Kupffer cells contain amorphous material in the cytoplasm (*arrows*). These Gaucher's cells occupied the liver sinusoid. Toluidine blue stain. ×450

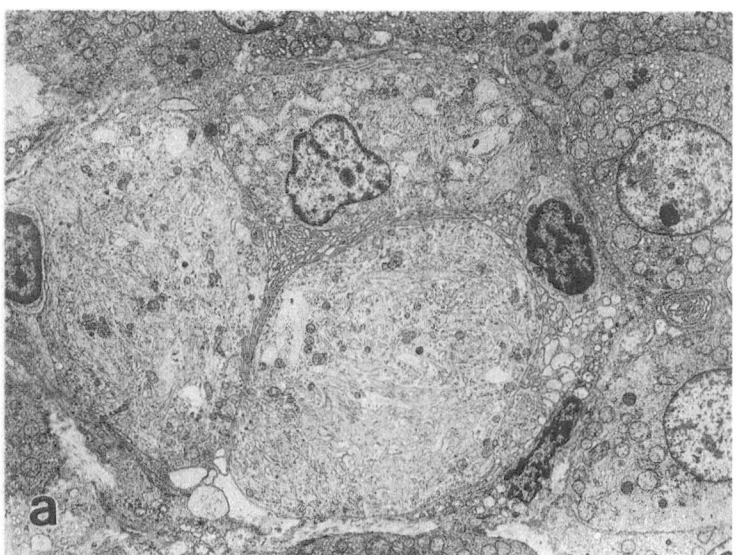

FIG. 4. Transmission electron micrographs of the liver (**a–d**) and the spleen (**e**) of a patient with Gaucher's disease. **a** ×2500; **b** ×6000; **c** ×31 000; **d** ×27 000; **e** ×3900

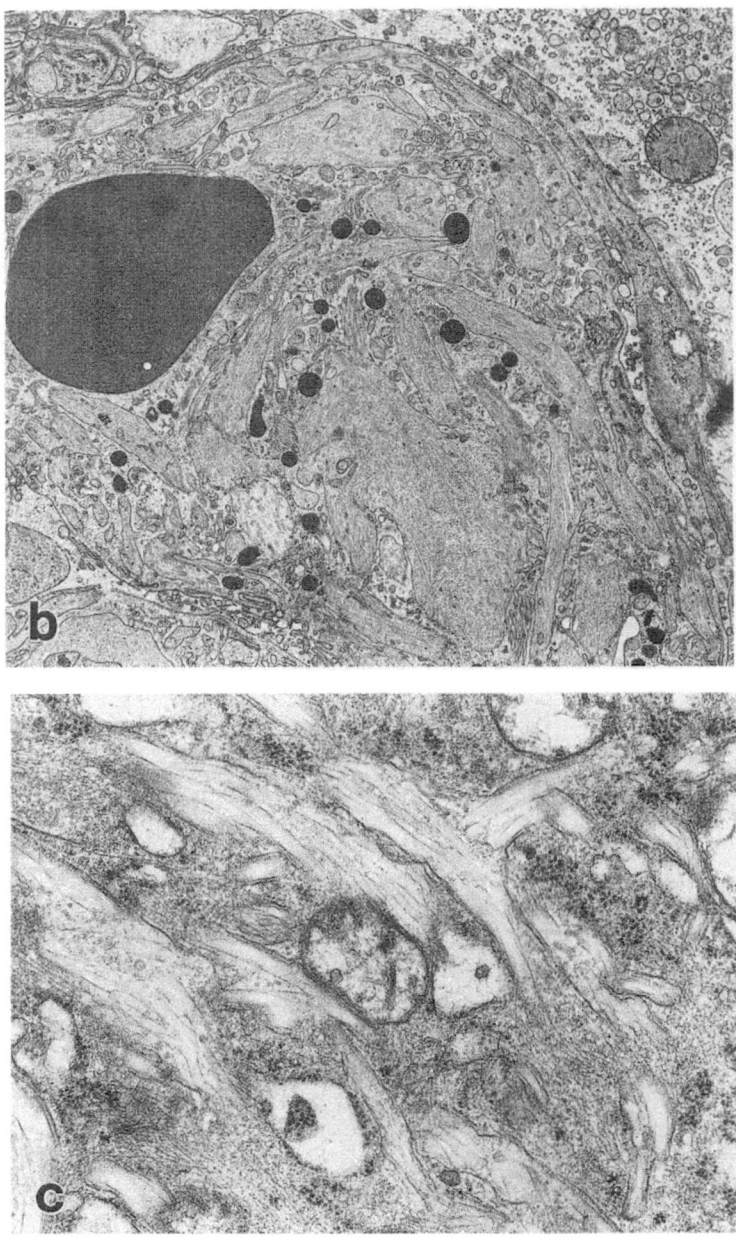

FIG. 4. *Continued*

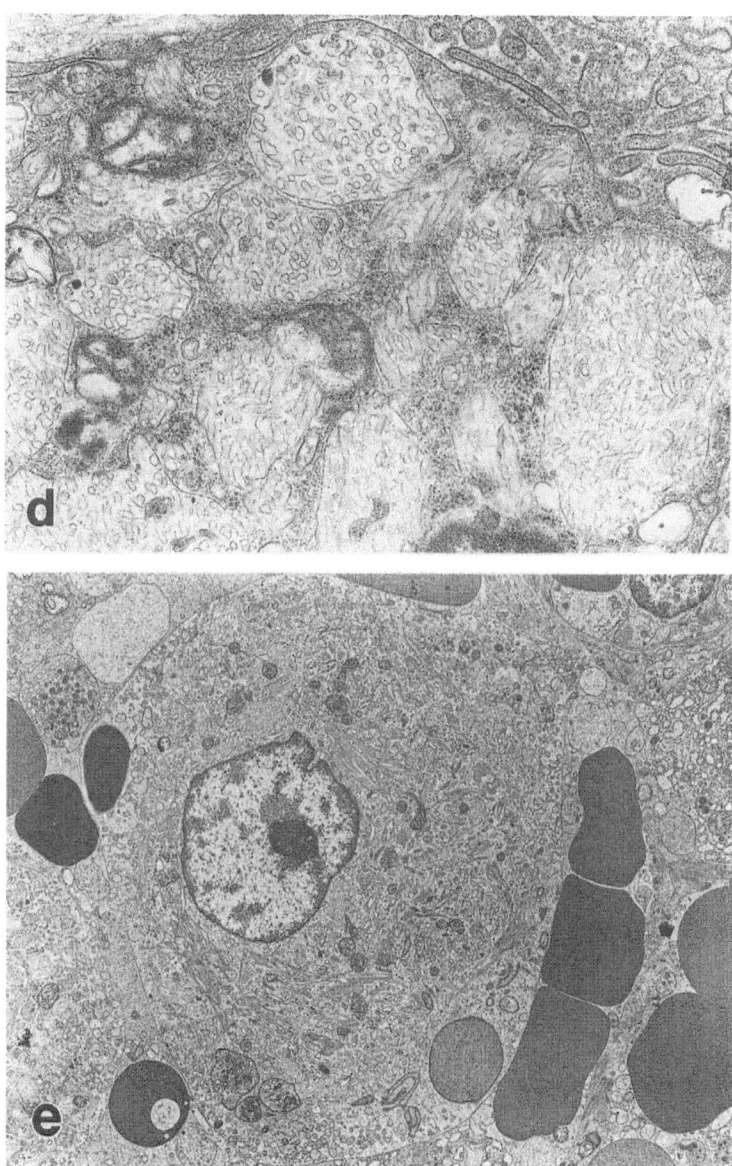

FIG. 4. *Continued*

## Discussion

Biochemical analysis, including leukocyte $\beta$-glucocerebrosidase activity and serum ACE level, light microscopy, and EM suggested Gaucher's disease. The gene locus responsible for the disease is found on chromosome 1 [2]. Gaucher's disease is autosomal recessive and is the most prevalent lysosomal disease, primarily because of the high prevalence (1 in 600) of type 1 disease in Ashkenazi Jews. Patients have an enzyme defect in $\beta$-glucocerebrosidase, so that glucocerebrsoide accumulates in macrophages of various organs such as the bone marrow, liver, and spleen. The leukocyte and erythrocyte membranes are the major source of glucocerebroside. Three clinical variants are described. They differ in the course of the disease, particularly type III, but cannot be distinguished by levels of enzyme activity. Type I, or chronic nonneuronopathic disease, usually causes hepatosplenomegaly in late childhood or adolescence, but was first detected in patients as old as 80 years. Pancytopenia is common, and thrombocytopenia is observed in more than 50% of patients, leading to mild hemorrhagic phenomena, as seen in the present case [2].

Although Brady first proposed enzyme replacement therapy in 1966, success was not obtained until 20 years later. The treatment is sequential deglycosylation of the secondary branches to form the purified enzyme isolated from human placenta. This exposes the mannose at the end of the primary carbohydrate side chains, which is preferentially taken up by the mannose receptor of macrophages, where the glucocerebroside is stored. The product is available as aglucerase (Ceredase), with which clinical responses are obtained with intravenous administration every 2 weeks. Clinical improvement was noted in blood counts and organomegaly in 12 patients. Bone marrow and liver transplantation have not yet resulted in significant improvements [2]. The present case has a rather slow progression with mild or no bone lesion, but the patient remains a candidate for that therapy owing to severe hepatomegaly and low albuminemia, that suggests progressive liver lesion. Recently, in Japan, recombinant glucocerebrosidase has been used. We have decided to start this enzyme therapy on this patient next month.

## References

1. Abramov A, Schorr S, Wolman M (1956) Generalized xanthomatosis with calcified adrenals. Am J Dis Child 91:282–286
2. Bockus Gastroenterology. 5th edn. (1995) In: Haubrich WS, Schaffner F, Berk JE (eds) Inherited metabolic disorders of the liver sharp HL. W.B. Saunders, Tokyo, pp 2362–2363
3. Fredrickson DS (1963) Newly recognized disorders of cholesterol metabolism. Ann Intern Med 58:718. Abstract
4. Gaucher P (1882) De l'épithélioma primitif de la rate. Thesis, Paris

# Key Word Index

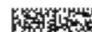